Psychopathology of the Situation in Gestalt Therapy

Reaching beyond standard textbook logic, this collection explores the impacts of difficult life situations on human development, experience, and functioning, through a phenomenological field-oriented lens.

Each author offers a Gestalt-centered perspective on the circumstances of those whose lives are lived in pain – a situational window, which includes the therapist and avails itself of tools configured to modify the entire experiential field. Through clinical case studies and theoretical reflections, the book examines the experience of children, difficult childhood situations (such as separations, abuse, neurodevelopmental disorders, adolescent social closure), the experience of dependency, couples and family therapy, the condition of the elderly and the end of life, interventions for degenerative diseases, and the trauma of loss and mourning, all of which are considered according to two cardinal points: first, the description of the relational ground experiences of those who are in pain, and second, a field perspective which allows the presence of the therapist to be modulated.

Psychopathology of the Situation in Gestalt Therapy: A Field-oriented Approach is essential reading for Gestalt therapists as well as other mental health professionals with an interest in Gestalt approaches and the relationship between individuals and society.

Margherita Spagnuolo Lobb, PsyD, is a Gestalt psychotherapist, director of Istituto di Gestalt Human Communication Center Italy (www.gestaltitaly.com); Scientific Director of International Training Programs in "Gestalt Therapy Psychopathology and Development"; and "Gestalt Therapy Supervisors". Editor of the Journal *Gestalt Therapy Journal*, and of the *Gestalt Therapy Book Series* (Routledge). Author of *The Now for Next in Psychotherapy: Gestalt Therapy Recounted in Post Modern Society*. She has received the Lifelong Achievement Award from AAGT (2018).

Pietro Andrea Cavaleri, PhD, PsyD, is a Gestalt Psychotherapist and Trainer at Istituto di Gestalt HCC, Italy. He has taught at the University of Palermo, at LUMSA University and at the Pontifical Faculty of Educational Sciences "Auxilium". He has been psychologist in chief at the Public Health Service and counselor for social policies of Caltanissetta. Author of *Living with the Other*: *Contribution for a Culture of Relationship; The Depth of Surface: Introduction to Gestalt Psychotherapy*.

The Gestalt Therapy Book Series

The Istituto di Gestalt series of Gestalt therapy books emerges from the ground of a growing interest in theory, research and clinical practice in the Gestalt community. The members of the Scientific and Editorial Boards have been committed for many years to the process of supporting research and publications in our field: through this series we want to offer our colleagues internationally the richness of the current trends in Gestalt therapy theory and practice, underpinned by research. The goal of this series is to develop the original principles in hermeneutic terms: to articulate a relational perspective, namely a phenomenological, aesthetic, field-oriented approach to psychotherapy. It is also intended to help professions and to support a solid development and dialogue of Gestalt therapy with other psychotherapeutic methods.

"The world situation for us clinicians and those whom we treat has taken on urgency in the face the global pandemic. This book is a blend of practical wisdom and thoughtful insights as Gestalt psychotherapists address this urgency at the psychological, anthropological, sociological, phenomenological, and neurobiological levels – all within a phenomenological, aesthetic and field perspective, the hallmarks of a contemporary approach."

Dan Bloom, *JD, LCSW, Psychotherapist, Fellow,*
Past-President, New York Institute for Gestalt Therapy

The series includes original books specifically created for it, as well as translations of volumes originally published in other languages. We hope that our editorial effort will support the growth of the Gestalt therapy community; a dialogue with other modalities and disciplines; and new developments in research, clinics and other fields where Gestalt therapy theory can be applied (e.g., organisations, education, political and social critique and movements).

We would like to dedicate this Gestalt Therapy Book Series to all our mentors and colleagues who have sown fruitful seeds in our minds and hearts.

For a full list of titles in this series, please visit www.routledge.com/Gestalt-Therapy/book-series/GESTHE and www.gestaltitaly.com

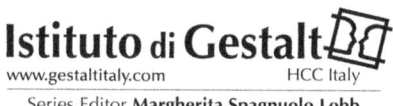

Istituto di Gestalt

www.gestaltitaly.com HCC Italy

Series Editor **Margherita Spagnuolo Lobb**

Psychopathology of the Situation in Gestalt Therapy

A Field-oriented Approach

Edited by
Margherita Spagnuolo Lobb and
Pietro Andrea Cavaleri

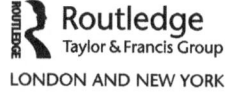

Routledge
Taylor & Francis Group

LONDON AND NEW YORK

Designed cover image: Rafael Megall, The Shelves of Kaspar Utz, (detail) 2020 Triptych

Oil, acrylic on canvas, 260 x 510 cm (260 x 170 cm each one). Courtesy of the Artist and MoMA, Moskow. Copyright Rafael Megall, Yerevan

First published 2023
by Routledge
4 Park Square, Milton Park, Abingdon, Oxon OX14 4RN

and by Routledge
605 Third Avenue, New York, NY 10158

Routledge is an imprint of the Taylor & Francis Group, an informa business

© 2023 selection and editorial matter, Margherita Spagnuolo Lobb and Pietro Andrea Cavaleri; individual chapters, the contributors

Translated by Joyce Myerson

The right of Margherita Spagnuolo Lobb and Pietro Andrea Cavaleri to be identified as the authors of the editorial material, and of the authors for their individual chapters, has been asserted in accordance with sections 77 and 78 of the Copyright, Designs and Patents Act 1988.

British Library Cataloguing-in-Publication Data
A catalogue record for this book is available from the British Library

Library of Congress Cataloging-in-Publication Data
Names: Spagnuolo Lobb, Margherita, editor. | Cavaleri, Pietro Andrea, editor.
Title: Psychopathology of the situation in Gestalt therapy: a field-oriented approach/edited by Margherita Spagnuolo Lobb and Pietro Andrea Cavaleri.
Other titles: Psicopatologia della situazione. English
Description: First English edition. | New York, NY: Routledge, 2023. | Series: Gestalt Therapy Book Series | "First Italian edition published by FrancoAngeli 2021" – title page verso. | Includes bibliographical references and index.
Identifiers: LCCN 2022047728 (print) | LCCN 2022047729 (ebook) | ISBN 9781032322032 (hardback) | ISBN 9781032322025 (paperback) | ISBN 9781003313335 (ebook)
Subjects: LCSH: Gestalt therapy.
Classification: LCC RC489.G4 P7913 2023 (print) | LCC RC489.G4 (ebook) | DDC 616.89/143 – dc23/eng/20221007
LC record available at https://lccn.loc.gov/2022047728
LC ebook record available at https://lccn.loc.gov/2022047729

ISBN: 978-1-032-32203-2 (hbk)
ISBN: 978-1-032-32202-5 (pbk)
ISBN: 978-1-003-31333-5 (ebk)

DOI: 10.4324/9781003313335

Typeset in Times New Roman
by Apex CoVantage, LLC

To our friend Georges Wollants,
to whom credit is due for having recognised and described
the unique relationality of Gestalt Therapy

Contents

Acknowledgments   xiv
Foreword   xv
SCOTT D. CHURCHILL

Editors' Introduction   1
MARGHERITA SPAGNUOLO LOBB AND PIETRO ANDREA CAVALERI

PART I
Psychopathology of the Situation   5

1 **Psychopathological Situations in a Post-Pandemic World:**
   Gestalt Therapy in Emergent Clinical Fields   7
   MARGHERITA SPAGNUOLO LOBB AND PIETRO ANDREA CAVALERI

2 **Working on the Ground, on Aesthetics, and on the "Dance":**
   Aesthetic Relational Knowing and Reciprocity   20
   MARGHERITA SPAGNUOLO LOBB

   Beyond Slogans: Connecting Individuals in a Community   43
   A COMMENT BY ERVING POLSTER

3 **Global Unrest and the Anthropological Perspective**
   of Gestalt Therapy   46
   PIETRO ANDREA CAVALERI

   The World Crisis and Gestalt Therapy: Response to Cavaleri   67
   COMMENT BY GARY YONTEF

4 Phenomenology and Gestalt Psychotherapy: New
  Challenges Under-the-Radar   70
  PIETRO ANDREA CAVALERI

5 The Gestalt Clinical Data Sheet: A Phenomenological,
  Aesthetic, and Field Instrument for Gestalt Psychotherapy
  and Supervision   81
  MARGHERITA SPAGNUOLO LOBB, ELISABETTA CONTE, AND
  MARIA MIONE

PART II
Psychopathological Situations in the Clinical Fields
of Human Relations   97

6 Ring-a-Ring O' Roses, a Pocket Full of Posies: Gestalt
  Psychotherapy and Childhood Suffering   99
  SILVIA TOSI AND ELISABETTA CONTE

7 Children of "Broken" Relationships: Repairing the Ground
  of the Parental Experience   119
  PAOLA CANNA AND MANUELA PARTINICO

8 Gestalt Psychotherapy and Complex Trauma in
  Preadolescence: How to Support the Integration of the
  Body, Emotions, and Words   133
  ROSANNA MILITELLO

9 To Be or Not to Be Autistic: From the *Camouflage* Effect to
  Élan Vital – A Gestalt Perspective   147
  ANTONIO NARZISI

10 Adolescents in Eclipse: Journey Notes From the Labyrinth
   of Social Withdrawal   159
   MICHELE LIPANI

11 Addiction as Persistent Trauma of the Ground Experience:
   Neuroscience and Gestalt Psychotherapy   173
   GIANCARLO PINTUS AND MARIALUISA GRECH

12 Conflict in Couple Relationships as Space for Recognition:
    An Opportunity that is Still Possible in the Post-Pandemic World   190
    PIETRO ANDREA CAVALERI

13 Working with the Family in Gestalt Psychotherapy   207
    GIUSEPPE SAMPOGNARO

14 Gestalt Psychotherapy and Ageing   222
    ALESSANDRA MERIZZI

15 Gestalt Psychotherapy in the Relationship with the Chronic
    Patient: Accepting and Supporting the Experience of Loss
    Through an Aesthetic Gaze   238
    ALESSANDRA VELA AND DONATELLA BUSCEMI

16 For Whom the Bells Do *Not* Toll: The Processing
    of Bereavement in Our Time   252
    CARMEN VÁZQUEZ BANDÍN

    Afterword   269
    SANTO DI NUOVO

    Biographical Notes   271
    Appendix   276
    Index   285

Acknowledgments

This text is the final outcome of a creative process that involves not only the Istituto di Gestalt HCC Italy, but also the extended international Gestalt community and the tightly interwoven network of contacts with colleagues representing other therapeutic models. We feel the need to thank firstly the authors of the individual chapters, who have worked to produce a text consistent with a shared epistemology. In addition, each colleague from our Institute, even if not a participant author, has afforded us support and useful suggestions. We are also grateful to our students, local and international, who through their questions, curiosity, and fresh vitality may be considered the implicit interlocutors from whom the idea and the structure itself of the book have arisen.

From the bottom of our hearts, we thank Erving Polster and Gary Yontef, who wrote a commentary on our theoretical chapters. Their words are a significant foundation of the efforts our Institute has made over the years to develop the Gestalt psychotherapy model. It is a good feeling to be supported by the words of those who have paved the way of the Gestalt therapy model for our soul.

Special thanks goes out to the author of the preface to the Italian edition (afterword in this English edition), professor Santo Di Nuovo, chair of the Italian Association of Academic Psychologists, and to professor Scott D. Churchill, University of Dallas, whose preface to the English edition and incredibly in depth and generous feedback have better grounded us into the tradition of phenomenological psychology.

We also thank those friends and colleagues who have supported this book with their endorsements – Dan Bloom, Peter Cole, Ruella Frank, Malcolm Parlett, Gordon Wheeler – Michael Clemmens, for his review that has allowed to improve the final edition of this book, and the Editorial Board of the Gestalt Therapy Book Series – first of all its coordinator, Stefania Benini. We are also grateful to Serena Iacono Isidoro, who has done a great job in supporting authors and checking all references – and the New York Institute of Gestalt Therapy – for their constant creative support to our work in the Gestalt therapy community.

Foreword

What a nice invitation, to write this foreword to such a fine collection of articles devoted to a rejuvenation of the classical ideas of Gestalt Therapy – in dialogue with kindred thinkers writing around the time of the advent of the Gestalt movement, as well as practitioners who have further developed and applied the early principles of Perls *et al.* (1951/1994) in their own work.

Situated in contemporary times where relationality is being emphasised in everything from psychoanalysis to neurophenomenology, this book represents a shift in Gestalt thinking from its more classically understood "client-centered" foundation toward a focusing on the encounter itself as the primary ground for psychotherapeutic understanding and change. It is reminiscent of the way in which the neo-Freudians began to re-examine their roots in classical psychoanalysis, bringing forth what was called "the interpersonal school" of psychoanalysis through the collective work of Horney (1939, 1945, 1950), Sullivan (1953, 1954), and Fromm (1947, 1956) – which in turn led to the "relational" school of psychoanalysis (Mitchell, 2000). Horney and Sullivan helped to remind us that what classical psychoanalysis had conceptualised as "intrapsychic" conflicts only ever manifested themselves within the interpersonal encounter of analyst and patient. (Of course, Freud was quite aware of the relational nature of the analytic situation, especially insofar as transference became one of the defining principles of his technique of therapy.) I am sure the same could be said for the founders of Gestalt Therapy: Perls *et al.*, the Polsters, Kempler, and others in the early days of this approach certainly saw that the encounter itself was the place where therapy occurred. But what is new here is the working through of conflicts not just with the therapist or the empty chair as a "stand-in" for someone else with whom the client is having conflict; rather, the relationship between *this* client and *this* therapist as a pivotal relationship in its own right (including its own conflicts), is now being revealed as an important "situation" within which psychotherapy can occur.

The concept of "situation" has held a central position within the thought of the existential phenomenologists. Taking his lead from Heidegger, Jean-Paul Sartre (1939/1948) wrote emphatically that the aim of phenomenological psychology is to understand "*man in situations*" – a phrase he used to differentiate the interest of the psychologist from that of the transcendental philosopher (p. 19). Indeed, Sartre was so enamored with the deep meaning that the term *situation* was given in Heidegger's writings that he entitled every volume of his own autobiographical writings "*Situations* I, II, III, IV, . . ." For Heidegger (1927/1962), the term "situation" had two important meanings: first, he used it to signify the "*there*" where each of us finds ourself lost and fallen and *from out of which* we become resolved to improve our relation to the world and to others (pp. 343–345). When in Gestalt therapy we talk about the client's need to "work" on the self, we are talking about confronting whatever it is that is holding us back from what Heidegger called our "ownmost potentialities for Being." In order to be *free for* authentic living, we need to *free ourselves from* the personally challenging "situations" – the existential circumstances and psychopathological conditions – that we bring to the work of therapy.

The second meaning of "situation" for Heidegger was to refer to the totality of a researcher's *presuppositions*, which he delineated as our "fore-having, fore-sight, and fore-conception" (pp. 191, 275). Collectively, these refer to everything the researcher or therapist brings with them to the encounter with a client. Heidegger called this the "hermeneutical situation" (p. 275). For example, it is my own "having been there before" (fore-having) that enables me to resonate with the client's feelings.

In the vignettes included in this book, the reader is given a palpable sense of the kinds of life circumstances that bring clients to the therapeutic encounter. It becomes clear that the problems people face are not something to be found "inside them" but rather in the social worlds that they inhabit. The fundamental nature of human persons according to Heidegger (1921–1922/2001, 1927/1962) is that above all else, we are "relational" beings who, in our relationality, find ourselves *thrown* into a world with others, *falling* away from ourselves, with the hopes of *projecting* ourselves into an open field of possibilities. Each of these "movements" occurs in relation to our own specific situation, and in this sense the movements that we exhibit in everyday life as well as in the therapeutic field are truly *our own*. For Sartre, we define ourselves in the various modes of our concrete relations with others. These relations always involve our embodiment, and for this reason Sartre (1943/1956) placed great emphasis on the ontological modes of the body (p. 400 ff). He believed that the body was "the psychological object *par excellence*," and in this sense our *character* becomes visible for other to see – in the real world as well as in the therapeutic encounter. This book helps us to appreciate *how it is* that a therapist has a foundation for perceiving, experiencing, and resonating with the client. Therapeutic presence is shown to be an *embodied presence* to the relational style of the client. The client's general *relationality* is revealed in *the particular bodily expressions and movements that occur in the field* opened up by the therapist.

What moves me in reading this book is the careful attention to the *particularity* of the individuals whose situations are disclosed to us. There is no "one-size-fits-all" approach to therapy that can work for everyone, and in each clinical vignette we find ourselves face-to-face with *encounterings* that take place in the particular field that is opened up between *this* client and *this* therapist. In the various chapters of this book, Gestalt therapists write about their experiences in bringing their clients to a better self-awareness, by grounding them in the "here and now" encounter in order to prepare them for the "soon to be" – a process described by Spagnuolo Lobb (2013) as the "now-for-next".

Beyond its contributions to the therapeutic literature, there is also a contribution to the history and theory of Gestalt therapy, insofar as these experienced practitioners make an effort to return to the founding ideas generated by Perls *et al.* (1951/1994) and breathe new life into them. Old expressions are given fresh meanings; more importantly, the language of Gestalt therapy is brought into dialogue with ideas drawn from the earlier Gestalt psychologists as well as the emerging field of neurophenomenology.

This book will be welcome reading for students and novice therapists who are looking to gain a deeper understanding of both the early foundational literature of the Gestalt movement in psychotherapy, as well as for the seasoned practitioners looking to enlighten and edify their understanding of the relational processes between themselves and their clients.

Scott D. Churchill,
University of Dallas

References

Fromm, E. (1947). *Man for himself. An inquiry into the psychology of ethics.* New York: Rinehart.

Fromm, E. (1956). *The art of loving.* New York: Harper.

Heidegger, M. (1962). *Being and time* (J. MacQuarrie & E. Robinson, Trans.). New York: Harper & Row. (Original work published 1927)

Heidegger, M. (2001). *Phenomenological interpretations of Aristotle: Initiation into phenomenological research* (R. Rojcewicz, Trans.). Bloomington: Indiana University Press. (Original lecture course given 1921–1922 and published 1985)

Horney, K. (1939). *New ways in psychoanalysis.* New York: Norton.

Horney, K. (1945). *Our inner conflicts.* New York: Norton.

Horney, K. (1950). *Neurosis and human growth.* New York: Norton.

Mitchell, S. (2000). Relationality: From attachment to intersubjectivity, New York: Analytic Press.

Perls, F., Hefferline, R. F., & Goodman, P. (1994). *Gestalt therapy: Excitement and growth in the human personality.* New York, NY: The Gestalt Journal Press, or.ed. 1951.

Sartre, J.-P. (1948). *The emotions: Outline for a theory.* New York: Philosophical Library. (Original work published 1939)

Sartre, J.-P. (1956). *Being and nothingness: An essay in phenomenological ontology* (H. Barnes, Trans.). New York: Philosophical Library. (Original work published 1943)

Spagnuolo Lobb, M. (2013). *The now-for-next in psychotherapy: Gestalt therapy recounted in post-modern society.* Siracusa: Istituto di Gestalt HCC Italy Publ. Co., www.gestaltitaly.com.

Sullivan, H. S. (1953). *The interpersonal theory of psychiatry.* New York: Norton.

Sullivan, H. S. (1954). *The psychiatric interview.* New York: Norton.

Editors' Introduction

*Margherita Spagnuolo Lobb and
Pietro Andrea Cavaleri*

Initially conceived to celebrate the seventieth anniversary of the birth of Gestalt psychotherapy, which came about with the publication of the text, *Gestalt Therapy*, by Perls, Hefferline, and Goodman, this book developed out of the desire on the part of a group of psychotherapists and trainers – belonging to the postgraduate School of Gestalt Psychotherapy of the Istituto di Gestalt Human Communication Center Italy – to re-examine the foundations of Gestalt psychotherapy in relational terms. The onset of the pandemic has brought about new challenges so central to our profession that we have been compelled to modify the orientation of the chapters in order to offer clinical tools more suitable to the times we are living through.

Our goal is to provide observations and new practices consistent with the epistemological principles of Gestalt therapy, in support of psychotherapists and caregiving professionals, who are performing a crucial task in the alleviation of the suffering caused by the pandemic.

We know that psychotherapy and society exist in a figure/ground relationship (Spagnuolo Lobb *et al.*, 1996; Lichtenberg, 1990). The problems which patients bring to therapy emerge out of the context of social, cultural, economic, and political situations, besides that of the specific stories of attachment in their primary and intimate relationships. Consequently, in society's various historical moments, psychotherapists are called upon to intervene in difficult situations. With this book, we wish to provide psychotherapists with relational keys to insight and intervention, useful for manoeuvring through the difficult and demanding state of affairs we are daily forced to confront. We are employing a phenomenological, aesthetic, and field perspective, and it represents a contemporaneous development in Gestalt psychotherapy.[1] In a desire to go beyond a manualised approach, we have not focussed on classical forms of psychopathology but have turned our attention to difficult life *situations*, to experiential fields of suffering within which we are working, rather than to the individuals in pain. We refer to the studies and exchanges we have had over the years with Gestalt psychotherapy colleagues, for instance Jean Marie Robine, Georges Wollants, Malcolm Parlett, Gordon Wheeler, and many others. This means we are observing the therapeutic situation

DOI: 10.4324/9781003313335-1

more than the symptom, and this involves considering complex interactions and resonances not only of individual psychopathological manifestations. In essence, it entails paying attention to the field of encounters. And it is for this reason, out of a passion for the field concept, duly embraced by all of our authors, that we have chosen to dedicate this volume to "psychopathological situations in the clinical fields of human relations". This represents a certain kind of relational compass in which to position the experiences of patients and the felt sensations of the therapist, as well as the unicity of their reciprocal interaction.

We have thus taken into consideration: the experience of children, some difficult childhood situations (such as separations, abuse, neurodevelopmental disorders, adolescent social closure), the experience of dependency, couples and family therapy, the condition of the elderly and the end of life, interventions for degenerative diseases, and the trauma of loss and mourning. These are all circumstances in which we think that it may be necessary to consider the intentionalities of contact of the individuals involved and the possibilities for change presented in the field, besides individual functioning, which could be neurotic, borderline, psychotic, traumatised, etc. (see Spagnuolo Lobb, 2016). A second volume will address the psychopathological experiences specific to our own time, and will attempt to reorganise the spectrum of the psychopathologies in the light of social developments and emerging suffering, especially due to the collective trauma generated by the pandemic. It is in this way that we would like to primarily offer up a view of the problematic experiential fields and a new reading of specific types of suffering.

We are delighted to present this first volume, which opens a Gestalt psychotherapy window on the life circumstances of those lives lived in pain – a situational window which includes the therapist themself and which avails itself of tools configured to modify the entire experiential field, not only the individual experience.

All the clinical studies and instruments presented in this book have been set up subject to an internal sense of cohesion. They begin with concrete situations, described according to the experiential ground of the patients, and provide examples of clinical work, which includes the feelings of the therapist, and which also aims to give a sense of relational security from which to build an integrated, well-oriented, and in a word, spontaneous sense of self.

These tough moments under consideration are dealt with according to two cardinal points: first, the description of the ground of these experiences; second, a field perspective which allows the presence of the therapist to be modulated. We use the concept of *aesthetic relational knowing* to orient the mutual intentionalities and the therapeutic movements during the session (the "dance steps" model, see Chapter 2).

The first five chapters, Part I, unveil the basic fundamentals of the book. An introductory chapter by the two editors, Margherita Spagnuolo Lobb and Pietro Andrea Cavaleri, defines the concept of the psychopathological situation, offering a new ethical position between the individual and society, one which allows the function of psychotherapy to evolve today. What follows is a chapter by Margherita Spagnuolo Lobb on contemporary treatment, with a focus on reciprocity and the therapeutic "dance" as a hermeneutic figure of therapeutic change, suited to today's need for relational rootedness. A third chapter by Pietro Andrea Cavaleri examines the anthropological model of Gestalt therapy and traces its development. These first chapters represent the specificity of the approach out of which the book emerges and continues its present-day perusal of the organism/environment field, including not only the therapeutic relationship but also the global social situation. For this reason, it seemed important for us to add the commentary of two luminaries of Gestalt therapy, Erving Polster and Gary Yontef. It was with great pleasure that we were able to detect some resonances with our approach. The fourth chapter, by Pietro Andrea Cavaleri, guides us to investigate "under the radar" phenomena as an epistemological orientation for the reader.

The fifth chapter finally describes the tool by means of which the book's clinical cases are presented, or at least studied – a clinical data sheet, developed in our Institute and as of now used by various other institutes and international psychotherapists. This tool is introduced by Margherita Spagnuolo Lobb, Maria Mione, and Elisabetta Conte.

Part II of the book deals with widespread clinical situations linked to various professional settings particularly affected by the pandemic. They pertain to traumatic situations and those of fragility requiring new types of expressly designed and effective professional tools, chiefly of the relational kind.

Silvia Tosi and Elisabetta Conte have dedicated their chapter to an examination of the new ways in which children are suffering. They describe a specific therapeutic setting and outline a clinical case. Marital separation, seen from the perspective of the couple's parental intentionality, is addressed by Paola Canna and Manuela Partinico. Rosanna Militello gives us an in-depth and vivid clinical deliberation on the complex trauma in preadolescence. Antonio Narzisi concentrates on the autistic spectrum disorder, referring particularly to the *Camouflage* effect. Michele Lipani introduces one of the most common types of malaise in Western society: social phobia among adolescents. The experience and treatment of addiction is described by Giancarlo Pintus and Marialuisa Grech. Pietro Andrea Cavaleri devotes the seventh chapter to the conflict within the couple as a "place of mutual recognition", whereas in the subsequent chapter, Giuseppe Sampognaro narrates in a most engaging manner the process of Gestalt therapy with a family. Alessandra Merizzi revisits from a Gestalt therapy standpoint the theme of ageing in today's world, in the time of the pandemic, with all of its stereotypes, its strengths, and its beneficial results. Donatella Buscemi and Alessandra Vela deal with the relationship with the chronic patient, in which the ability to accept and support on the part of the therapist becomes essential. The last chapter is an original contribution of Carmen Vázquez Bandín entirely dedicated to the grieving process in our time.

Note

1 You can read this particular development in Cavaleri, 2003, 2019, 2020; Spagnuolo Lobb, 2013, 2017a, 2017b, 2019.

References

Cavaleri, P. A. (2003). *La profondità della superficie. Percorsi introduttivi alla psicoterapia della Gestalt* [The depth of the surface. Introductory paths to Gestalt psychotherapy]. Milano: FrancoAngeli.

Cavaleri, P. A. (2019). Gestalt anthropology for businesses: How to face globalisation, solitude and production. In M. Spagnuolo Lobb & F. Meulmeester (Eds.). *Gestalt approaches with organisations* (pp. 67–86). Siracusa, Italy: Istituto di Gestalt HCC Italy Publ. Co., www.gestaltitaly.com.

Cavaleri, P. A. (2020). A Gestalt therapy reading of the pandemic. *The Humanistic Psychologist*, *48*(4), 347–352. DOI: 10.1037/hum0000214.

Lichtenberg, P. (1990). *Community and confluence. Undoing the clinch of oppression.* Highland, NY: Gestalt Press.

Spagnuolo Lobb, M. (2013). *The now-for-next in psychotherapy: Gestalt therapy recounted in post-modern society.* Siracusa: Istituto di Gestalt HCC Italy Publ. Co., www.gestalt italy.com.

Spagnuolo Lobb, M. (2016). Self as contact, contact as self. A contribution to ground experience in Gestalt therapy theory of self. In J.-M. Robine (Ed.). *Self. A poliphony of contemporary Gestalt therapists* (pp. 261–289). St. Romain la Virvée, France: L'Exprimerie.

Spagnuolo Lobb, M. (2017a). From losses of ego functions to the dance steps between psychotherapist and client. Phenomenology and aesthetics of contact in the psychotherapeutic field. *British Gestalt Journal*, *26*(1), 28–37.

Spagnuolo Lobb, M. (2017b). Phenomenology and aesthetic recognition of the dance between psychotherapist and client: A clinical example. *British Gestalt Journal*, *26*(2), 50–56.

Spagnuolo Lobb, M. (2019). The paradigm of reciprocity: How to radically respect spontaneity in clinical practice. *Gestalt Review*, *23*(3), 234–254. DOI: 10.5325/gestaltreview.23.3.0232.

Spagnuolo Lobb, M., Salonia, G., & Sichera, A. (1996). From the "discomfort of civilisation" to "creative adjustment": The relationship between individual and community in psychotherapy in the third millennium. *International Journal of Psychotherapy*, *1*(1), 45–53.

Psychopathology of the Situation

Chapter 1

Psychopathological Situations in a Post-Pandemic World

Gestalt Therapy in Emergent Clinical Fields

Margherita Spagnuolo Lobb and
Pietro Andrea Cavaleri

1. The Ethical Position of the Psychotherapist in the Post-Pandemic Period: The End of Narcissistic Solitude

Over the months and years to come, we will be dramatically changing our perspective on psychotherapeutic values as well as creating new tools. Humanistic values, traditionally focussed on supporting human potential and individual creativity, are evolving towards the value of a relational co-creation of a sense of security in our patients' ground experience.

Gestalt psychotherapy is contributing to this turning-point by focusing on the unfolding of experience of both patient and therapist in the here-and-now of their encounter and by using aesthetic tools capable of diagnosing[1] and helping the client by means of the knowing provided by the senses (in line with the phenomenological and humanistic tradition of Husserl; Merleau Ponty, Gendlin, and others); concentrating moreover on the "dance" between the therapist and the patient, made up of intentional reciprocal movements and supported by the therapist's relational aesthetic. Trusting the "dance" allows the patient to perceive the therapist's presence as deeply connected to their spontaneous movements and to feel the secure ground that grows out of this relationship. The pandemic spread of COVID-19 has influenced the perception of our contact with the environment, our relationship with the world, and our sense of self. The feeling of having a safe and secure ground – already precarious before coronavirus (Spagnuolo Lobb, 2013) – is lacking. People need to rediscover the sense of being able to count on the environment and on themselves in order to be open to a creative accommodation with the other.

We are daily experiencing our own *vulnerability* and that of the other. This can become an antidote to narcissism and a basis for the building of social solidarity (Cascio, 2020). Habitual narcissistic dissociation that leads us to blame or admire the other (Kohut, 1971; Lachmann, 2008) is put to the test. We have lost our isolated and narcissistic power (Lasch, 1978); we have understood that we cannot save ourselves by ourselves. We can imagine that salvation will come from our ability to be fully present and embrace our diversity, rather than through an

DOI: 10.4324/9781003313335-3

individual hero who performs righteous deeds. This new awareness can lead us to a deep and durable sense of belonging to the human community and allow us to accept our vulnerability, at the same time nurturing the growth of our humanity and our ethical values. The pandemic emergency can, in this way, guide us towards the very essence of our existence and towards a feeling of belonging.

In order to be a psychotherapist, one does not need to make "the right move" or blame oneself for not being empathic or creative no matter what. What is essential is an ecstatic and aesthetic attitude towards the experience of oneself and the patient. It entails having a humble and ethical attitude which does not deny limits and places reciprocity of presence in the foreground (Levinas, 1985; Ricoeur, 2005; Orange, 2017, 2018; Spagnuolo Lobb, 2018, 2019).

In this current period, exemplified by stressful social circumstances and lack of support, the ability of therapists to take care of their own well-being assumes an even greater value. We, too, are part of this society and just like our patients, we have been hit by a collective trauma. More than ever in this period, it is important for us, as psychotherapists, to maintain an equilibrium between our bodily sensations and our self-definitions. We must stay focussed on what we want to do as people, citizens, and professionals. Attaining a meaningful dialogue with other colleagues and belonging to a community are fundamental prerequisites for achieving this goal.

2. The Lack of Ground in a Desensitised Society

The evolution of primary relationships over the course of the last 70 years has directed us towards a very different ground experience than that of our predecessors, who inhabited the society in which most of the modern psychotherapies, including Gestalt psychotherapy, were born. In the Fifties, the experiential boundaries were clear. The gender roles, like the generational ones, for example, were (although superficial) well-defined (Irigaray, 1985; Recalcati, 2013). Becoming a grown-up meant taking responsibility, and a young person saw this passage as a proof of his own growth. Someone who did not conform to this "normalcy" was excluded and forced into a morass of pain and suffering, which created an unfair dichotomy (Ehrenberg, 2010). This injustice became the banner for the struggle of social minorities, being so central as it was to the human rights cause and to the values of humanistic therapies (Nota *et al.*, 2019).

It was precisely this destructuration of the previous reference points and of the social dichotomies that gave way to a loss of certainties (Vattimo and Rovatti, 2013). People at the time had to come to terms with a less clear definition of self, and with more fluid parental, filial, and social roles (Bauman, 1999). It was however important to feel fulfilled. Social rules were perceived as an obstacle to self-realisation as they were considered equal to the imposition of dictatorial regimes (Adorno, 1978). The freedom to express one's ideas, a basic victory of civil rights, was encouraged, as was the right to do whatever it takes to feel good (Berne, 1975; Rogers, 1978; Perls, 1942). The faith in the self-regulation of one's children motivated parents to confide in them, rather than take care of them, and to offer them a freedom that often resulted in confusing messages. This society, which was deemed narcissistic (Lasch, 1978), generated a crisis in relational and family ties, in favour of individual development. Subsequent generations had to deal with professionally fulfilled parents, who – trusting in the value of freedom – expected to have gifted offspring without the patience that the care of youngsters requires or the perception that this might be indispensable in their role as parents. This generation grew up lurching between admiration from their parents and the sense of being a sham, experiencing the absence of some type of enclosure that could truly make them feel seen and contained. The economic boom and the possibility of having everything that one could want on a consumer level often created more distance. This generation gave rise to insubstantial and fluid primary bonds. Their sons and daughters developed a sense of emptiness and personal instability. They had to physically desensitise themselves since they were unable to cope with the lack of containment of their energy. The most common clinical disorders were desensitisation, dependencies, depression, anhedonia, anxiety disorders, the difficulty to relate, eating disorders, and the struggle to focus in children. The pandemic fastened itself onto this relational set of emotional circumstances and became a collective trauma that intensified certain afflictions to do with individual/world relations (Taylor, 2020; Bocian, 2020).

The lack of containment in primary relationships and the uncertainty characterising previous generations have produced a crucial change in people's way of life. Our patients do not suffer so much because of their inability to separate themselves from important relationships (a problem of their personality-function: who am I in this relationship?) but more because they are uncertain about who or what they are, what they want, and if it is worth living, given that they don't know if they will be alive tomorrow. The embodied sense of security is compromised. There is a new existential condition that people are experiencing: they need to know whether they will continue to live tomorrow, whether they will be decapitated by fundamentalists or killed by an invisible virus, knowing that everything will happen for reasons beyond their control. There is an existential fear of not being able to control their entering into contact with the environment. All of this has given rise to a generalised experiential condition of desensitisation and a lack of a relational security that can be taken for granted.

Over the years, the need to work on the ground experience of patients has emerged more and more within psychotherapeutic treatment, certainly more than the work on the figure patients bring to therapy (Wheeler, 2000). The most famous Gestalt techniques, such as the empty chair, the exaggeration and expression of a sensation, etc., have for quite some time proven inadequate with respect to the need for the relational grounding of patients. We remember a demonstration session during a conference, in which the patient, one of the students of the therapist, kept asking the therapist/trainer "what do you think?" with respect to her problem of whether to stay or not in a relationship about which she felt ambivalent. The therapist continued to say to her that she had to take responsibility for her emotions and consequently for her choices, but the patient/student persisted: "I've come here to find out what YOU think." Working on the ground would entail responding to the need for this young woman's relational rootedness, for example by asking: "What do you feel when you ask me that question?" It is about working on the processes of their being in contact, in the here-and-now. It is possible for this person to find an answer if she feels comfortable with the therapist, if she works on the bodily processes that are activated in his presence (does she feel trust and thus breathes deeply, or shame and anger and thus stiffens, unable to open herself up to other feelings?), and she will then perceive a mutual correspondence in the therapist (will she feel him to be accepting and trusting or dismissive?). Today, in fact, patients do not need to find themselves within a relational autonomy (like during the time of the founding of Gestalt psychotherapy), but to feel their own presence and that of the therapist on the contact boundary between them. It is here that the experience of feeling seen and recognised by a significant other may be born. It is from here that a more vital and well-directed sense of self can emerge.

There is a widespread need today to work, as Porges (2017) underscores, on the co-creation of a safe ground, more than on the understanding of conflictual dynamics (do I have to stay in this relationship or not?).

3. The Social Ground: The Fear of Death and the Need to Feel Rooted

What can we say then about the ground experience which is common to everyone today?

The general impression is that there is a fear of death on the one hand and a need for rootedness on the other (Spagnuolo Lobb, 2016a). If we look at the socio-political movements of the Western world in the last few decades, we see that they have imposed their economic values on the poorer continents, promising an improvement in terms of welfare and democracy (Cavaleri, 2020). This imposition, however, has generated rampant poverty and drawn-out debilitating wars, "mass proletarianisation", corruption, and ever-growing inequalities between the few in power and the rest of the population (Bauman, 2001). A greater number of people have become poor, and there are more wars but less democracy. Now this movement is backfiring against the rich Western world, with mass migrations, loss of jobs and poverty, especially in the nations of the South. This has created a sense of ambivalence and uncertainty on both the social and clinical level. To what extent must we open our doors to foreigners? In the Fifties and Sixties, there was also, in the Western world, a large migratory wave following economic disaster created by the world wars. However, at that time, the ground experience of people in society was different: there were clearer points of reference and a more certain sense of self ("I know who I am, what I feel, what I believe in, and where I want to go") (Bauman, 1999).

Next to the experience of migratory flows, there is also the experience of terrorism and unexpected malicious acts, in which the enemy could be anyone who crosses our path. Our senses or feelings are not capable of perceiving who is a terrorist and who is instead a friendly and reliable person. Terrorism next door produces a sense of impotence and existential turmoil: not one of us can be sure of coming home alive when he goes out. Indeed, we cannot know if our neighbour is a terrorist or not. At the same time, technological development has greatly contributed to the globalisation of communication. Anyone, especially children, can find anything anywhere, although with a "non-grounded" sense of agency. What experience of agency can a child be expected to have if one can buy something or meet someone from another part of the world with a simple "click"? More often than not, this child has no idea what he/she is doing, only knowing that this "click" will produce a result. Sometimes this becomes too much for the child, and they are forced to become desensitised to their anxieties and fears. Life is full of surprises, and the child is not capable of connecting them with a sense of self, with their very own power to make contact (Rosa, 2016).

Another new aspect within our ground experience concerns climate change and natural disasters. Even though we are dealing with a real threat, if not the main one, we are not yet mindful enough of this danger in terms of our existence and that of our descendants. Courageous youngsters like the Swede, Greta Thunberg (2018), or colleagues like Donna Orange (2017), have brought to our attention the need to do something soon. The earth is no longer safe and yet we are desensitised vis-à-vis this issue just as we have probably become to the experience of the unreliable other.

4. Brilliant Ideas and Evolving Contradictions

Gestalt psychotherapy was founded in 1951. Since then, many things have changed, in society, in the patients as well as in the psychotherapeutic models.[2] But the novelty advanced by the founders at the time, one which remains at the heart of the approach, is the choice to focus on the here-and-now of the encounter between therapist and patient, on the contact, which they co-construct in the moment in which one seeks help from a concrete person and the other identifies him/herself in the role and intentionality of giving help. The founders' choice was for phenomenology (the here-and-now aimed towards the "soon-to-be"), for the aesthetics (the use of the senses as the chief tool of therapeutic knowledge), for the organism/environment field (that single and unrepeatable experience that is created when both the patient and therapist participate with their senses open, with full awareness, in their encounter which is firstly human and then professional). This relational, procedural, and field spirit that is so present in the original book did not immediately emerge, perhaps due to an obvious paradox. The authors, in fact, introduced, by means of the book, concepts, which were radically new for the beginning of the Fifties (for example "contact" and "contact boundary", "the self as a function of the organism/environment field" etc.), but at the same time used conceptual categories largely borrowed from psychoanalysis and in particular from the defence mechanisms analysed by Anna Freud. Not having an adequate terminology at their disposal (and not having devoted the time necessary for the development of new terms), they found themselves paradoxically almost forced to describe the phenomenology of the relational field by utilising concepts in vogue at the time, borrowed from an intrapsychic perspective, very different from their own. As Wollants states (2012), we would have to identify ourselves with the relational, contextual, and situational perspective, described in the first part of the book by Perls *et al.* (1951/1994), and afterwards, in the last chapters, not coherently developed.

After its establishment in the era of the New Age, Gestalt therapy proved attractive for its techniques, for the creativity with which it upheld individual freedom, for the vitality for which it advocated within psychopathological symptoms, and in short, for the free spirit which it managed to sustain within a generation, which, after the dictatorships and the trauma of war, needed to find the freedom and the power to be itself.

5. The Relational Turning-Point in Psychotherapy and the Field

In the complex post-modern society of the Eighties, it was necessary to re-emphasise the value of the relationship as intimately integral to humankind. It was important to find oneself not by freeing oneself from bonds (as propagandised in the previous decade by the aforementioned narcissistic society) but on the contrary, by the mutual constitutive mirroring provided by one's ties (Zambrano, 2000; Pulcini, 2001). In this way relational epistemology inherent within Gestalt psychotherapy was restored and developed.

Linking itself to neuroscientific research (Rizzolatti *et al.*, 1996; Gallese *et al.*, 2007; Damasio, 2010; Panksepp and Biven, 2012; Porges, 2011), to the evolutionary perspective of relational psychoanalysis (for instance Benjamin, 2017) and intersubjective psychoanalysis (Stern, 1985; Beebe and Lachman, 2002; and others), and obviously to the relational insights of colleagues of Gestalt therapy (Yontef, 2001; Frank, 2001, 2016; Robine, 2003; Jacobs and Hycner, 2009, Clemmens, 2020, to name only a few), The Gestalt Institute HCC Italy has done specialised research in psychopathology (Francesetti *et al.*, 2013), on development (Spagnuolo Lobb *et al.*, 2016), on groups and organisations (Spagnuolo Lobb and Meulmeester, 2019), and on the field (Francesetti, 2015; Spagnuolo Lobb, 2018, 2019; Macaluso, 2020a). The field perspective, which supports the input of the therapist's presence in the diagnostic and therapeutic process (Parlett, 1991; Spagnuolo Lobb, 2018; Macaluso, 2020b; Spagnuolo Lobb and Resnick, 2020), has enhanced and deepened clinical thought. Furthermore, the use of the senses, since the beginning central to the Gestalt psychotherapy approach, permits the Gestalt psychotherapist to grab onto the vitality still present within the psychic malaise and reinforce it during the therapeutic intervention.

When, in the 2000s, the loss of reference points in the post-modern era brought us to the collapse of existential, economic, and relational certainties, Gestalt psychotherapy was ready to take up the need to work on the ground more than on the figure (Wheeler, 2000; Spagnuolo Lobb, 2012, 2016b), in order to rebuild precisely those certainties once taken for granted, and which now seem to be lacking in our "liquid" society. By highlighting the importance of the ground, Wheeler has furnished a frame for moving the emphasis from an individualistic paradigm to a relational one (or one of the contact boundary) (Macaluso, 2015).

For example, if a client, feeling ashamed, says to us, that he was aggressive with his partner, the figure is the aggression (subject of the referral) or, in relational terms, the figure is the feeling of shame, for example, that the patient feels towards the therapist at the moment in which he tells her that he has been aggressive. The ground is the experience from which the shame emerges, the sense of security or uncertainty, which he senses and which makes him feel comfortable or not, the short or relaxed breath, the stiff or flexible posture. Working on the figure entails understanding the aggression (when it is presented, what does it remind him of, what does the patient feel when he tells the story to the therapist?). Working on the ground entails facilitating a sense of security taken for granted between therapist and patient, making the patient feel that he is in a safe place to the extent that he will express fear and shame with all of himself to the therapist. It means asking the patient what he sees, how he perceives the therapist. It means inviting him to breathe, giving him those neurophysiological supports that promote the ventro vagal sensation of security.[3] For Gestalt psychotherapy, the self is contact (Perls *et al.*, 1951/1994), and the process of the figure/ground formation expresses the modality with which it happens. The organism/environment field is the experiential unity from which both change and growth emerge. As the founders state: "the energy for the figure-formation comes from both poles of the field, both the organism and the environment." (Perls *et al.*, 1951/1994, p. 181).

The organism and the environment are in a reciprocal relationship with each other. This relationship is not to be understood in the sense that first there is a person and then there is a world, but both are inseparable and interdependent parts of a dynamic totality. This interweaving of interactions between a human being and his or her environment is defined by Robine (2003) and Wollants (2012) with the term situation, which they prefer to the term field, often used in other fields and with other meanings. Thinking in terms of situation allows us to avoid many dichotomies and to better understand the processes that take place in the field.

The situation is "prior" to the subject/object distinction. To conceive of the human being as a "situational being" is to affirm the impossibility of separating the two parts. The self is always "engaged in the situation" and "there is no feeling of self and other objects outside the experience we have of the situation" (Perls *et al.*, 1951/1994, p. 155). The id of the situation is the (preverbal, prepersonal, implicit) way in which the body experiences its situation (Robine, 2003).

The therapist's feeling is part of the field. Their awareness, if it emerges from the full presence at the contact boundary with the patient, becomes an important tool for both therapeutic insight and therapeutic intervention. The construct of *aesthetic relational knowing* (Spagnuolo Lobb, 2018), which will often recur in this book, signifies a process that occurs between the therapist and the client by means of which the therapist comes to know in a bodily felt manner the meaning being expressed in the field (Gendlin, 1968). It is a clinical construct that has been validated (Spagnuolo Lobb *et al.*, 2022) in order to make the therapeutic activity as specific as possible, tailoring it to the patient's particular experience and contextualising it within a specific therapeutic field (see Chapter 2).

6. The Gestalt Institute HCC Italy and Studies on Development, Psychopathology, and the Field

For more than 15 years, the Gestalt Institute HCC Italy has been working on the concept of psychopathology and development in a field perspective (Francesetti and Gecele, 2009; Spagnuolo Lobb, 2012, 2013). Over and above the "translation" of the concepts of classical psychopathology and the clinical classifications of the DSM in Gestalt therapy terms (Francesetti *et al.*, 2013), the Institute has developed the possibility of including the evolution of a person, the establishment over the years of an existence that is now manifested in a given way in the here-and-now of the therapeutic session (Spagnuolo Lobb, 2016a). Working on the patient's developmental aspects (something that, in Gestalt therapy before the year 2000 was often considered a distraction from the here-and-now) has provided concrete instruments for addressing therapeutic intervention on the ground experience, which is especially weakened today. Many of us have developed what Heidegger (1921–1922) has extensively written about: "the relationality and its vicissitudes". Concepts such as the *polyphonic development of domains* (Spagnuolo Lobb, 2012), the *aesthetic relational knowing* (Spagnuolo Lobb, 2018), the *now-for-next* (Spagnuolo Lobb, 2013), the *dance of reciprocity* (Spagnuolo Lobb, 2017a, 2017b, 2019), have represented concrete tools for tackling contemporary clinical examples of suffering. As Wollants claims (2012, Chapter 2), the psychopathology of development should try to understand psychological problems within the totality of the context of development.

In fact, it is from this safe ground that a unified sense of self can emerge. Without it, the experience of self-in-the-world becomes fragmented, subject to traumas, dissociated, desensitised, and even violent. The concept of psychopathology in Gestalt psychotherapy is defined as a loss of spontaneity, engendered by the anxiety with which certain modes of contact are learned, for example, introjecting with anxiety (Spagnuolo Lobb, 2013, p. 66).

This is our Gestalt therapy contribution to this epoch-making turning-point which we are living through: to go from the advocacy of freedom and individual integrity to the creation of a sense of security and self-rootedness that emerges from the co-created field of the therapeutic relationship.

7. The Challenges of the Pandemic

The pandemic experience was appended to this precarious organism/environment balance, and to a widespread sense of uncertainty and fragility. This has been a devastating landmark event that quickly turned into a collective trauma. The collapse of the myth of modern science, of the power of being interconnected with the entire globe, the inability to have faith in the air we breathe, and the necessity of considering others as potential viral spreaders have generated the sudden vulnerability of an unexpectedly treacherous and uncertain present. The pandemic is revealed on the planetary level not only as an unstoppable health crisis, but above all as a political and ethical crisis, as it sheds light on unresolved contradictions and ones still awaiting adequate as well as radical answers.

Common to every traumatic experience, the effects of the pandemic will become clear only after a profound "post-traumatic processing" of what happened takes place. Now, from a planetary perspective, we all need to reflect together on our present way of life and plan the future. The time has come to place the environment at the centre of our lives. However, we do not mean only the natural environment, but the ecosystem, and resource management, but also the human environment, comprised of relationships, of the attention to the dignity of all, of the recognition of the needs of others, of the fight against injustice, of the resistance to inequalities and to the many forms of poverty as well. In this complex and laborious "post-traumatic processing", every psychotherapist is called upon to do their part and in so doing, discover the rich political and social value of the approach they endorse.

In a world deeply wounded by the pandemic and by what we might call the "spirit of war", it is first of all necessary to take care of ourselves, heal our ground experience in order to be able to offer up a sound and stable presence to our patients. Unlike other traumatic situations confronted in therapy, in the case of this pandemic, those who are giving the care are exposed to the same risks as those being treated. This situation radically alters the way in which we do psychotherapy. It creates a field of profound humanity, in which it makes no sense to behave with the detachment of someone who does not wish to get involved with the patient's pain. We have been able to concretely experience that what we need to treat our trauma (we cannot think that we have not been influenced by it) is to dialogue and debate with colleagues, to listen to their pain and express our own, to feel that we are not alone in this loss of our previous certainties. It is by feeling on safe ground that we can be ready to forge a stable and welcoming environment for our patients.

This book is the result of the exchange of a group of psychotherapy trainers "impacted" by the pandemic currents.

Notes

1   The etymology of the word "dia-gnosis" comes from knowing (gnosis) through (dia).

2   For an analysis of clinical suffering and the corresponding social experiences in various decades, see Spagnuolo Lobb, 2013, 2016b, 2017c, 2017d; Cavaleri, 2019.
3   For an in-depth study of the clinical concept of the experiential ground, see Chapter 2.

References

Adorno, T. (1978). *Minima Moralia: Reflections from damaged life*. London: Verso.
Bauman, Z. (1999). *La società dell'incertezza* [The uncertainty society]. Bologna: il Mulino.
Bauman, Z. (2000). *Missing community*. Cambridge: Polity Press.
Bauman, Z. (2001). *Community. Seeking safety in an insecure world*. Cambridge: Polity.
Beebe, B., & Lachmann, F. M. (2002). *Infant research and adult treatment: Co-constructing interactions*. Hillsdale, NJ: The Analytic Press/Taylor & Francis Group.
Benjamin, J. (2017). *Beyond doer and done to: Recognition theory, intersubjectivity, and the third*. New York: Routledge.
Berne, E. (1975). *Transactional analysis in psychotherapy*. London: Souvenir Press Ltd.
Bocian, B. (2020). Fear, self-support, and "good introjects". *The Humanistic Psychologist*, *48*(4), 363–368. DOI: 10.1037/hum0000206.
Cascio, A. R. (2020). Le eredità del Covid-19: la necessità di un pensiero psicologico nei nostri ospedali [The legacies of Covid-19: The need for psychological thinking in our hospitals]. *Piazza Futura*. https://piazzafutura.it/2020/04/04/eredita-covid-19-ospedali/.
Cavaleri, P. A. (2019). Gestalt anthropology for businesses: How to face globalisation, solitude and production. In M. Spagnuolo Lobb & F. Meulmeester (Eds.). *Gestalt Approaches with Organisations* (pp. 67–86). Gestalt Therapy Book Series. Siracusa, Italy: Istituto di Gestalt HCC Italy Publ. Co., www.gestaltitaly.com.
Cavaleri, P. A. (2020). A Gestalt therapy reading of the pandemic. *The Humanistic Psychologist*, *48*(4): 347–352. DOI: 10.1037/hum0000214.
Clemmens, M. C. (Ed.). (2020). *Embodied relational Gestalt: Theories and applications*. Abingdon, UK: Routledge, Taylor & Francis Group Ltd.
Damasio, A. (2010). *Self comes to mind: Constructing the conscious brain*. New York: Pantheon.
Ehrenberg, A. (2010). *The weariness of self: Diagnosing the history of depression in the contemporary age*. Montreal: McGill-Queen's University Press.
Francesetti, G. (2015). From individual symptoms to psychopathological fields. Towards a field perspective on clinical human suffering. *British Gestalt Journal*, *24*(1), 5–19.
Francesetti, G., & Gecele, M. (2009). A Gestalt therapy perspective on psychopathology and diagnosis. *British Gestalt Journal*, *18*(2), 5–20.
Francesetti, G., Gecele, M., & Roubal, J. (2013). *Gestalt therapy in clinical practice. From psychopathology to the aesthetics of contact*. Gestalt Therapy Book Series. Siracusa, Italy: Istituto di Gestalt HCC Italy Publ. Co., www.gestaltitaly.com
Frank, R. (2001). *Body of awareness. A somatic and developmental approach to psychotherapy*. Highland, NY: Gestalt Press.
Frank, R. (2016). Moving experience: Kinaesthetic resonance as relational feel. In M. Spagnuolo Lobb, N. Levi, & A. Williams (Eds.). *Gestalt therapy with children. From epistemology to clinical practice* (pp. 87–99). Gestalt Therapy Book Series. Siracusa: Istituto di Gestalt HCC Italy Publ. Co., www.gestaltitaly.com.
Gallese, V., Eagle, M. N., & Migone, P. (2007). Intentional attunement: Mirror neurons and the neural underpinnings of interpersonal relations. *Journal of the American psychoanalytic Association*, *55*(1), 131–175.

Gendlin, E. T. (1968). *Focusing*. New York: Bantam.

Heidegger, M. (1921–1922). *Phenomenological interpretations of Aristotle: Initiation into phenomenological research*. Indiana University Press, 2001. https://doi.org/10.2307/j.ctvswx8nz.

Irigaray, L. (1985). *Speculum of the other woman*. Ithaca, NY: Cornell University Press.

Jacobs, L., & Hycner, R. (Eds.). (2009). *Relational approaches in Gestalt therapy*. New York: A Gestalt Press Book.

Kohut, H. (1971). *The analysis of the self: A systematic approach to the psychoanalytic treatment of narcissistic personality disorders*. New York: International Universities Press.

Lachmann, F. M. (2008). *Transforming narcissism: Reflections on empathy, humor, and expectations*. New York: The Analytic Press.

Lasch, C. (1978). *The culture of narcissism: American life in an age of diminishing expectations*. New York: W.W. Norton & Co.

Levinas, E. (1985). *Ethics and infinity*. Pittsburgh: Duquesne University Press.

Macaluso, M. A. (2015). Beyond the perls-goodman model: From the organism-environment field to the relational field. *Gestalt Review*, *19*(3), 233–250. DOI: 10.5325/gestaltreview.19.3.0233.

Macaluso, M. A. (2020a). Deliberateness and spontaneity in Gestalt therapy practice. *British Gestalt Journal*, *29*(1), 30–36.

Macaluso, M. A. (2020b), Il concetto di "campo" in psicoterapia della Gestalt. Sviluppi e implicazioni [The concept of "field" in Gestalt psychotherapy. Developments and implications]. *Quaderni di Gestalt*, *XXXIII*(1), 57–73. DOI: 10.3280/GEST2020-001005.

Nota, L., Mascia, M., & Pievani, T. (2019). *Diritti umani e inclusione* [Human rights and inclusion]. Bologna: il Mulino.

Orange, D. M. (2017). *Climate crisis, psychoanalysis, and radical ethics*. New York, NY: Routledge.

Orange, D. M. (2018). My other's keeper: Resources for the ethical turn in psychotherapy. In M. Spagnuolo Lobb, D. Bloom, J. Roubal, J. Zeleskov Djoric, M. Cannavò, R. La Rosa, S. Tosi, & V. Pinna (Eds.). *The aesthetic of otherness: Meeting at the boundary in a desensitized world, proceedings* (pp. 19–32). Siracusa, Italy: Istituto di Gestalt HCC Italy Publ. Co., www.gestaltitaly.com.

Panksepp, J., & Biven, L. (2012). *The archaeology of mind: Neuroevolutionary origins of human emotion*. New York: W.W. Norton & Company Inc.

Parlett, M. (1991). Reflections on field theory. *British Gestalt Journal, 1*, 68–91.

Perls, F. (1942). *Ego, hunger and aggression: A revision of Freud's theory and method*. New York: Random House.

Perls, F., Hefferline, R. F., & Goodman, P. (1994). *Gestalt therapy: Excitement and growth in the human personality*. New York, NY: The Gestalt Journal Press, or.ed. 1951.

Porges, S. W. (2011). *The polyvagal theory: Neurophysiological foundations of emotions, attachment, communication, and self-regulation*. New York: W.W. Norton & Company, Inc.

Porges, S. W. (2017). *The pocket guide to the polyvagal theory. The transformative power of feeling safe*. New York: W.W. Norton & Company, Inc.

Pulcini, E. (2001). *L'individuo senza passioni. Individualismo moderno e perdita del legame sociale* [The individual without passions. Modern individualism and loss of the social bond]. Torino: Bollati-Boringhieri.

Recalcati, M. (2013). *Il complesso di Telemaco. Genitori e figli dopo il tramonto del padre* [The Telemachus complex. Parents and children after the decline of the father]. Milano: Feltrinelli.

Ricoeur, P. (2005). *The course of recognition*. Cambridge: Harvard University Press.

Rizzolatti, G., Fadiga, L., Gallese, V., & Fogassi, L. (1996). Premotor cortex and the recognition of motor actions. *Brain Research. Cognitive Brain Research, 3*(2), 131–141.

Robine, J.-M. (2003). Intentionality in flesh and blood: Toward a psychopathology of forecontacting. *International Gestalt Journal, XXVI*(2), 85–110.

Rogers, C. (1978). *Personal power: Inner strength and its revolutionary impact*. New York: Little, Brown Book Group.

Rosa, H. (2016). *Resonanz. Eine Soziologie der Weltbeziehung*. Berlin: Suhrkamp.

Spagnuolo Lobb, M. (2012). Toward a developmental perspective in Gestalt therapy, theory and practice: The polyphonic development of domains. *Gestalt Review, 16*(3), 222–244.

Spagnuolo Lobb, M. (2013). *The now-for-next in psychotherapy: Gestalt therapy recounted in post-modern society*. Siracusa: Istituto di Gestalt HCC Italy Publ. Co., www.gestaltitaly.com.

Spagnuolo Lobb, M. (2016a). Self as contact, contact as self. A contribution to ground experience in Gestalt therapy theory of self. In J.-M. Robine (Ed.). *Self. A poliphony of contemporary Gestalt therapists* (pp. 261–289). St. Romain la Virvée, France: L'Exprimerie.

Spagnuolo Lobb, M. (2016b). Gestalt therapy with children. Supporting the polyphonic development of domains in a field of contacts. In M. Spagnuolo Lobb, N. Levi, & A. Williams (Eds.). *Gestalt therapy with children. From epistemology to clinical practice* (pp. 25–62). Siracusa: Istituto di Gestalt HCC Italy, www.gestaltitaly.com.

Spagnuolo Lobb, M. (2017a). From losses of ego functions to the dance steps between psychotherapist and client. Phenomenology and aesthetics of contact in the psychotherapeutic field. *British Gestalt Journal, 26*(1), 28–37.

Spagnuolo Lobb, M. (2017b). Phenomenology and aesthetic recognition of the dance between psychotherapist and client: A clinical example. *British Gestalt Journal, 26*(2), 50–56.

Spagnuolo Lobb, M. (2017c). Psychotherapy in Post Modern Society. *Gestalt Today Malta, 1*(2), 45–55.

Spagnuolo Lobb, M. (2017d). Die Psychotherapie in der postmodernen Gesellschaft. *Gestalt Therapie, 31*(1), 3–25.

Spagnuolo Lobb, M. (2018). Aesthetic relational knowledge of the field: A revised concept of awareness in Gestalt therapy and contemporary psychiatry. *Gestalt Review, 22*(1), 50–68. DOI: 10.5325/gestalt review.22.1.0050.

Spagnuolo Lobb, M. (2019). The paradigm of reciprocity: How to radically respect spontaneity in clinical practice. *Gestalt Review, 23*(3), 234–254, 2019. DOI: 10.5325/gestaltreview.23.3.0232.

Spagnuolo Lobb, M., Levi, N., & Williams, A. (2016). Introduction: From dental aggression to suffering of the "between". In M. Spagnuolo Lobb, N. Levi, & A. Williams (Eds.). *Gestalt therapy with children. From epistemology to clinical practice* (pp. 13–20). Siracusa: Istituto di Gestalt HCC Italy Publ. Co., www.gestaltitaly.com.

Spagnuolo Lobb, M., & Meulmeester, F. (Eds.). (2019). *Gestalt approaches with organisations*. Siracusa (Italy): Istituto di Gestalt HCC Italy Publ. Co., www.gestaltitaly.com.

Spagnuolo Lobb, M., & Resnick, R. W. (2020). *The presence of Gestalt therapist in the field. Dialogue on Isadore from's lesson*. Free access articles, www.gestaltitaly.com, www.gestaltitaly.com/contents/freeaccess/20201130_dialogue_Spagnuolo_Lobb_Bob_ Resnick.pdf.

Spagnuolo Lobb, M., Sciacca, F., Iacono Isidoro, S., & Hichy, Z. (2022). A measure for psychotherapist's intuition: Construction, development, and pilot study of the aesthetic relational knowledge scale (ARKS). *The Humanistic Psychologist*, *50*(1). DOI: 10.1037/hum0000278.

Stern, D. N. (1985). *The interpersonal world of the infant: A view from psychoanalysis and developmental psychology*. New York: Basic Books.

Taylor, M. (2020). Collective trauma and the relational field. *The Humanistic Psychologist*, *48*(4), 382–388. DOI: 10.1037/hum0000215.

Thunberg, G. (2018). *Our house is on fire: Scenes of a family and a planet in crisis*. Broadway and New York, NY: Penguin Random House.

Vattimo, G., & Rovatti, P. A. (2013). *Weak thought*. Albany, NY: State University of New York Press.

Wheeler, G. (2000). *Beyond individualism: Toward a new understanding of self, relationship, and experience*. Hillsdale, NJ: The Analytic Press.

Wollants, G. (2012). *Gestalt therapy. Therapy of the situation*. London: Sage.

Yontef, G. M. (2001). Relational Gestalt therapy. In J.-M. Robine (Ed.). *Contact and relationship in a field perspective* (pp. 79–94). Bordeaux: L'Exprimerie.

Zambrano, M. (2000). *Persona e democrazia* [Person and democracy]. Milano: Bruno Mondadori.

Chapter 2

Working on the Ground, on Aesthetics, and on the "Dance"

Aesthetic Relational Knowing and Reciprocity

Margherita Spagnuolo Lobb

1. Introduction

As Hanna Arendt has said, *the presence of others that see what we see and hear what we hear reassures us of the reality of the world and of ourselves.*

We have advocated for the importance of psychotherapy to be concerned with the ground experience of patients, an aspect of the sense of self-in-relation-to, something which happens to be especially fragile at this time. This need is, and will be, even more crucial during and after the pandemic, and the war in Ukraine, given that a collective trauma is drastically threatening our basic sense of security, and therefore the ground experience with which people perceive and define themselves in their contact with others.

In this chapter, I will attempt to call our attention as psychotherapists firstly to the ground experience of people taking part in our style of treatment; secondly, to the therapist's field sensitive presence; and thirdly, to the "dance of reciprocity" between therapist and patient as the space for therapeutic change.

In all likelihood, our entire psychotherapeutic culture will have to become increasingly focussed on the ground in the coming years, in order for us to more deeply understand people and their processes of change. In addition, this work on the ground will require intervening in different, less classical settings. We will place our psychotherapeutic skills at the disposal of situations in which a sense of self is being constituted, just as it is in schools, in primary relationships, in adolescent groups, and in the work environment.

A teacher, for example, of a class of pupils who cannot stay still and concentrate effectively on what she is explaining, can be helped to better carry out her work if she understands certain psychological aspects of the pupils' ground experience. In order to remain still and concentrate, they need to feel safe, and not have to embark on emergency functions (see Tucci *et al.*, 2018), such as escaping, or being hyper-attentive to other collateral stimuli. Before approaching a lesson, the teacher, seeing that the class is hyperactive and little inclined to concentrate, could initiate a physical exercise that facilitates a deep physiological sense of security, and therefore the possibility of feeling rooted and unthreatened.[1] If this sensation of safety does not exist, as Porges states (Porges and Dana, 2018), it is not

DOI: 10.4324/9781003313335-4

possible to set in motion the learning process. This is true not only in a school setting but also for the productive processes within the work environment and for therapeutic change. It is especially so, in the case of psychotherapy, that achieving a deep feeling of security within oneself, in the moment of entering into contact with the other, becomes the goal of intervention itself, the fundamental sense of neuroceptive and relational security.

2. What Does it Mean that Psychotherapy Must Concern Itself With the Ground?

The ground includes the way in which we have learned to make contact with our surroundings, what we have learned and have unconsciously put into practice in the here-and-now of our being-with the environment. A very simple example is our seated posture when in the living-room with friends. It is about the physiological and motor adjustments with which we have learned to exhibit our body in a group, which in turn encompasses our history, with respect to the ease or unease of being with our body that has been forged over countless experiences (Reich, 1933; Lowen, 1958). For instance, it is possible that our body did not fall prey to serious illnesses, or instead, it could have been subjected to painful adjustments. It includes being male, female, or non-binary in the face of the world, and the way in which we define ourselves socially: timid, or able to engage others, agreeable, in spite of our problems, or disturbing, aside from feeling sympathy for them.

From these examples, we can understand how the ground positions us in the world, depending on the various situations in which we find ourselves (Clemmens, 2020). Contrary to what was highlighted in the Fifties by the here-and-now approaches, today we can state that, in order to understand a person, we cannot disregard previous experiences, not in causal terms, but rather for how they establish and support this person's presence now, nor can we operate without the situational context in which we find ourselves with him/her.

For example, in order to understand a patient who says he wants help to separate from his wife, we have to ascertain how he has learned to be in the world with his body and the way in which he defines himself (with the subtle and complex neurobiological and relational processes), if he cannot breathe when his wife accuses him, or if he feels guilty for not making her happy. And we also have to grasp how he expects the world to react to his suffering.

In terms of a very interesting principle of phenomenology, a reality does not exist disconnected from the present experience of the persons involved (cfr. Husserl, 1910/1980). Perls *et al.* (1994) describe it in a vivid way when they refer to their "contextual" method:

> Thus the reader is apparently confronted with an impossible task: to understand the book he must have the "Gestaltist" mentality, and to acquire it he must understand the book.
>
> (Perls *et al.*, 1951/1994, p. XXIV)

We cannot understand a patient in the abstract; we can only *express our experience in the here-and-now of our encounter with him/her*. And it is there that all of our art is implemented. For us, reality is always in the here-and-now, even when we ask for something to be simulated. The patient's reality is one in which he lives. We have no other realities except those of the here-and-now.[2] In the specific case of the therapeutic session (whether individual, couple, family, or group), its reality is made, above all, by a patient who has significantly invested in the coming to therapy, and who has his/her own specific story of the evolution of a sense of self, at a bodily and social level. It is from this ground that the patient becomes determined to be with us, deciding in the fleeting moment of the present what to say and not say to the therapist, and "keeping hold of the helm" of his/her request for help from the therapist in a way that is more or less clear and defined. This process of identifying oneself on the basis of a ground, motivated by contact intentionality, is the patient's masterwork of integration (regardless of the gravity of the disorder). The therapist is successful in capturing this "beauty" if he turns his attention not only to what the patient does or asks but also to *how* he asks it, and to his/her *own feeling* in the role of therapist in that situation.

In order to enter into a dialogue with the patient's "masterwork", the therapist works on three levels, integrating (1) what they know about the patient (diagnostic and anamnestic elements), (2) what they observe of the patient's way of making contact with them, (3) their spontaneous resonance when facing that specific patient (see figure 2.1).

Referring to the previous example of a seated posture in the context of a session – I am aware of simplifying for the sake of explanation – the patient could have learned that his sexual feelings are not "normal" for the other, and this could

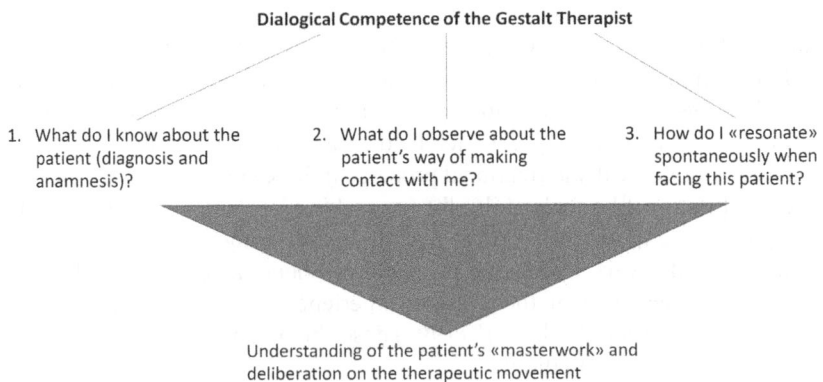

Dialogical Competence of the Gestalt Therapist

1. What do I know about the patient (diagnosis and anamnesis)?

2. What do I observe about the patient's way of making contact with me?

3. How do I «resonate» spontaneously when facing this patient?

Understanding of the patient's «masterwork» and deliberation on the therapeutic movement

*masterpiece = unitary typical of the patient's experience

Figure 2.1 Dialogical competence of the Gestalt therapist

have led him to experience these emotions with excitement, without the support of oxygen, of a deep breath, that is with a feeling of anxiety (first level: according to the DSM-5, this could be diagnosed as generalised anxiety disorder). This is visible to the therapist by the embarrassment that he notices in the way in which the patient makes contact with him (second level: according to a Gestalt diagnosis, we are able to notice that the patient creatively adjusts to the perceived loss of the other's support, to his own excitement, retroflecting his contact energy), but also by exploring himself, his own feeling when faced with this patient (third level: the therapist could feel disillusioned by this patient who is unable to overcome his timidity, thus reproducing the unitarity typical of that patient's experience: feeling embarrassed in front of the other who expects rather than supports).

3. The Relational Turning-Point in Gestalt Psychotherapy: The Field and the "Dance"

As outlined in Chapter 1, our lens as Gestalt psychotherapists widened after the relational turning-point of the 1990s. We look not only at the client but also at the co-creation between therapist and client, and we see the therapist's feelings as part of the client's experiential field (Spagnuolo Lobb, 2019). Perls' slogan, "Lose your mind and come to your senses" is now seen as coming to the "senses of the field." Both the client's perception and the therapist's are considered not as isolated phenomena but as individual perceptions which, insofar as they emerge from a given situation, have something in common: both of them contribute to create a shared reality.

It is from the Perls and Goodman model (Perls *et al.*, 1951/1994) – which, if on the one hand explores what happens in the "between", and on the other, is still, for many aspects, centred on the individual (cf. Wheeler, 2000; Wollants, 2012) – that we moved forward to the dynamic and creative organisation of the experience co-created in the space and time of the encounter with the other (Spagnuolo Lobb, 2013a). We are not dealing with organismic self-regulation, in terms of the traditional humanistic perspective of the Sixties, but with the self-regulation of a situational field of contacts (Parlett, 1991; Bloom, 2003; Stemberger, 2018; Spagnuolo Lobb, 2017a, 2017b; Wollants, 2012). We are not looking at the self-regulation of a person, but at the self-regulation of the experiential field between therapist and patient, of their being together.

The primary space of the psychological experience, upon which psychotherapeutic theory and practice must turn their attention, is precisely the contact, in other words, the space in which the self and the environment enact their encounter and become involved with each other. Any type of contact has a creative and dynamic character (cf. Spagnuolo Lobb, 2016b).

The contact boundary is therefore the place in which the experience occurs, where differences and their integration emerge; on the other hand, the field expresses in a unitary way the reality of the organism and its environment.[3] For example, in the case of a couple coming into therapy because of continuous fights surrounding decisions involving their son, the contact boundary is the quarrel about the son's education, and the field is the tension both are experiencing in their desire to achieve what is best for the child. The psychological intervention should focus on supporting this shared intentionality, more than on the dispute. In a field perspective, any definition of making contact has to consider the experience of the partners in contact. It makes no sense to look at the patient without considering the therapist. The same patient with a narcissistic experience (someone who, for instance, must avoid the anxiety generated by an intense closeness) could become inaccessible to a therapist who possesses a warm style but available and open to another who has a detached style. The same patient can trigger different reactions when faced with different therapists. In truth, even if we have been repeating this concept for many years, the fundamental idea of observing the patient rather than the experience of both therapist and patient is still what guides our actions.

This chapter attempts to develop and promote those competencies for working on what happens in the field experience. The concept of the aesthetic knowing, which I will discuss later on, is aimed to support the intuition of the therapist – including the counter-transferential processes – in field terms. I have described it elsewhere (Spagnuolo Lobb, 2018a, p. 61) as "the sensorial intelligence of the shared phenomenological field". We become acquainted with the other through our senses, which also transmit any experiential change. The relational approach leads us to focus on the reciprocity of our interaction with the patient, rather than simply on how the patient makes contact with us (see Spagnuolo Lobb and Resnick, 2020; Müller, 1993), because it is there, in the "dance" between us, that we find the possibility of revitalising the contact boundary where the self is co-created. For that patient with narcissistic experience, the possibility of feeling accepted and acknowledged resides in the "dance" that he and that particular therapist will be able to create, regardless of whether the therapist is warm or detached. Besides looking at the experiential ground, by means of which patients present themselves to us, we pay attention to the figure, and to the "dance" with which we co-create our therapeutic contact (see paragraph 5.3).

The fact that we concentrate on the "dance" allows us to stay faithful to the concept of *vitality*, crucial for the Gestalt therapy founders (Perls *et al.*, 1951/1994, p. 61 ff). Thanks to the therapist's own resonance in the situation shared with the patient, the therapist can seize upon what he could not develop, that vitality, which the patient had to stifle, in order to creatively adapt to difficult situations. In the case of the patient with narcissistic experience, the therapist can take hold of his need to be acknowledged for his self-sacrifice, in order to be responsible towards others.

4. Psychopathological Situations

In Gestalt therapy, we consider psychopathology as a *creative adjustment in a difficult situation* (Perls *et al.*, 1951/1994, p. 209; Wollants, 2012, pp. 35–48). It is precisely thanks to the field perspective that we can think back on psychopathology as a way of facing the world in difficult life situations, a way that satisfies important needs and reduces or avoids the anxiety that accompanies them. To function in a healthy way, an individual needs input from the world, from society: a healthy solipsistic functioning cannot exist. Gestalt psychotherapy is challenging traditional psychopathology by stating that the so-called "mental disorders" represent "disorders in the reciprocal relationships of a person and his/her phenomenal surroundings" (Wollants, 2012, p. IX), in which the symptoms are better understood as significant attempts to cope with these disorders. Defining a behaviour as "healthy", "mature", or on the contrary, "pathological" or "immature" implies a reference to a norm external to the person's experience, set by someone not immersed in the situation (and for this reason considered "objective") (Spagnuolo Lobb, 2013a, p. 36).

Psychopathology is basically the lack of spontaneity in the act of contacting the environment, a loss of parts of the functioning of the self, and is tied to both the condition of the ground and the modality with which the figures are co-created (Spagnuolo Lobb, 2016a; Macaluso, 2015, 2020). The usual interruptions of contact lead to an accumulation of incomplete situations (interrupted spontaneity results in open Gestalts and incomplete situations), which subsequently continue to interrupt other processes of meaningful contact. The *anxiety* which accompanies the primary interruption of contact (that with the repetition of situations becomes habitual) is the consequence of an excitement that has not had sufficient support on the physiological (adequate breathing) and relational level (lack of recognition of intentionality) (Spagnuolo Lobb, 2001a, 2001b, 2013a, p. 93).

> Psychopathology must be conceived in the *full* context of human development, as a non-fit between the needs of the person and the requirements of his/her environment. It is about the complex result of all the protective forces and of risk factors involved in the total situation.
>
> (Wollants, 2012, p. 34)

5. Clinical Perspectives and Instruments

In order to support the vitality of the ground experience of the client, and to re-create a "dance of reciprocity" with them, I find it useful, during therapeutic interventions, to let myself be impacted by three clinical perspectives: (1) working on *the ground experience*; (2) working in a *field perspective* using my own aesthetic knowing; (3) switching the locus of therapy from the individualistic paradigm (the experience of the client) to the *paradigm of reciprocity* (what heals is the "dance" between therapist and client).

I will now approach each of these three perspectives, considering also their related clinical instruments.

5.1 Working on the Ground Experience

The current phenomenal state that forms the patient's process of contact with the therapist in the here-and-now carries with it the history of previous contacts.

What we are interested in is the development of the intentionalities for contact and of the processes by which the person has attempted to fulfill them. It is above all a question of seeing the experience and the assimilated contacts from a positive anthropology, in which the creative adjustment to difficult situations is the lens through which to look at the patient's symptoms, as well as their relational resources. What is generally defined as a disease, in our approach, can be viewed as "active expressions of vitality" (Perls *et al.*, 1951/1994, p. 25). Resistances in Gestalt therapy are considered "assistances", like Laura Perls used to say: an adjustment that resolves a situation (Wollants, 2012, p. 60).

Let us look, for example, at the suffering of an adolescent who spends his life in his room, with apparently no interest in seeing (real, not virtual) friends or in exploring the world outside. Our curiosity generates some questions: Where is his vitality now? What is the story behind this? When did he start to renounce his interest in friends and physical activity? How (with what physiological reaction) and when (in which circumstances) did he lose his joy of being in the world? His ground experience is made up of physiological adjustments and self-definitions. For instance, did a humiliating sentence expressed by a friend create a feeling of shame and so did he subsequently feel confused about what he had previously deemed as a positive reaction from the other? His spontaneity towards this other no longer appropriate, did he withdraw his bodily enthusiasm, and negatively define himself, as he waited for a new way to be? Then probably other humiliations followed and he couldn't find a new way to be what he wanted to be. Perhaps a sense of solitude then ensued and he took refuge in a lonely world, where only virtual reality was admitted. If this is the case, in the moment he is in a therapeutic situation, he needs to experience a contact though which he can be himself and can be met by another who can recognise his intentionality (instead of diminishing him). In this way, he can experiment his sense of agency with the other and rely on safe ground when he meets others.

This is one of many examples of relational sufferings and of related therapeutic diagnosis and intervention on the ground experience. We help our clients to stay with the experience of senses-in-contact. Of course, we need first to feel *our own* experience of senses-in-contact. Feeling that they can *rely on* the other and on the ground where they stand seems the most appropriate form of therapeutic support today, in a post-pandemic world. Let's approach now two aspects of the ground experience during the therapeutic session.

5.1.1 Neurobiology of the Relational Sense of Safety

The ground experience we deal with today has to do with a basic perception on the part of the patient that they can feel safe and secure in the session with us. According to the polyvagal theory of Stephen Porges (2007), a neurobiological approach, the sense of safety is an important moderator that influences the efficacy of psychotherapy. It is experienced via what he calls "neuroception": the primordial sense of safety or danger. Often, clients do not have access to this kind of bodily process, and they lack this basic sense of security.⁴ Now, if the patient is triggered into a defensive response, one cannot accomplish the work of psychotherapy. Consequently, the therapist has to learn to intuit the neurobiological defensive states and elicit regulated states in the patient. As Gestalt therapists, we need to develop therapeutic skills to provide the perception of safety and build on that when suggesting our experiments. The work of a few Gestalt therapy colleagues can specifically help to foster this therapeutic skill. The Nervous System Energy Work (NSEW) developed by James Kepner and Carol DeSanto enhances the capacity for regulating arousal and sustaining bodily conditions of safety in contact and growth (see Kepner, 1995; DeSanto and Kepner, 2002). Taylor (2014) reminds us to consider the "window of tolerance," (Siegel, 2010) pertaining to our client's experience, something for the most part taken for granted years ago, and to propose interventions that support patient resilience. Ruella Frank (2001, 2016a, 2016b) works on support for the basic relational movements that establishes a sense of self as well as spontaneity in contact-making. This is crucial when we – especially Gestalt therapists – work with anger and arousal. Our traditional way of dealing with these feelings is to trust that they can be managed by the patient, and that they can be expressed without the risk of the patient self-fragmenting. But today we need to take this risk into account, since people cannot easily rely on a safe and secure ground and on a whole sense of self. Today, it is more appropriate to work on what the person feels when they communicate *to us* anger or other hyperactive feelings. Today, the question is no longer to let the anger out (so that the person can re-own it). We rather wonder whether the patient is able to face us with his/her anger (or be able to tolerate it).

Psychophysiological studies of attachment delve into these concepts from the biological standpoint, and confirm that relationships influence and are influenced by the underlying biological processes. Research on animals and on humans demonstrates that the quality of early primary relationships shapes the individual unique physiological and behavioural responses to stress (Cassidy and Shaver, 2016). Current clinical and experimental attention on how these affective processes are interactively and implicitly regulated, involving the body in a fundamental way, has directed the theory of attachment towards a theory of regulation (Schore, 1994; Schore and Schore, 2007).

This research has led us to linger on our patients' micro-movements, and to focus on the primary support that we as caregivers are called upon to provide for their self-regulation.

5.1.2 The Polyphonic Development of Domains5

In my understanding, the ground can be considered a "Polyphonic Development of Domains": a complex weaving of vital, acquired ways of introjecting, projecting, retroflecting, and so on, with more or less anxiety. Not only can the so-called "losses of ego functions" (Perls *et al.*, 1951/1994) be seen as modalities of contact, ways through which the organism has creatively adjusted to difficult situations (see Polsterand Polster, 1973; Müller-Ebert *et al.*, 1988), but they can also be viewed as acquired competencies for contacting, as parts of the ground that intertwine to create the experience of the ground, that in the here and now supports the process of contact.

Our clients have a bodily memory of introjecting, projecting, retroflecting, etc. as acquired competencies. These acquired competencies for being in the world create an organisation of domains,[6] which make the ground of their experience. The way the client sits, moves, looks at the therapist, considers himself when facing the therapist, is made up of previously acquired contacts. The here-and-now experienced by the patient is a creative Gestalt that summarises the bodily and socially relational schemas assimilated in the preceding contacts (the being-with through the body – id-functioning – and through the social definition – personality-functioning – of the self) and the intentionalities (the excitement for contact) that support the present contact that the patient makes with the therapist (ego-functioning of the self). It thus becomes fundamental to make reference to a developmental perspective, in order to read the development of the modalities of contact with the significant other and with the environment in general (Spagnuolo Lobb, 2012).

Going back to the adolescent who doesn't leave his room, the question is: how has he learned the capacity to introject, to project, to retroflect, etc.? If we take for instance his capacity to introject, did he swallow rules and definitions instead of chewing them? To what aspect of his primary environment was he adjusting creatively? What kind of vitality was he bringing into that field? For instance, has he experienced his parents as absorbed by difficult situations (poor marital relationship, or financial problems, or psychiatric burdens?). Did he not want to stress that situation even more with his questions and desire to understand? Where did he experience that retroflection in his body (and did it result in symptoms like tics, nightmares, eating problems)? And how did he define himself? As a good and self-sacrificing son? Or as an ineffective and closed-off kid? All these micro-learnings in his development reinforce his presence *now* when he faces us. How did withdrawal from contact represent a collapsed or resilient modality of contact and what physiological supports (breathing, control of the diaphragm, etc.) can he still rely on?

What is helpful to us has to do with supporting his vitality, it is not seeing whether the patient has reached certain goals (this is just one of many aspects), but *how* he has fulfilled the intentionality of contact adjusting creatively to difficult situations. The development is always a process of self-regulation of the organism/environment field, a melody that becomes more and more complex and articulated, and which must be appreciated and supported, not subjected to measures of comparison (Tronick *et al.*, 1978; Stern, 1985, 1990).

The complexity of individual development is the result of many conditions, as they decline themselves in contacting the environment. This developmental complexity may be better respected if we consider the present moment as a transversal plane of the development of the various domains (see Figure 2.2), which interweave differently at each moment, giving rise to the Gestalt of the contact in the here-and-now.

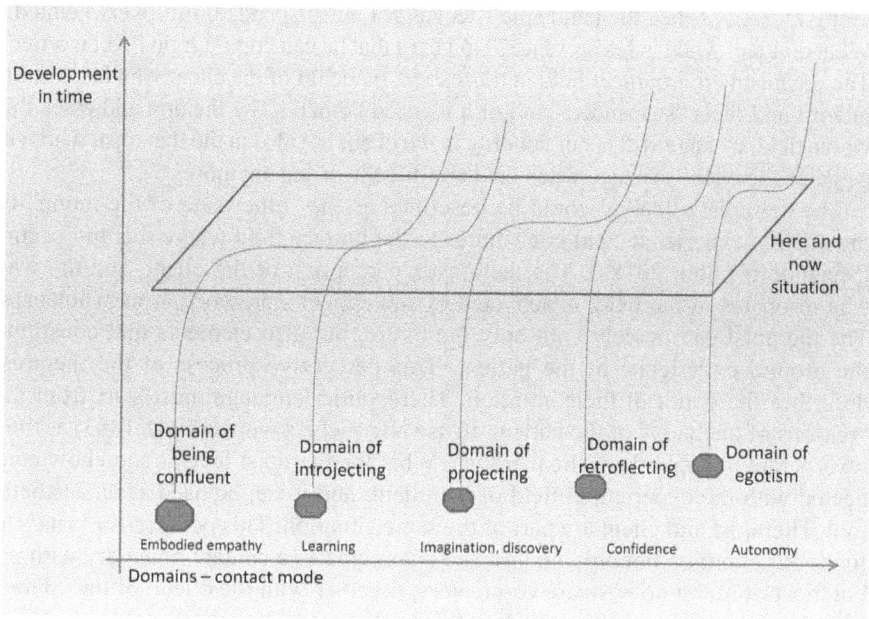

Figure 2.2 The Gestalt map of the polyphonic development of domains, or assimilated contacts (adjusted from Spagnuolo Lobb, 2013a, p. 115)

5.2 The Field and the Co-Created Experience: The Aesthetic Relational Knowing

As Perls *et al.* (1951/1994) have written: "the field is activated every time there is a contact boundary" (p. 35). The organism/environment field is a unitary experience (Perls *et al.*, 1951/1994, p. 4 ff.). A child's feeling – for instance in the case of stomach cramps – becomes an experience according to the environmental reaction, if for instance the mother comes to their aid with a smile and feeds the child, or does not come at all. The experience is formed in contact-making with the other. When we apply this contextualised perspective to the patient's experience, we realise that what *we* do and feel is part of the client's experience. What resonance does the experience of being with that client have for us? What is the emotion activated in the field that we co-create with them? Our field-oriented perspective prompts these specific questions:

What do I feel when facing this person?
What movement do I perceive in the other and in myself?
What energy do I feel in the field?

For instance, the client tells me: "I don't feel any interest in what I do at work nor really in my kids. . . . Since the pandemic I feel as if I am suspended. I'm overwhelmed." What do I feel when in his presence? Do I trust that he can cope? Or do I feel worried? The organism/environment field in this case is made up of the client who has lost his interest and feels "suspended" and of a worried "other". The therapy addresses this whole field. Change will occur not only in the client but also in the therapist, who will perceive the client's change when he doesn't feel worried anymore.

The therapist's feeling could be described as the "other side of the moon" of the client's experience, and contributes to the unitary field where therapy occurs (Spagnuolo Lobb, 2018a). The therapist's perception of the client, and the way s/he resonates in the field, is activated by the patient's presence in its wholeness. The therapist can perceive not only the figure, but also elements that constitute the ground experience of the patient. This perceptive process of the therapist describes the depth of their intuition. Therapeutic language must start from the "reasons of the body" of the patient, to use Nietzsche's words (1961/1883) as they reverberate in the body of the therapist. What the therapist feels is somehow connected with the experiential field of the client, and it can be used as an aesthetic tool. Therapist and client are part of the same situation. This perspective brings to focus our attention not only on how the client creates a contact boundary with us, but most of all on how *we* are co-creators, together with the client, of the contact boundary. We are not just partners with our clients, we are co-creators.

Drawing on Stern *et al.*'s (1998) concept of "Implicit Relational Knowledge", which expresses the ability of the child and mother to get to know each other through non-verbal means, such as movement, tone of voice, interactive patterns, and procedural aspects of interaction, I have tried to describe a tool to discover the patient's interest/curiosity/love (Polster, 1987, 2021), drama, and resilience, using the therapist's felt sense of the field. The aesthetic (not implicit) knowing of the therapist includes the capacity to know via their senses and to "vibrate" in the presence of the patient (see Spagnuolo Lobb, 2018a). I have called this process *aesthetic relational knowing*. Precisely because we take part in it, we come to know the client's experience via both our *embodied empathy* – feeling in our body what the patient feels (see Heidegger, 1996; Marleau Ponty, 1962; Gallese, 2009) – and our *resonance* – to respond synchronically to the patient's motion (see Tschacher *et al.*, 2014). This makes a specific therapeutic action possible, tailored to that particular experience of the client, and contextualised in that therapeutic field.

Not only are we empathically sensitive to our patients, we can also be empathically sensitive towards field phenomena, which include the feeling of the other with whom the experience has been co-created. For example, we might feel in our body the humiliation the client feels when he tells us that he has lost his interest, and we might also feel disappointed, like the "other side of the moon" experience of the client, the experience of the "other" that makes humiliation possible for the client. The way I resonate with a specific client in a specific moment is like waves that "resonate" with his presence. Lynne Jacobs (2018) expresses it well when she speaks of staying in the play as part of the therapeutic situation. Resonance is the contribution of the therapist (a meaningful other) to the situation.

All this contextualised and embodied understanding of the patient's relational suffering is important to reactivate their integrative capacity, providing a caring situation where a specific support is possible.

When we use our aesthetic knowing in a field perspective, we can support the client to activate or reactivate their ability to interact with the environment so that they can be spontaneous and function as a whole, and feel like an agent of their own growth. For instance, in the face of a patient who doesn't feel interest in his/her professional and affective life, we might resonate with a feeling of ambivalence: we admire this client and at the same time we feel angry and disappointed in him/her. If we consider these feelings as belonging to a whole situation, we can understand that our ambivalence is somehow "supporting" the lack of interest. Our diagnostic competence and knowledge about attachment theory will help us to understand the situation. And we can become the therapist of the situation (see Wollants, 2012), rather than of the patient, and support the patient to reach us (the other) in a more spontaneous way. We give, for instance, the patient feedback on how able he/she is to reach us in a bold and unique way. In this way we co-create together a new situation, where the patient can experiment with a new and more positive contact, where the other is not ambivalent. Thanks to their sensitivity to the field of experience that opens up to them, the therapist is able to support the client's intentionality and creative adjustment, with a specific interpersonal support addressed to their ground experience and to the field.

Here is *an experiment*: imagine a client of yours that you would like to understand better. Relax and breathe while you remember him/her in a therapeutic situation. Now try to remember a movement of that client, even an almost imperceptible one, which is typical of that person when he is in your presence. Now think of a movement with which you might wish to respond. Draw the two movements on a piece of paper and see what impresses you in this dance. Are you comfortable? What could you do to feel more comfortable in that situation?

5.3 The Paradigm of Reciprocity: A Turning Point in Clinical Practice

As we have seen, focus has been put on the *experiential field* that therapist and client co-create, and on their *reciprocity* or the act of moving-toward-the-other in the therapeutic process. In Gestalt therapy terms, we do not aim to solve individual needs but to *co-create a new experience* of contact that makes spontaneous movement possible. *Mutual synchronisation*, already pointed out by the models of precocious interactive regulation, from Winnicott (1991) to Odgen (1989) to Fogel (1992, 1993) and Beebe *et al.* (1992), is a useful criterion of observation for us: we re-cognise ourselves in the contact with the other; the self is a process of contact (cf. Spagnuolo Lobb, 2005) which is formed at the boundary. And vice versa, developmental blocks coincide with a blocked bodily process, which always implies a reduction (or loss) of sensitivity (of being fully present to one's own senses), and hence the reduced ability to tune in to the other.

Research on the relational mind (Seikkula *et al.*, 2015), in the neurosciences (Gallese, 2009), psychophysiology (Porges, 2007), epigenetics (Spector, 2013), new approaches on therapeutic alliance (Tschacher *et al.*, 2014; Tschacher *et al.*, 2015; Tschacher and Pfammatter, 2016; Flückiger *et al.*, 2012), and intersubjectivity (Stern, 2010; Beebe and Lachmann, 2002) have drawn the attention of psychotherapists to what happens between therapist and client, and to how they regulate one another, rather than to one or other of the partners of the therapeutic situation (Spagnuolo Lobb, 2016c).

Considering the mutual perceptions and the intentional movements in the process of contact between client and therapist, the therapeutic process becomes a "dance" of reciprocity, made up of movements intended to achieve a fuller and more spontaneous sense of self of the client (Spagnuolo Lobb, 2019, 2020).

Every significant bond translates into a mutual "going towards" the other (Frank, 2001, 2016b). What creates the therapeutic change is not only the focus on the being-with of the client, but on the reciprocity of the mutual being-with of client and therapist. It is a relational dimension that generates a sense of secure ground in the client and avoids narcissistic splits (Lachmann, 2008; Orange, 2018; Spagnuolo Lobb, 2018b) in both therapist and client (see Chapter 1).

When we focus on the "dance" of reciprocity between therapist and client, therapeutic change is supported by a harmonious and fluid figure-ground dynamic. The "dance" is made up of mutual perceptions and reactions to the perception of the other, supported by the vitality that each one places in being with the other.

5.3.1 The "Dance of Reciprocity" Model[7]

Based on the epistemological principles of Gestalt therapy, such reciprocity can be observed metaphorically as "the dance between therapist and client," taking into account nonverbal aspects of their interaction (e.g., movements, intentionalities, excitement for contact, relaxation when the contact goal is achieved, breathing, time of contact) and their place in a process.

To describe this dance in terms of the intentionality of their "being-with" throughout the time of the meeting, I offer *eight dance steps*, each associated with appropriate intentional behaviours. So far, this dance has been described in terms of two main intimate interactions: *caregiver/child* (Spagnuolo Lobb, 2016a) and *therapist/client* interactions (Spagnuolo Lobb, 2017a, 2017b). In the case of caregiver/child interactions, an observational tool of their being-in-contact has been created and validated. Its purpose is to support parents with their children, to facilitate a more spontaneous and functional meeting of their wishes, or to study primary interactions in specific populations (e.g. autistic children and their parents). Regarding therapist/client interactions, we use self-reports filled in by therapist and client at the end of the session. A measurement of synchrony concerning their experience will give the therapist a sense of their reciprocity.[8] These two clinical tools can also be used in research to study different populations and/or validate our method. I will now briefly describe the "dance steps", referring to specific publications when a more detailed and contextualised discussion in the clinical treatment is necessary (Spagnuolo Lobb, 2016a, 2017a, 2017b). The "dance steps" are described as a sequence of intentional movements related to different contact aspects. Even if they are thought of as part of a sequence, they do not have to occur in sequence. They are procedural and spontaneous actions of contact between child and caregiver, or between therapist and client:

1.   *Building together the sense of the ground*

This step has no movement yet: it is the pre-defined feeling of the other and of the situation.

The more the primary ground provides a secure feeling, the more this domain is fluid and produces contactful (good) forms. Contact takes place with spontaneity and clarity: the organism moves towards the environment with energetic and well-oriented   determination, and the movement towards the other is clear and spontaneous. If this "step" is experienced with anxiety within the contact between therapist and client, there is a risk of developing delusional ideas in which intuition gives way to anxiety and fear for one's survival. For instance, a thirty-year-old man shouts: "They are coming for me now, and they want to kill me". The therapist asks: "Who is coming for you?" He replies: "They are. It's a conspiracy." The therapist demonstrates attunement with the client's great impotence and at the same time resonates with a strong sense of solitude in the field, so he answers: "You sense that you are powerless in the face of the solitude around you." The resonance of the therapist provides a wider awareness of what is in the field, and the client calms down, with the feeling that his pre-defined intuition has been acknowledged.

2.   *Perceiving one another*

This describes the activation of mutual perception in the experiential concreteness created by the contact senses. The self of the psychotherapist and the self of the client are in the mutual act of perceiving one another. For example, during a therapy session, do therapist and client become active in response to the movements of the other, or are they perceptively rigid, almost independent from the movement of the other, insensitive towards the uniqueness that each of them brings to the field and their attempts to generate change in their contact? Plus, what do each of them do when the other does not activate or appear to respond to them? Do they keep trying to be noticed by the other or do they retreat within themselves in a defeated attitude?

3.   *Acknowledging one another*

This step consists of recognising and acknowledging the intentionality of contact in the other that brings any movement to the relational sense of that contact-making: "I have a sense of what you are feeling and of where you are going and what is important for you". Beyond empathy, this 'step' implies the recognition of the movement-towards, of the now-for-soon to be, which makes the other feel deeply understood in a human sense. An example of a borderline client can be a good description of this step. The client says to the therapist at the beginning of a session: "I will never trust you anymore, because you didn't answer me when I called you last night. I felt really bad." The therapist answers: "I appreciate your dignity in saying that." Beyond her anger (from the night before, when she had tried to reach the therapist with a late-night phone call), the therapist acknowledges the wish of the client to reach him with all of herself. He adjusts to the client's perception (you were not there for me and I have the right to be angry at you) and also says how he resonates (the dignity) in the face of the client's wish to reach him with her whole self.

4.   *Adjusting to one another*

The ability to adjust to each other implies both being attuned to one another (feeling what the other feels) and resonating (responding with one's own presence and creative differentness). In fact, the complementary movements that make a spontaneous dance possible express the full presence of both persons.

Therapist and client modulate their movements in the session, and the therapist's competence in seeing how they adjust to one another may result in the client's letting go in the therapeutic process. The client always starts the dance; for instance, they may say they have been depressed all week. The therapist is sorry and verbalises that feeling. The client feels the presence of the therapist and feels encouraged to continue to describe his/her depressive mood, this time introducing something novel: a subtle smile. The way in which the therapist resonates lies in his/her absorbing the implied intentionality of that hint of a smile, which means: "I want to see if and how much you only believe in my depression or whether you also see my wish to be better". The therapist "dances" and says: "You really wish to be better." The client feels lighter and tells the therapist about what he/she had wanted to do during the week. Their adjusting to each other allows the balance between figure and ground to fluidly support the wish of the client to continue.

5.   *Taking bold steps together*

There are times when therapist and client do something together which unlocks a fixed Gestalt and directs them towards a third element, thus releasing them from an impasse. This concentration on something else, which attracts them both, is a courageous step to take, creating in turn something that transcends them. This step is what in Gestalt therapy is called an *experiment*: an attempt to include something novel in the field in order to expand contact possibilities and awareness. The therapist adapts to the rhythm of the client; she supports his more daring actions, and together they learn to surpass what had previously seemed to be their limit. Here is an example: In a session, a client is very sad and describes a painful time in childhood during which his parents continually fought with each other. The therapist, too, feels sad yet at the same time is aware of a sense of harmony in his body. He experiences an unusual desire to dance with the client. So he asks the client: "How would you like to express together what we are feeling through a dance that gives voice to your childhood situation, to all the people involved in that pain, and to your wish to love them?" The client and the therapist start to dance together, feeling the pain and also the beauty of the client's love for his parents and siblings. A magical feeling develops. All the pain seems to be integrated and alleviated in the dance. It is as if in the dance both therapist and client find a higher order of meaning in the suffering.

Obviously, this dance does not solve all the problems, but in the client's perception, the fighting between his parents will no longer be the sole hard and fast response to situations of tension. The bold step taken by client and therapist has given the client an important recognition of his harmonic capacities. What he will learn is the freedom to take a chance on new and creative solutions to problems (cf. Wertheimer, 1945). And to be effective, this has to be done with the freshness of spontaneous contact: should the behaviour become repetitive, it would be a sign of desensitisation.

6.   *Having fun*

Therapist and client can have good moments together, enjoy being in one another's presence, and experience moments of light-heartedness. Their attunement to each other is at the highest possible level and their resonance includes the ability to take bold steps together. They can each breathe and relax with the other, feel confident, and trust life. It is a new breath of life born out of suffering, a fleeting transition to another level, one which feels good to experience. This "we can have fun" moment makes life easier. The therapist takes pleasure in seeing the client, and the client comes to therapy with a sense of hope.

7.   *Connecting*

Is the therapist curious about the client? Is she interested in the client's state of mind? Or perhaps she is focused on her own state of mind and interacts with the client as if he were something extraneous? Does the therapist participate in the client's act of exploring his feelings and meanings? Does she support the novelty and risk that the client is taking in disclosing himself to her? From the client's perspective, is he curious about the therapist? Does he have the sense that the therapist is a person with her own feelings, values, etc.? Does he feel able to reach the therapist as a person with his stories?

The therapist verbalises the client's state of mind, saying perhaps: "You feel you were able to tell me this story as you have lived it". The client takes a deep breath, looks into the therapist's eyes and feels he has fully connected with the therapist and has fulfilled the goal of the session. This kind of interaction provides both client and therapist with a feeling of being reachable and being able to reach the other. The client becomes rooted in a sense of self which is safe and secure, appreciated by others, and from which he is able to take a chance on something new. This step also provides the client with a sense of *agency*.

8.   *Entrusting oneself to the other/Taking care of the other*

The client is capable of letting himself go, and the therapist feels able to take care of the situation in a spontaneous way. And now the dance can be over. The client ends the session with the feeling of having accomplished what he wanted to work on and the therapist is ready to turn her own attention elsewhere.

In conclusion, these "steps" can help to monitor the experience of therapist/client reciprocity. Observing the dance of reciprocity is useful to support the co-regulation of the therapeutic relationship, as well as the process of contact, beyond the single action of one or the other. Each therapeutic "dance" is a unique co-creation, which gives dignity to mutual regulative processes and qualitative aspects of clinical practice.[9]

6. The three "magic" questions

In order to orient psychotherapists towards the use of their *intuitions* in the thera-peutic field and support spontaneity in their "dance" with the client, I have identi-fied three questions, which may help them to reflect on their therapeutic process with a particular client and which may be applicable for supervision:

1.   What do you feel, as a therapist, in being-with this client?
2.   What meaning do you think your "feeling" has in the client's life?
3.   What should change in your experiential approach in order for the client to be more spontaneous?

These questions give the therapist (or the supervisor) a clear sense of how she is contributing to the field with that particular client and what kind of reciprocity the client has usually shaped with caregivers. They help to orient the therapeutic "dance" with that particular patient, in order to provide the best condition pos-sible for him to feel safe and vital while interacting under difficult or traumatic circumstances.

Let me give a concrete clinical example. I remember a client, a young man suffering from a severe anxiety disorder, with social withdrawal, and obsessive (even occasionally delusional) thinking. During the first lockdown, he felt better, somehow recognised by society in his fears and his need to protect himself. After the lockdown, it was difficult for him to decide whether he should return to regular sessions. On one occasion, during that time, he started an online session saying that the therapy was not helping him, and he wanted to end it. He was dismissive. In answer to the first question (What do you feel, as a therapist, when with this client?), I felt irritated. I felt that we had started the session without the feeling of a solid ground. Maybe some strong new intentional force was at work here, and it needed a ground upon which to forge our relationship. We were building a field in which he needed to be "grown up" in front of me, and I wanted him to be able to leave his house as a measure of his "normality". I didn't get into a tug-of-war with him, as this would have been the case with his family of origin. In terms of the second question (What meaning do you think your "feeling" has in the client's life?), this was how I reflected upon it: I knew that to split my "truth" from his need would have brought us to a worse end than the one that he had already decided upon. He needed to feel that I acknowledged his wish to decide by himself, and he could only do that by dismissing me.

In order to adjust to his "step", I asked him to tell me how he felt and how important it was for him to go forward alone. In my attempt to answer the third question (What should change in your experiential approach in order for the client to be more spontaneous?), I took a bold step, and so managed to go beyond my own habitual patterns. I gave him an account of all the positive traits which I had discerned in his behaviour: his capacity to find an intelligent solution even when he had felt alone and neglected by others. How he had learned to survive and maintain his autonomy even with a very low income. How he had chosen the company of three dogs when he was incapable of cultivating a relational life. I spoke of other things as well. His mood suddenly changed: he became gentle. He relaxed. And he whispered "thank you". This was a sign of our having a good time together, of enjoying each other's presence ('having fun'), and also of connectedness: He could reach me and I could reach him. The patient was able to root himself in a more secure sense of self (feeling recognised and acknowledged by me). From this, he was able to take a chance on something new, with a sense of agency. We interrupted our sessions for two months, and he had the opportunity to experiment a range of possibilities in his life as well as his fragilities. He was able to pursue a real social life in the actual presence of others. For my part, I had explored my own fragilities as a psychotherapist. We both felt that we had dealt with what he would have wanted and were ready to turn our attention elsewhere ("relying on the other/taking care of the other").

Our contact was very different when he came back. He was more detached and less delusional in his thinking. I felt compassionate. I also remained steady and constant at his side.

7. The Paradigm of Reciprocity in the Training of Psychotherapists for a Post-Pandemic Humanistic Ethic

Having tools to focus on the regulative processes of meaningful interactions is important in clinical practice as well as in training: students can be assisted in developing their relational mind in the process of learning psychotherapy. Moreover, the use of "dance steps" to supervise psychotherapists has proven to be essential in avoiding the risk of shame that often coincides with supervision. Finally, the "dance steps" can support the psychotherapist in trusting aesthetic and field-oriented feelings in their work; in trusting their capacity for being-with in spite of a narcissistic culture that upholds the notion of the therapist who must make the "right move" (Spagnuolo Lobb, 2018b).

And so the task of the therapist today is to co-construct with the patient a presence at the contact boundary so that they can have a sense of existing for someone. The therapist also has the responsibility of providing the patient with a feeling of being recognised and acknowledged in their intentionality of contact on the part of a significant other, and even finding within the other someone who is overseeing a containment wall that is curbing an energy sometimes perceived as at risk of becoming uncontrollable.

People need to regain the sense that they can rely on the environment and on themselves, to open themselves up to a creative adjustment with the other.

The pandemic has certainly increased our feelings of insecurity in terms of the ground, but it has also shaken to the foundations some perceptive inflexibilities of post-modern society, envisaging the emergence of new resources, which will take on a more defined form in the coming years.

In our clinical environment, we have to work so that the patient may (re)acquire a feeling of belonging to a community of human beings, and may become oriented towards their surroundings with determination, grace, and a relational sense of rhythm.

References

Beebe, B., Jaffe, J., & Lachmann, F. M. (1992). A dyadic systems view of communication. In N. Skolnick & S. Warshaw (Eds.). *Relational perspectives in psychoanalysis* (pp. 61–81). Hillsdale, NJ: The Analytic Press.

Beebe, B., & Lachmann, F. M. (2002). *Infant research and adult treatment: Co-constructing interactions*. Hillsdale, NJ: The Analytic Press/Taylor & Francis Group.

Bloom, D. J. (2003). Tiger! Tiger! Burning bright" – Aesthetic values as clinical values in Gestalt therapy. In M. Spagnuolo Lobb & N. Amendt-Lyon (Eds.). *Creative license. The art of Gestalt therapy* (pp. 63–78). Wien, NY: Springer.

Brownell, P. (2018). *Gestalt psychotherapy. Coaching for relationships*. New York: Routledge.

Cassidy, J., & Shaver, P. R. (Eds.). (2016). *Handbook of attachment. Theory, Research, and clinical applications* (3rd ed.). New York: Guilford Press.

Churchill, S. D. (2018). Explorations in teaching the phenomenological method: Challenging psychology students to "grasp at meaning" in human science research. *Qualitative Psychology*, 5(2), 207–227. DOI: 10.1037/qup0000116.

Clemmens, M. C. (Ed.). (2020). *Embodied relational Gestalt: Theories and applications*. Abingdon, UK: Routledge, Taylor & Francis Group Ltd.

De Simone, M. (2017). La pratica della mindfulness nel contesto formativo universitario: un apprendimento trasformativo? [Mindfulness practice in the university educational context: Transformative learning?] *Ricerche Di Pedagogia E Didattica. Journal of Theories and Research in Education, 12*(3), 97–133. DOI: 10.6092/issn.1970-2221/764.

DeSanto, C., & Kepner, J. (2002). *The highway of light: Energetic healing thru nervous system.* Long Island, NY – 2/23/2002 (6 CDs).

Flückiger, C., Del Re, A. C., Wampold, B. E., Symonds, D., & Horvath, A. O. (2012). How central is the alliance in psychotherapy? A multilevel longitudinal meta-analysis. *Journal of Counselling Psychology, 59*(1), 10–17.

Fogel, A. (1992). Co-regulation, perception and action. *Human Movement Science, 11,* 505–523.

Fogel, A. (1993). *Developing through relationships.* Chicago: University of Chicago Press.

Frank, R. (2001). *Body of awareness. A somatic and developmental approach to psychotherapy.* Highland, NY: Gestalt Press.

Frank, R. (2016a). L'esperienza del movimento: la risonanza cinestesica come sentimento relazionale. Intervista a Ruella Frank a cura di F. Maggio e S. Tosi [The experience of movement: Kinesthetic resonance as a relational feeling. Interview with Ruella Frank edited by F. Maggio and S. Tosi]. *Quaderni di Gestalt, XXIX*(1), 9–24. DOI: 10.3280/GEST2016-001002.

Frank, R. (2016b). Moving experience: Kinaesthetic resonance as relational feel. In M. Spagnuolo Lobb, N. Levi, & A. Williams (Eds.). *Gestalt therapy with children. From epistemology to clinical practice* (pp. 87–99). Siracusa: Istituto di Gestalt HCC Italy Publ. Co., www.gestaltitaly.com.

Gallese, V. (2009). Mirror neurons, embodied simulation, and the neural basis of social identification. *Psychoanalytic Dialogues, 19,* 519–536.

Heidegger, M. (1996). *Being and time. A translation of "Sein und Zeit".* Albany, NY: SUNY Press.

Husserl, E. (1910/1980). *Ideas pertaining to a pure phenomenology and to a phenomenological philosophy – third book: Phenomenology and the foundations of the sciences.* Dordrecht: Kluwer.

Jacobs, L. (2018). Comment to my other's keeper: Resources for the ethical turn in psychotherapy, by Donna M. Orange. In M. Spagnuolo Lobb, D. Bloom, J. Roubal, J. Zeleskov Djoric, M. Cannavò, R. La Rosa, S. Tosi, & V. Pinna (Eds.). *The aesthetic of otherness: Meeting at the boundary in a desensitized world. Proceedings* (pp. 37–40). Siracusa, Italy: Istituto di Gestalt HCC Italy Publ. Co., www.gestaltitaly.com.

Kepner, J. (1995). *Healing tasks: Psychotherapy with adult survivors of childhood abuse.* San Francisco: Jossey-Bass.

Lachmann, F. M. (2008). *Transforming narcissism: Reflections on empathy, humor, and expectations.* New York: The Analytic Press.

Lowen, A. (1958). *The Language of the Body.* New York: Macmilian Publ. Co.

Macaluso, M. A. (2015). Beyond the Perls-Goodman model: From the organism-environment field to the relational field. *Gestalt Review, 19*(3), 233–250. DOI: 10.5325/gestaltreview.19.3.0233.

Macaluso, M. A. (2020). Deliberateness and spontaneity in Gestalt therapy practice. *British Gestalt Journal, 29*(1), 30–36.

Merleau-Ponty, M. (1962). *Phenomenology of perception.* London: Routledge & Kegan Paul.

Müller, B. (1993). Isadore from's contribution to the theory and practice of Gestalt therapy. *Studies in Gestalt Therapy, 2,* 7–21.

Müller-Ebert, J., Josewski, M., Dreitzel, P., & Müller, B. (1988). Narzißmus. *Gestalttherapie*, *2*, 27–58.

Nietzsche, F. (1961). *Thus spoke Zarathustra*. Harmondsworth: Penguin Books (original published 1883).

Odgen, T. H. (1989). *The primitive edge of experience*. Northvale, NJ and London: Jason Aronson Inc.

Orange, D. M. (2018). My other's keeper: Resources for the ethical turn in psychotherapy. In M. Spagnuolo Lobb, D. Bloom, J. Roubal, J. Zeleskov Djoric, M. Cannavò, R. La Rosa, S. Tosi, & V. Pinna (Eds.). *The aesthetic of otherness: Meeting at the boundary in a desensitized world, Proceedings* (pp. 19–32). Siracusa, Italy: Istituto di Gestalt HCC Italy Publ. Co., www.gestaltitaly.com.

Parlett, M. (1991). Reflections on field theory. *The British Gestalt Journal*, *1*, 68–91.

Perls, F., Hefferline, R. F., & Goodman, P. (1994). *Gestalt therapy: Excitement and growth in the human personality*. New York: The Gestalt Journal Press, or.ed. 1951.

Polster, E. (1987). *Every person's life is worth a novel*. New York: W.W. Norton & Co.

Polster, E. (2021). *Enchantment and Gestalt therapy. Partners in exploring life*. London, UK: Routledge.

Polster, E., & Polster, M. (1973). *Gestalt therapy integrated. Contours of theory and practise*. New York: Vintage Books.

Porges, S. W. (2007). The polyvagal perspective. *Biological Psychology*, *74*(2), 116–143.

Porges, S. W., & Dana, D. (2018). *Clinical applications of the polyvagal theory. The emergence of polyvagal-informed therapies*. New York and London: W.W. Norton & Company.

Reich, W. (1933). *Charakteranalyse. Technik und Grundlagen für studierende und praktizierende Analytiker*. Wien: Selbstverlag des Autors.

Schore, A. N. (1994). *Affect regulation and the origin of the self: The neurobiology of emotional development*. Hove, UK: Psychology Press.

Schore, J. R., & Schore, A. N. (2007). Modern attachment theory: The central role of affect regulation in development and treatment. *Clinical Social Work Journal*, *36*, 9–20.

Seikkula, J., Karvonen, A., Kykyri, V.-L., Kaartinen, J., & Penttonen, M. (2015). The embodied attunement of therapists and a couple within dialogical psychotherapy: An introduction to the relational mind research project. *Family Process*, *54*, 703–715.

Siegel, D. J. (2010). *Mindsight. The new science of personal transformation*. New York: Bantam Books.

Spagnuolo Lobb, M. (2001a). The theory of self in Gestalt therapy. A restatement of some aspects. *Gestalt Review*, *5*, 276–288. DOI: 10.5325/gestaltreview.5.4.0276.

Spagnuolo Lobb, M. (2001b). From the epistemology of self to clinical specificity of Gestalt therapy. In J.-M. Robine (Ed.). *Contact and relationship in a field perspective* (pp. 49–65). Bordeaux: L'exprimerie.

Spagnuolo Lobb, M. (2005). Classical Gestalt therapy theory. In A. L. Woldt & S. M. Toman (Eds.), *Gestalt therapy. History, theory, and practice* (pp. 21–39). Thousand Oaks, CA: Sage Publications.

Spagnuolo Lobb, M. (2012). Toward a developmental perspective in Gestalt therapy, theory and practice: The polyphonic development of domains. *Gestalt Review*, *16*(3), 222–244.

Spagnuolo Lobb, M. (2013a). *The now-for-next in psychotherapy: Gestalt therapy recounted in post-modern society*. Siracusa: Istituto di Gestalt HCC Italy Publ. Co., www.gestaltitaly.com.

Spagnuolo Lobb, M. (2013b). Developmental perspective in Gestalt therapy. The polyphonic development of domains. In G. Francesetti, M. Gecele, & J. Roubal (Eds.). *Gestalt therapy in clinical practice. From psychopathology to the aesthetics of contact* (pp. 109–130). Siracusa, Italy: Istituto di Gestalt HCC Italy Publ. Co., www.gestalt italy.com.

Spagnuolo Lobb, M. (2015). The body as a "vehicle" of our being in the world. Somatic experience in Gestalt therapy. *British Gestalt Journal, 24*(2), 21–31.

Spagnuolo Lobb, M. (2016a). Self as contact, contact as self. A contribution to ground experience in Gestalt therapy theory of self. In J.-M. Robine (Ed.). *Self. A poliphony of contemporary Gestalt therapists* (pp. 261–289). St. Romain la Virvée, France: L'Exprimerie.

Spagnuolo Lobb, M. (2016b). Gestalt therapy with children. Supporting the polyphonic development of domains in a field of contacts. In M. Spagnuolo Lobb, N. Levi, & A. Williams (Eds.). *Gestalt therapy with children. From epistemology to clinical practice* (pp. 25–62). Siracusa: Istituto di Gestalt HCC Italy, www.gestaltitaly.com.

Spagnuolo Lobb, M. (2016c). Psychotherapy in post modern society. *Gestalt Today Malta, 1*(1), 97–113.

Spagnuolo Lobb, M. (2017a). From losses of ego functions to the dance steps between psychotherapist and client. Phenomenology and aesthetics of contact in the psychotherapeutic field. *British Gestalt Journal, 26*(1), 28–37.

Spagnuolo Lobb, M. (2017b). Phenomenology and aesthetic recognition of the dance between psychotherapist and client: A clinical example. *British Gestalt Journal, 26*(2), 50–56.

Spagnuolo Lobb, M. (2018a). Aesthetic relational knowledge of the field: A revised concept of awareness in Gestalt therapy and contemporary psychiatry. *Gestalt Review, 22*(1), 50–68. DOI: 10.5325/gestalt review.22.1.0050.

Spagnuolo Lobb, M. (2018b). Comment to my other's keeper: Resources for the ethical turn in psychotherapy, by Donna M. Orange. In M. Spagnuolo Lobb, D. Bloom, J. Roubal, J. Zeleskov Djoric, M. Cannavò, R. La Rosa, S. Tosi, & V. Pinna (Eds.). *The aesthetic of otherness: Meeting at the boundary in a desensitized world. Proceedings* (pp. 41–44). Siracusa, Italy: Istituto di Gestalt HCC Italy Publ. Co., www.gestaltitaly.com.

Spagnuolo Lobb, M. (2019). The paradigm of reciprocity: How to radically respect spontaneity in clinical practice. *Gestalt Review, 23*(3), 234–254. DOI: 10.5325/gestaltreview.23.3.0232.

Spagnuolo Lobb, M. (2020). Gestalt therapy during coronavirus: Sensing the experiential ground and "dancing" with reciprocity. *The Humanistic Psychologist, 48*(4), 397–409. DOI: 10.1037/hum0000228.

Spagnuolo Lobb, M., & Castaldi, L. (2021, May 20). *Questionari di processo sulla reciprocità fra terapeuta e paziente.* Protocollo di Ricerca – Istituto di Gestalt HCC Italy.

Spagnuolo Lobb, M., & Resnick, R. W. (2020). *The presence of Gestalt therapist in the field. Dialogue on Isadore From's lesson.* Free access articles, www.gestaltitaly.com, www.gestaltitaly.com/contents/freeaccess/20201130_dialogue_Spagnuolo_Lobb_Bob_ Resnick.pdf.

Spector, T. (2013). *Identically different: Why you can change your genes.* New York: Overlook Press.

Stemberger, G. (2018). Wie hätte sich die Gestalttherapie wohl auf gestalttheoretischer Grundlage entwickelt? Georges Wollants (1941–2018). *Phänomenal – Zeitschrift für Gestalttheoretische Psychotherapie, 10*(2), 33–39.

Stern, D. N. (1985). *The interpersonal world of the infant: A view from psychoanalysis and developmental psychology*. New York: Basic Books.

Stern, D. N. (1990). *Diary of a baby*. New York: Basic Books.

Stern, D. N. (2010). *Forms of vitality. Exploring dynamic experience in psychology and the arts*. Oxford: Oxford University Press.

Stern, D. N., Bruschweiler-Stern, N., Harrison, A., Lyons-Ruth, K., Morgan, A., Nahum, J., Sander, L., & Tronick, E. (1998). The process of therapeutic change involving implicit knowledge: Some implications of developmental observations for adult psychotherapy. *Infant Mental Journal, 19*(3), 300–308.

Taylor, M. (2014). *Trauma therapy and clinical practice. Neuroscience, Gestalt and the body*. Maidenhead, UK: Open University Press, McGraw-Hill Education.

Tronick, E. Z., Als, H., Adamson, L., Wise, S., & Brazelton, T. B. (1978). The infant's response to entrapment between contradictory messages in face-sto-face interaction. *Journal of the American Academy of Child and Adolescent Psychiatry, 17*, 1–13.

Tschacher, W., Haken, H., & Kyselo, M. (2015). Alliance: A common factor of psychotherapy modeled by structural theory. *Frontiers in Psychology for Clinical Settings, 6*, 421.

Tschacher, W., & Pfammatter, M. (2016). Embodiment in psychotherapy. A necessary complement to the canon of common factors? *European Psychotherapy, 13*, 9–25.

Tschacher, W., Rees, G. M., & Ramseyer, F. (2014). Nonverbal synchrony and affect in dyadic interactions. *Frontiers in psychology, 5*, 1323.

Tucci, J., Weller, A., & Mitchell, J. (2018). Realising "deep" safety for children who have experienced abuse: Application of polyvagal theory in therapeutic work with traumatized children and young people. In S. W. Porges & D. Dana (Eds.). *Clinical applications of the polyvagal theory: The emergence of polyvagal-informed therapies* (pp. 89–105). New York: W.W. Norton & Company.

Wertheimer, M. (1945). *Productive thinking*. New York: Harper and Bros.

Wheeler, G. (2000). *Beyond individualism: Toward a new understanding of self, relationship, and experience*. Hillsdale, NJ: The Analytic Press.

Winnicott, D. W. (1991). *Playing and reality*. Hove, UK: Psychology Press.

Wollants, G. (2012). *Gestalt therapy. Therapy of the situation*. London: Sage.

Beyond Slogans
Connecting Individuals in a Community

A comment by Erving Polster

I think your chapter is an excellent corrective for stereotypes of Gestalt therapy. The chapter offers an advance beyond the individualistic aspects of living. Instead, it provides new perspective on how we all live together, forming many varieties of relationship. It is well written, beautifully thought out and offers a wide view of what matters both in the therapy experience itself and in the society at large. It is very timely, given the incredible splits in the world we live in. It moves beyond the sloganisms of the Gestalt prayer, aboutism, narrow immediacy, prohibition of the question "why" and other shorthand complaints about human error. It goes into what it is like to be human and to be connected to the society of everyday experience. I am happy to see this and I believe it is not only timely but fits Gestalt therapy's original principles.

Today, 70 years after its birth, Gestalt therapy is still distorted by many slogans and stereotypes that prevent us from grasping its worldliness and interpersonal connectedness. It is much broader than the empty chair, which can be used selectively and must be introduced in a way that makes sense to the patient. Many are totally confused and need to understand how the empty chair may be an important experiment. This empty chair technique must not overshadow the relationship with the therapist. That relationship is indispensable. I remember when, working with a patient who was angry with him, Fritz Perls would say: "Put Fritz in the empty chair and speak to him." Well, ok, that might be quite useful, but what about having direct response from the patient concerning his anger with Fritz? By bypassing the actual relationship, Fritz exemplified a technique-oriented perspective. But we are not all Fritz and we must find a way that his generalities can help us individualistically rather than imitatively.

First of all, we need to be less insistent on certain language or understandings. For example, it is absurd to exclude words like "about" or "it", and other interesting but exclusionary concepts. You can't get around using those concepts, and they must be well said with implications and complexities accommodated. What I mean is this: while the word "it" can be a depersonalised thought, "it" is only problematic when it actually depersonalises. Some discrimination is required. The same is true of other slogans. At the same time, these simple exclusionary beliefs that Perls promulgated swept Gestalt therapy into a narrow language. That language had a missionary simplicity in the mid-20th century, but it is out of date because it doesn't cover the full function. The book by Perls, Hefferline and Goodman, on the other hand, was much more free of slogans and difficult to understand for many readers who would cut out the full meaning in order to get a narrow understanding.

Well, the bottom line is that I think your chapter does a real service in honoring relationship in its implications for an expanded view of what life is about. Your illustrations of specific events or conversations are illuminating. I also feel the importance of your emphasis on a long-neglected aspect of Gestalt therapy: its social implications.

The lines of progress in Gestalt therapy, especially on a relational level, move forward into a communal connectedness of people to each other in the everyday world. That is, individuality should not be overriding the community but rather, individuality should be indivisible from the community. To do that, we need to provide communal groups for people to join together with each other to explore their lives and make them, first of all, meaningful, and second of all, faithful to the needs of the community. I have described that to some extent in the formation of Life Focus Groups,[10] the hint of which was a very dear part of the emotionally-based early Gestalt training experiences. In addition to this theoretical shift, there is the need for Gestalt therapy to form a world-wide community where people in one place know what's going on in another. I know there are international conferences and that is a great plus, but these are usually theme oriented and they do not substitute for honoring the variety of Gestalt therapy training places. That is a big ticket and very hard to accomplish, but it would be a considerable benefit.

Another concern is that we pay more attention to standards of leadership and even to standards for training. I don't have an easy answer for that but I know that the looseness on such matters has been both a benefit by inclusiveness but also a barrier created by people who represent Gestalt therapy either mistakenly or narrowly.

The formation of Life Focus Groups, if there are a sufficient number of them, and if they successfully explore what life is about, would address such issues as morality, belong, ambition, passivity, conflict, joy, expectation, and all the many human phenomena that populate our lives. We should become heir to religion in orienting and guiding the population in what life is about.

You should be very pleased with what you have written. It is an antidote to the Perlsian frame-of-mind, and I believe it will be an important contribution to the arousal of the Gestalt community, as it broadens.

Notes

1 See for instance the experience of the use of mindfulness or meditation in classes before the lesson begins (De Simone, 2017).
2 For a description in a post-modern key to the phenomenological attitude to clinical practice and the art of teaching it, see Churchill (2018).

3 For the concept of field in Gestalt psychotherapy, see Chapter 4.
4 "The term neuroception was introduced to emphasize a neural process, distinct from perception, capable of distinguishing environmental and visceral features that are safe, dangerous, or life-threatening. . . . Feature detectors . . . sensitive to the intentionality of biological movements . . . might be involved in the process of neuroception" (Porges and Dana, 2018, p. 58).
5 See Spagnuolo Lobb (2012, 2013a, 2013b, 2015, 2016a) for a more detailed description of the evolutionary perspective in Gestalt therapy to which I am referring.
6 The domain is an area of processes and competencies by which the various functions – related to various developmental areas – mutually integrate. While the stages are cumulative, so that each presupposes the competencies of the preceding one, the concept of domain clearly differentiates competencies, which have their own development in the whole course of life, and which mutually interact giving rise to the harmony (we might say to the gestalt) of the person's present competency (Spagnuolo Lobb, 2012, p. 226).
7 For a more detailed description, supported by research, see the model of "dance steps" (Spagnuolo Lobb, 2016a, 2017a, 2017b). I use the word "dance" in a metaphorical way.
8 This clinical procedure is supported by qualitative research supervised by professor Luisa Castaldi of the University of Vigna del Mar (Santiago, Chile) (see Spagnuolo Lobb and Castaldi, 2021).
9 An example of a therapeutic session observed with these "dance steps" can be found in Spagnuolo Lobb, 2017b.
10 See Polster, 2015 and his most recent book Polster, 2021 (e.n.).

References

Polster, E. (2015). *Beyond therapy: Igniting life focus community movements*. New Brunswick, NJ: Transaction Publishers.
Polster, E. (2021). *Enchantment and Gestalt therapy. Partners in exploring life*. London, UK: Routledge.

Chapter 3

Global Unrest and the Anthropological Perspective of Gestalt Therapy

Pietro Andrea Cavaleri

1. A Story Like Many Others

Face buried in the sand, a red t-shirt, blue shorts, shoes still laced up. The small body lies there, defenceless and now lifeless, lapped by the waves of the sea on the shore of a beach in Bodrum. A grim Turkish police officer, visibly moved with emotion, bends down to gather up the body in his arms and take it away. A time-less moment, immortalised by a series of snapshots taken on September 2nd, 2015, which would soon be seen around the world, rousing international public opinion from its indifference.

The lifeless little body was that of Aylan Kurdi, a three-year-old Kurdish boy who had fled his home in Kobane, a city in the north of Syria, to escape the dev-astation of a bloody war that had reduced the city to a pile of rubble and killed thousands of other children his age. A body washed up by the sea, together with the corpses of his mother and younger brother, after a tragic sea crossing made in the hope of bringing the family to safety on the nearby island of Kos, in Greece, to then join relatives in Canada. Their story is told by the father, the sole survivor, overcome with hopeless despair.

The sad story of the young Aylan is disturbing in many ways. But its implica-tions go beyond the episode itself, reaching out and touching each of us to the core of our hearts and compelling us, still today, to reckon with the deeper questions of the mystery of human nature, with its disturbing cynicism and it recurrent and cruel contradictions, and with the intricate complexities of a crisis that for several years now has gnawed at us without respite, constantly on new fronts.

Why, despite our initial and sporadic signs of concern and emotion, has inter-national public opinion proved completely "desensitised" to the drama of Syrian refugees? Why, when faced with the challenges of globalisation, has humankind continued to regress in its response, resorting to the same old and inadequate strategies of adaptation, such as war, exploitation, exclusion, and cynical indi-vidualism? Why do we feel overwhelmed by a Great Unrest that we are incapable of governing, and which in no time is wiping out the most elementary of human rights? What are the incalculable "human costs" produced by this Great Unrest[1] in us and around us? These are the questions that the following pages will seek

DOI: 10.4324/9781003313335-5

to explore, beginning with an in-depth look at the many different social contradictions unleashed by *economic globalisation*,[2] to then move on to suggest an *anthropological model* for understanding the phenomenon, a model built entirely on Gestalt Therapy.[3]

2. Desensitisation as a Response to Complexity

Western society has been unable to turn globalisation from an essentially economic phenomenon – imposed from on high with inequalities and injustices – into a cultural and political phenomenon, created from the bottom through social cohesion, the defence of human rights, a real and authentic international cooperation, the valorisation of different traditions, and the creation of new, more complex forms of interaction among people.

Faced with an upset social order that needs more adequate and complex forms of coexistence among different people, human beings so far appear completely "antiquated", with a dangerous tendency to "regress".[4] They respond to the complex challenges of globalisation by not seeing, not hearing, desensitising themselves, regressing to archaic behaviours, obsolete and primitive forms of social adaptation such as war, exploitation of their peers, non-recognition of the other, and finally the most absolute and cynical *indifference*. Conversely however, we know that the "human form" of every new social order can only be born from an experience of mutual recognition, by the respectful solidarity of accepting the other (Cavaleri, 2007). The question of culture and human nature is looked at similarly in Lichtenberg's work (1969, 1990). On the basis of these considerations, it would not be wrong to see the evolution of our civilisation as the human race's strenuous search for increasingly appropriate and complex "forms of recognition" in terms of supportive cooperation, social cohesion and peaceful coexistence (Molinari, Cavaleri, 2015). Anything that does not take mutual recognition into account turns into regression, social involution and a growing inability to perceive and recognise the other (Erikson, 1968). The philosopher Gunther Anders (1956), who has long speculated about Nazism and more generally, about the effects that modern technology has on mankind, clearly states this (Galimberti, 1999).

He regards contemporary man as "antiquated", in other words stuck to "pre-technological" thinking patterns, still unable to cope with and manage in a complete way the complex results of the technology he has created over time. Consequently, a dangerous "gap" has formed between human beings and their own products. This is a grave inadequacy, which Anders calls a *promethean gap*; in other words, the asynchronisation, growing day by day, between man and the world of its products (Anders, 1956).

Today, man's capacity to create technology is so advanced that it surpasses their imaginative power which, in contrast, is still very limited. This limited imaginative power does not allow man to adequately assess the effects of the technology he develops. When chats were invented, nobody thought that, within a few years, all teenagers and most adults would become addicted to this kind of virtual communication but unable to notice who is standing next to them in the physical reality of things. In every field (industrial, commercial, administrative), imagination is also limited by the gradual fragmentation of production processes, which prevents human beings from fully understanding their complex structure, thus losing the sense of what they are doing but also the sense of responsibility for their own actions. The consequences of the fragmentation of production processes are well-known to the business world: it is one of the most common demotivation and non-identification factors that affect employees with productive goals.

The extreme complexity of technology does not only inhibit the imagination of us human beings but also our very perceptive abilities. In fact, while *technical production* and other organisational systems connected to it become more complicated by the day, our ability to understand the processes of which we have, at last, become passive components and their final outcomes, of which we remain oblivious more and more often. The increasing gap between *technical production* on the one hand and *human imagination and perception* on the other makes our "feeling" in relation to our own behaviours inadequate.

So, the imagination and perception deficit immediately turns into a deficit of the feeling, which makes us "emotional illiterates", unable to recognise our own and others' emotions and feelings.

We are desensitised to such an extent that we find ourselves cold and detached, no longer able to grasp the effects that our actions have on our neighbours. This makes the business climate more detached from emotions and focussed on the task, to the detriment of the relational background which, as we know, is indispensable to the creation of a serene and constructive work environment.

This is how, nowadays, a small financial and economic oligarchy has become able to control – in an almost "feudal" way – much of the globe's wealth with utter, cynical indifference, in other words without any perception of the concrete effects that their choices will have on millions of human beings: creating material poverty, destroying the creativity that is intrinsic to human beings, and bringing about social inequality. Every day, financiers, entrepreneurs, technocrats speculate on the stock market, relocate productions, lay workers off without feeling anything for the ones who are subjected to their decisions, without identifying with what they do, without imagining or perceiving the "human cost" of their actions. But the very same perceptual deficit and indifference are blurring the sight of much of the Western world, which witnesses every day, without blinking, the deaths of thousands of African people per day due to malnutrition, the unstoppable impoverishment of the "internal proletariat" and the desperate exodus of the "external proletariat".

As "antiquated men" who are still unable to handle the complexity of the *globalisation* processes, we react by becoming *indifferent*, by neutralising every emotional reaction, by blurring our own ability to perceive and feel. The absence of feelings, however, soon turns into a lack of responsibility. In this respect, Anders (1964) warns that "the inadequacy of our feelings" is not a flaw like many others, but by far the worst. By becoming *indifferent*, by not "feeling" anymore the consequences of our actions, we run the risk of endlessly repeating the dehumanising actions we are capable of, without having to feel even slightly responsible for them. Thus the perfect rationality with which technology organises its research, industrial production, and economic and financial management systems, becomes stifled within itself, as well as blatantly irrational and inhumane.

The small elite that holds the reins of economic-financial globalisation is not the only one that loves to hide within its own "cocoon",[5] indifference, the inability to perceive and hear what is happening all around, and, in a nutshell, the most cynical and ferocious individualism. The vast multitude of people who are passively subjected to its decisions also shares the same generalised attitude. Zygmunt Bauman (2013) calls it "modern individualism" and regards it as the real key to understanding the end of the modern era and the crisis of our times. He believes that, in our society, it is inappropriate to keep the traditional distinction between middle class and proletariat as, for several years, both classes have been in fact unified and replaced by a new one: The "precarious class". What characterises the precarious class is a condition of *solitude*, the most helpless, solitary form of social fragmentation. What makes the category of precarious workers cohesive and unified is their "atomisation", their "pulverisation", which makes them unable to escape solitude and isolation, to connect with each other and fight the small elite that keeps them hostage, blackmails, exploits and despises them (Bauman, 2013).

Faced with the challenges and complexity of globalisation, both the precarious class and the small elite of the powerful surrender to the "charm of regression", manifesting the typical behaviour of the "antiquated" human beings who cannot perceive the effects of their actions. The individualism that "desensitises" and makes "indifferent" the elite of the powerful also inhibits the perception of the multitude of precarious workers, preventing the most elementary expressions of solidarity between them; it makes relationships more fragile and unstable in private, with the family, in the city, fuelling violence, and infinitely multiplying the possible forms of addiction, psychic suffering, mental illness and social discomfort.[6] We often find ourselves working as social or mental health workers, or business consultants in this environment, and the challenge for us, and for what we want our intervention to bring, is interesting to say the least.

3. The Novelty of Gestalt Therapy Anthropology

Trying to read from a "Gestalt therapy point of view" all the anthropological and social issues we have represented so far, how can we explain them? How can we interpret the obvious contradiction of a human being who sacrifices their dignity to the logic of *production* and who, facing the complex challenges of *globalisation*, desensitises themself, shuts themself up in a "shell" of *solitude* and *indifference*, resorting to antiquated adaptive strategies? What hypothesis can we use to understand the dynamics of a seemingly evolved civilisation, such as the western one, which, however passively, surrenders once again to the irrationality of reason?

Let us start from the founding text by Perls *et al.* (1951/1994). The authors dedicate the sixth chapter, one of the richest and most original, to human nature and the "anthropology of neurosis" (which today we might expand as psycho-pathology of our time). Here we can find the arguments we need to formulate a plausible answer to the aforementioned questions.

Anthropology, according to the authors, usually focuses on the "evolutionary steps" that have led our species to our present-day civilisation and behaviour. In contrast to this line of thought, the founders instead suggest an "alternative anthropology", capable of understanding the pole which is opposite to the one usually highlighted, focusing its attention "not on the increased power and achievement gained by each step of human development, but on the dangers incurred and the vulnerable points exposed, that then have become pathological in the debacle" (Perls *et al.*, 1951/1994, p. 89).

Human beings, in their progressive transformation from simple animals into social animals, in other words a person, acquire without a doubt a number of "new powers", which are added to the previous ones, already experienced and in their possession. But these "new powers require more complicated integrations, and these have often broken down" (Perls *et al.*, 1951/1994, p. 89). Perls and Goodman here outline their evolutionary perspective,[7] but above all their extremely original anthropological model, which differs radically from Hobbes', more commonly associated with the psychoanalytic tradition (Freud, 1922, 1930). As we know, Hobbes (1983, 1986) regards the animal dimension of man as opposite to the social. In their anthropological theory, *homo homini lupus*, man is irreparably wolf to man; furthermore, men are determined to create a civil society, a "civilisation" based on shared rules and institutions, for the sole purpose of not destroying each other while still remaining wolves in their most intimate essence. In the anthropological model by Perls and Goodman, however, the social dimension, with its "new powers", does not exclude or contradict the animal dimension; instead, it adds something new, in continuity with it. The social dimension and the animal dimension do not inevitably and irreducibly collide, they are not in rigid contrast to each other: instead, they are part of an inclusive logic within which each one is called to "integrate" with the other through increasingly "complex" forms. Along the course of evolution, in fact, "new powers require more complicated integrations" which, however, are not always completely implemented, resulting in a sort of failure or defeat, creating "pathological dangers" and making man more and more vulnerable.

Therefore, the hidden danger of evolution lies in the fact that, on the one hand, a self emerges and grows, one which is increasingly capable of complex and sophisticated integrations; on the other hand, however, the same self and its basic functions become more vulnerable to "defeat", "illness", "pathology". It follows that mental suffering, psychological or social discomfort are not the outcome of a perennial conflict between nature and culture, as classical psychoanalytic anthropology asserts, but rather the expression of a partial integration – or lack thereof – of different dimensions of human vitality, which spontaneously tend towards a "dynamic unity"; of a lacking functionality of self which is unable to give a complete, integrated form to the ever-increasing and increasingly demanding complexity which evolution keeps generating.

It is now evident that the anthropological theory of Perls and Goodman is very distant from Freud's. The latter, in fact, is based on the irreconcilable contrast between nature and culture, on a rigid *aut-aut*. Nature *or* culture. Nature instead of culture and vice versa. Conversely, Gestalt anthropology supports the continuity between nature and culture, their compatibility and integrability, outlining in strong detail the unitary perspective of the "together-with", of the *et-et*.[8]

4. Evolution and Its Pitfalls

As originally pointed out by Erving Straus (1952), Perls and Goodman consider the animal's transition to the upright stance as one of the key turning points along the long and troubled evolutionary path that led to the appearance of the human species. In their view, the upright stance, the freedom of hands and head granted great benefits to the animal species, allowing its power of orientation and manipulation to evolve greatly. These remarkable improvements, however, exposed animals to multiple disadvantages and negative consequences:

> the head is removed from close-perception, and the "close" senses, smell and taste, atrophy somewhat. The mouth and teeth become less useful for manipulation; as such, in an intensely manipulating animal, they tend to pass from felt awareness and response. . . . In brief, the entire field of the organism and its environment is immensely increased . . ., but the closeness of contact is more problematic. . . . The back is less flexible, and the head is more isolated from the rest of the body and from the ground.
>
> (Perls *et al.*, 1951/1994, pp. 89–90)

Re-examining the "stages of evolution leading to modern man and our civilisation", we realise how animals gradually learned to "distinguish a greater number of shapes" and to differentiate more objects in their "perceptual field". Over time, they learned the refined ability to discriminate between the different elements of an experience, and to act on them. Their ability to create "connections between different impressions and their deliberate selection" grew exponentially. Their brain grew, their awareness became clearer, their memory improved, and they became capable of relevant abstractions.

But evolution has pitfalls, negative consequences in this case, too:

> there is now likely to be occasional loss of immediacy, of the sense of ready flow with the environment. Images of objects and abstractions about them intervene: the man pauses, with heightened consciousness, for a more

deliberate discrimination, but then may forget or be distracted from the goal, and the situation is unfinished. A certain pastness that may or may not be relevant increasingly colors the present. Finally, one's own body too becomes an object – although later, for this is perceived very "closely".

(Perls *et al.*, 1951/1994, p. 90)

While evolving with extraordinary creativity, human beings built permanent tools as extensions of their limbs, and "their instinctive, situational cries" became an increasingly sophisticated and complex "indicative language". Imitation intensified, social bonding became closer and richer in meanings (Morris, 1967). But even behind these undeniable elements of evolution, there are more than a few pitfalls and numerous dangers. The pre-existing "original unity" felt by human beings between "object, person, instrument, word" weakened, they became high-level abstractions, "the original ground for contact".

Even personal relationships became "verbal for the most part". As the evolution progressed, something changed in a radical, dangerous way: "The differentiation that existed 'along with' the underlying organisation now exists *instead* of it. Then contact diminishes, speech loses feeling, and behavior loses grace" (Perls *et al.*, 1951/1994, p. 91). Additionally, it is possible to identify an evolutionary turning point which, more than others, spurred these fundamental changes: "the separation between the muscle-motor and the mind-sensory nerve centers".[9] In this regard, Perls and Goodman believe that

in neurosis this same division is fateful, for it is seized on in order to prevent spontaneity; and the ultimate practical unity of sense and motion is lost. The deliberation occurs "instead of" rather than "along with": the neurotic loses awareness that the smaller motions are taking place and preparing the larger motions.

(Perls *et al.*, 1951/1994, p. 92)

Human beings, over the course of their unique evolution, moved from a stage in which the self is "felt and not differentiated" to one characterised by "a feeling of 'self' that mirrors other people". It was a "human sense", "a bond between people". Social relations were outlined. People now "were formed by their social contacts, . . . they identified with society as a whole" (Perls *et al.*, 1951/1994, p. 123). These fundamental evolutionary steps made possible the birth of the human society culture as a legacy that is passed on from one generation to another. Again, this brings to the table unquestionable "advantages" for the whole human species, together with obvious "disadvantages" upon which it would be advisable to reflect.

In the newborn human society, in fact, taboos and laws "constrain the organism with the interests of the super-organism".

Controlled by taboos, the imitations become unassimilated introjections, society contained inside the self and ultimately invading the organism; the persons become merely persons *instead* of also animals in contact. . . . The inherited culture can become a dead weight that one painfully learns, is forced to learn by the duteous elders, yet may never individually use.

(Perls *et al.*, 1951/1994, p. 93)

Nowadays, man is constantly exposed to a context which is mostly made up of symbols, complex abstractions and verbal ambiguities of various kinds. In this context, which has become much more complex than before, man has to face many difficulties, ambiguities and deceptions. For example, it would be deceptive to think that individuals existed before society, "for there is no doubt that the existence of individuals comes about as the result of a very complicated society" (Perls *et al.*, 1951/1994, p. 93).

Similarly, as it cannot be denied that a man is first of all a person, "the expression 'animal' contact cannot mean 'merely' animal contact" (Perls *et al.*, 1951/1994, p. 93). People, in fact, are "reflections of an interpersonal complex", and everyone's personality can be better understood if seen as an expression of a self which forms within a shared social context (Köhler, 1925; Schütz, 1932; Berger and Luckmann, 1966; Marcuse, 1970; Russeau, 1968). The self, however, can never be "reduced" or completely assimilated to such a context. It represents at all times a unique and unrepeatable reality. In fact, "the self, as the system of excitement, orientation, manipulation, and various identifications and alienations, is always original and creative" (Perls *et al.*, 1951/1994, p. 93).

The complexity of human evolution is expressed above all in the appearance of an increasingly sophisticated verbal language, in the creation of very varied abstractions and symbols. Man is essentially unique because he lives in a world of symbols. "He symbolically orients himself as a symbol to other symbols, and he symbolically manipulates other symbols" (Perls *et al.*, 1951/1994, p. 94). This exceptional evolutionary process, on the one hand, has produced enormous development, greatly expanding the field of action and the manipulative power of mankind; on the other hand, it has led to a great deal of "further dangers" and, in particular, it has made possible the creation of a world of symbols that sometimes is an end in itself, in which "there is no animal satisfaction and may not even be personal satisfaction" (Perls *et al.*, 1951/1994, p. 94).

We have to accept that the world of symbols and abstractions, created by human beings to increase their power of orientation and manipulation of the environment, has tragically backfired. This world of symbols and abstractions has ended up constraining them, inhibiting and silently suppressing the "dynamic unity" of their person, without which neither mental well-being, nor mental balance, nor any state of "grace" are possible.

5. Regression as a Reaction to Complexity

In what way, with what survival strategy do human beings react to the painful frustration described in the preceding paragraphs, to such an alienating and inadequate state of life? Simply put, they respond by regressing, going back-wards, retracing the stages of evolution, in other words by managing in archaic, "antiquated" ways their organism-environment contact. In this regard, Perls and Goodman state bitterly: "In these conditions it is not surprising that persons toy with the sadomasochism of dictatorships and wars, where there is at least control of man by man instead of by symbols, and where there is suffering in the flesh" (Perls *et al.*, 1951/1994, p. 95).

Resorting to wars and dictatorships is not the only strategy with which human beings can react to the frustration of being prisoners of abstractions and sym-bols, of feeling without body, flesh, and bones. Faced with the ongoing threat of watching their "unity" and "full functioning" compromised, the human organism has learned to fall back on a few effective "security mechanisms", which at least allow them to maintain a minimum balance, essential to their very survival. Some of these "security mechanisms" are: hallucination, isolation, escape from oneself and from others, the *regression* towards further, archaic forms of contact with the environment.

By using such "antiquated" adaptive strategies "man essays to make "living on his nerves" a new evolutionary achievement" (Perls *et al.*, 1951/1994, p. 95). In fact, even if in the early stages of human evolution a healthy organism would fully succeed in the crucial task of "integrating" new developments with pre-existing ones, harmonising them into a new unitary complex and creating "new forms", in successive ages, the process of integration would become more and more com-plex and sophisticated, making this task harder and more difficult to carry out.

With time, the original and "healthy" integration perspective of *et-et* and *together-with*, has been progressively replaced by one of "neurotic scission", of *aut-aut* and fragmentation, that is the negation of unity, in other words complete form, *Gestalt*. The inability to open up to the accelerated complexity of novelty creates a "neurotic turning point" in human evolution, a powerful backward pull towards an outdated, but safer, form of adaptation. Regression then becomes an "unhealthy" way of returning to the most archaic evolutionary stages in search of a lost balance, of a "whole form" that has progressively "disintegrated" under the weight of complexity.

We could describe regression as a kind of backward "escape route" towards archaic forms of life in which the self, minimising its field of orientation and manipulation as much as possible, is relieved of the overwhelming task of inte-grating the pressing complexity of a body that has remained animal but from which, in the meantime, has emerged a mind capable of increasingly intricate and bewildering abstractions.[10] The many addictions of our time, together with old and new forms of psychic suffering, fulfil the challenging task of relieving the self of the stress of having to assemble in a *Gestalt* – a coherent and meaningful unity – the numerous elements of a process of adaptation to a reality which is hard and often contradictory (Cavaleri, 2013b, 2014). This is how the "escape route" of regression can make people feel relieved of the heavy task of reconstructing, after a painful shattering, the "dynamic unity" of a person, especially if the social and relational context in which one lives does not provide enough appropriate means of support and recognition.

In this involutional movement caused by regression,

> it is as if neurotics went back and singled out the vulnerable points of the past development of the race: the task is not to integrate erect posture into animal life, but to act on the one hand as if the head stood in the air by itself and on the other hand as if there were not erect posture or no head at all.
>
> (Perls *et al.*, 1951/1994, p. 95)

To contain the devastating effects of a culture which is no longer complementary to nature, of a society which is unfit to support individual potential, of a technology no longer at the service of mankind and of a head that has been irreparably separated from the heart and the gut, man intensifies separation and lack of integration in two ways. He can, in fact, either "forget to be a body" so much as to desensitise himself; or he can relearn how to live "without a head", becoming capable of a completely irrational and destructive kind of rationality.[11]

6. Evolutionary Stalemate and the Vitality of Human Nature

As they begin to bring their anthropological reflection to a conclusion, Perls and Goodman wonder "whether or not this neurotic turn is a viable destiny for our species" (Perls *et al.*, 1951/1994, p. 96). Beyond any possible evaluation, however, they still regard such a change as "human nature's response", one that might still have "a vital social future". At the time Perls *et al.* (1951/1994) wrote the first edition they were looking back on the first half of the 19th century, when the "neurotic turn" represented, so to speak, the ultimate adaptive strategy of the human species. It became widespread in an "epidemic" way and is considered "normal" everywhere (Horney, 1937; Rollo, 1950). The forms of adaptation that the neurotic turn has produced "employ the new power 'instead of' the previous nature, which is repressed, rather than 'along with' it, in a new integration" (Perls *et al.*, 1951/1994, p. 96).

The reflection of the founders dates back to the early 1950s, marked on the one hand by the profound wounds of the Second World War which had just ended, and on the other by a significant economic and industrial recovery. Compared to then, the context has radically changed, perhaps for the worse. Today, we face the contradictions of a globalisation to which we respond – most of all, in the working world – by adopting "neo-feudal" organisational patterns, dramatically failing to address the challenges of the new society, together-with the best of the past, for example the workers' rights acquired over the last century. The "neurotic turn" seems to replicate, condemning us once again to an evolutionary stalemate.

That being the case, will the human species continue to be held hostage by the neurotic turn for the time being? Is this man's last evolutionary horizon? Or is it possible to imagine different, more evolved "human forms"? Can human beings finally get rid once and for all of the irreconcilable conflict between nature and culture and between individual and society? To answer these questions, our two authors make a preliminary but very important reference to the role played by what they call "the excitement of the hunt." In this regard, they write: "Civil security and technical plenty, for instance, are not very appropriate to an animal that hunts and perhaps needs the excitement of hunting to enliven its full powers" (Perls *et al.*, 1951/1994, p. 96).

In other words, this means that human beings will never be satisfied with the "neurotic turn", which is capable of providing social and technical security in abundance but cannot grant them a full integration of all their potential powers. As a "hunting animal", man will always feel the irrepressible need to be "excited" by what is complicated and unknown, by what represents a challenge, by what implies uncertainty, research, exploration, and discovery. Only from such a point of view, in which so much of man's potential is waiting to emerge in a creative way, can all of his "powers" fully come to life and integrate with each other. If, with the ultimate victory of one of the two poles, the conflict between nature and culture and between individual and society should come to an end, in that very moment the "human excitement", the creative energy that makes possible the evolution and regeneration of new "human forms" would be forever extinguished with it.

It is very likely that, in the current evolutionary stage of the human species, the conflict between "social harmony" and "individual expression" is particularly rooted and hard to bridge.

> On the other hand it is also likely . . . that these 'irreconcilable' conflicts have always been, not only at present, the human condition; and that the attendant suffering and motion toward an unknown solution are the grounds of human excitement.
>
> (Perls *et al.*, 1951/1994, p. 96)

They believe that human nature is a continuous "potential", but it is only possible to talk with certainty about what it has produced to date, perhaps looking at the spontaneity of children, the achievements of heroes, the community life of normal people and the feelings of lovers (Perls *et al.*, 1951/1994, p. 128). As to the rest, everything remains unknown, open and uncertain. It is evident, however, that the secret of human nature does not lie in the conflict between nature and culture, between individual and society, but rather in the creative potential contained therein, in all the things that "can be" and "aren't yet", in all the "human forms" that it can generate but are still hidden: "'human nature' is a potentiality" (Perls *et al.*, 1951/1994, p. 98).

As we know, in Aristotelian thought, which is certainly not alien to Gestalt theory, the concept of *potentiality* refers to a latent developmental ability in the moment before the full manifestation or accomplishment of something. Aristotle[12] (1966), in fact, rethinks the idea of "becoming" in an original way, that is in terms of "power" and "act". Specifically, power is the ability of matter to take a certain form, while the act constitutes the realisation of such a possibility. As a consequence, potential is the ability to take different forms, to change, to become something else and, for this very reason, it is a powerful reading key which is needed to fully understand the dynamics of evolution in their more creative and generative salient aspects (Erikson, 1968).

If conceived in creative and generative terms, the conflict between nature and culture, between individuals and society ceases to be the infinite source of all neuroses, and instead takes the shape of an inexhaustible source of potential, "human excitement" and vital energy, capable of integrating human powers into ever newer and more evolved forms. Starting from a negative criticism of the society of their time, our founders developed a creative solution which is free from clichés, positive at its heart, full of faith and hope in the potentiality of man. Perhaps what prevents us from fully understanding the social discomfort and the psychic suffering of our time is not conflict *per se*, the clash between nature and culture, but rather the "adaptive strategy" with which it can be faced and kept under control.

In every company, for instance, there comes the time when the interests of the entrepreneur and their executives clash with those of their employees. In some cases, this is to avoid bankruptcy by unloading the costs of the rescue operation on the workforce; in other cases, the aim is to increase profits or competitiveness by imposing unacceptable working conditions (wage reduction, underpaid overtime, altered pay slips, etc.). From that Gestalt perspective of 1951, the conflict that develops between company and workers can be managed through two different forms of "adaptation": *psychopathological* and *creative*. It is possible to handle the conflict by having one of the parties prevail on the other, usually the one that, at the moment, has the power to force their own needs and point of view on the other. Alternatively, it is possible to face the conflict by having both parties acknowledge one another, each one recognising the other's point of view and "hunting" for new solutions with which to create new contractual relationships and innovative organisational formulae. In the first case, the adaptive strategy will be *neurotic* and therefore "regressive"; in the second the adaptation will be *creative* and therefore "generative".

Perls and Goodman tell us that "neurotic adaptations" turn conflict into a sterile, suffocating prison and give rise to regression and involution, while "creative adaptations" turn conflict into a new opportunity for integration, a fertile incubator for change, a space for conflicting parties to acknowledge one another, a generator of "human excitement"; in short, an inexhaustible source of vital energy.[13] So the problem is not the conflict *per se*, but the way it is faced and experienced, even in the controversial era of *globalisation*. There is a saying that might help us express more accurately what we are describing: "If the wind blows strong, do not build thick walls, but robust windmill sails".

At this point, we cannot deny how numerous and stimulating are the ideas that emerge from Perls' and Goodman's anthropological reflection, from which clearly arises the precious invitation to read the contradictions and challenges of globalisation in a "generative" way – not only the "unrest" caused by the global economy, the disturbing tension between the global elite and the global precarious class, but also the manifold and multifaceted conflicts that, in our time, continue to create all kinds of social discomfort and psychic suffering, without ever making the transition into potential spaces for mutual recognition.[14] Perhaps conflicts and breakups are part of the very nature of man; perhaps it is not in our power to rid human nature of these conflicts and the traumatic breakups that follow them. However, we can most likely learn to "repair" both in a generative way. In every social context the possibility of turning a conflictual experience into a "generative" one depends on the *tension to mutual recognition* of the parties involved.[15]

7. Gestalt Anthropology at the Time of the Pandemic

The macro-conflicts in the world today, as well as the micro-conflicts that have upset and keep upsetting our relationships, and the precarious balance of the people we hold dear, can lead to radically different outcomes, according to the strategies we adopt when facing them. We can hide behind thick walls, which only create separation and an illusory sense of security, or we can invent robust windmill sails capable of capturing the powerful energy of the wind and turning every frustrating limit into a fascinating, extraordinary possibility.

Therefore, our hope is that the current crisis can finally be interpreted and addressed in "evolutionary" rather than "regressive" terms, radically transforming not just the working world and the reorganisation of productive systems, but also the worlds of politics and economics, starting with the inalienable centrality of human beings and their dignity and the courageous recovery of indispensable conceptual categories, such as "relational well-being" and "common good" – the only grounds on which the *humanisation* of work and the necessary regeneration of human civilisation can be founded (Rifkin, 2014).

The original perspectives that emerged from gestaltic anthropology have so far helped us to better understand some great contradictions of the global economy and guess how to counter them. These same perspectives, similarly, can now help to read what has happened on our planet following the COVID-19 pandemic. Richard Horton (2020), director of *The Lancet*, the authoritative English scientific journal, argues that the global response to the pandemic has turned out to be one of the greatest political and scientific failures in our recent history.

The pandemic has resulted in a global crisis that now needs global responses capable of rethinking our future, giving more dignity to human beings and greater care for our planet. The "collective trauma" caused by the pandemic can only be overcome if all together we understand what happened and, consequently, agree on how to orient our future choices. To this complex "post-traumatic elaboration" the Gestalt model and its anthropology can contribute through the reading keys given in this chapter.

7.1 Figure and Ground, Symptom and Disease

A first aspect of the pandemic that Gestalt therapy can help shine a light on is the figure-ground dynamic (Cavaleri, 2003) that stands between the novel corona virus – that could be singled out as the terrible enemy to be defeated as quickly as possible – and all that lies behind it and of which it might be a product, a final outcome. As is always the case, from a Gestalt perspective, the figure emerges from a ground and it is there that we need to look to identify the key elements that can help us understand and make sense of the figure (Spagnuolo Lobb, 2013, 2016). We need to grasp that complex and essential dynamic if we want to understand the experiential field, of which we are co-agents and co-constructors.

In the collective imagination, the pandemic immediately emerged as the dominant figure, where fighting the pandemic has become all-out war, and the coronavirus the great enemy to be defeated. But is that really the case? Are we really so sure that COVID-19 is the true enemy to be targeted? Or, rather, does it represent the symptom of a much more complex disease, one we urgently need to learn to recognise and counter for the benefit of the entire planet?

It seems that intensive (and highly polluting) animal farming on the industrial scale has given rise to a number of pandemic diseases, which in the near future could jump species to infect humans, bringing with them scenarios even more dramatic than what we are witnessing now (Barbera *et al.*, 2020; Pievani, 2019). From the other side, in large urban centres and in high-density industrial areas, the coronavirus has been spread by particulate matter, as well as by the higher rate of immunodeficiency and respiratory diseases in the population (Travaglio, 2020). If the aforementioned studies are correct, an evident correlation might appear to exist between farming, industrial production, pollution, respiratory diseases, immunodeficiency, and pandemic. Moreover, the coronavirus would appear to have spread more rapidly in areas where health care and prevention services are less widespread and lacking in coverage (Capobianco *et al.*, 2020). In countries where health care is public, but dysfunctional (like Italy or Spain), due to disinvestment in recent years, treatment has been denied to elderly patients. The effects of the pandemic are of course correlated, besides other aspects, to the economic management of a nation, social inequality and material poverty.

From the facts and reflections exposed so far, the coronavirus appears as the non-random outcome of a complex chain of causes; it emerges as a "figure" with a sick planet as its "background". Perhaps the real problem to be solved is not only the figure (Covid-19), but above all, the background (sick planet) from which it emerges. Finding a vaccine will not suffice to resolve our problems and cheerfully restore us to the security of our former "normality" – we probably need to focus on more structural changes in the management of the planet. The essential lesson that we can learn from the pandemic is that of realising new possibilities of social justice and solidarity, centred on the human being and the natural environment we live in.

7.2 Emergency and Vulnerability as a Permanent Human Condition

When you think you are invincible and believe the society you live in is safe and secure, being faced suddenly with the exact opposite is for many an experience of discontinuity that is extremely traumatic, especially for people with a high level of emotional fragility and the need for stable contexts (Frewen and Lanius, 2015; Taylor, 2014).

Confronted with a traumatic event, the human brain often reacts by interrupting the neural circuits that connect the more archaic and instinctive areas of the brain with its more rational and evolved areas (Van der Kolk, 2014). An impending threat to our very existence leaves us no time to reason, as the autonomic nervous system takes hold and with its instinctive reactions and archaic automatisms seeks to keep our life "safe" (Panksepp and Biven, 2012; Porges, 2017; Taylor, 2014). And so it happens that, with a pandemic in full swing, for all the technological advancement of our society and the enormous strides made by scientific progress, we unconsciously consign ourselves to the most instinctive irrationality (Anders, 1956; Galimberti, 1999). How is all this possible? Is our society really so "safe"? Maybe, generally speaking, people intuit that they are not safe in this society.

The Gestalt therapy approach and its vision of human existence can help us, in no small way, to orient ourselves in the actual situation. To understand the experience of "emergency", we need to understand its opposite – namely, the experience of "normality". As Michel Foucault (2008) has written, by attributing omnipotence to science and to individual genius, modern culture – of which we are all a product – has led us to believe, until now, that everything can be controlled, predicted, and steered by scientists. The illusion that normality is solid and scratch-proof is fuelled by the deeply rooted conception in our dominant culture that all of nature, that which surrounds us and in which we live, can be kept under control by scientific knowledge (Galimberti, 1999). If we consider that the human condition has always had its (sometimes tragic) fragilities, it would be wiser to take emergencies more into account when we think about our normality.

In order to understand in concrete terms how fragile and vulnerable human beings are, it is sufficient to look at the ecosystem we live in – to the problems tied to pollution, to climate change, to deforestation, and to continuing natural disasters (Pievani, 2019), but also to wars and migration flows (Braga *et al.*, 2020) and to pandemics themselves, such as the pandemic that is shaking the tranquillity of our lives. To develop a wider awareness of our human limits, let's try to rethink what is meant by "normality" and what is meant by "emergency" (Foucault, 2008). In the narcissistic horizon of modern culture (Lasch, 1978), emergency is all that which only momentarily or fortuitously escapes the omnipotent control of science. The life of our human species has always been a continuous becoming, a constant emergency that is never normalised and which exposes us to continuous and frustrating vulnerability. But what can the vision of humanity developed by Gestalt therapy tell us in this regard?

Following closely in the footsteps of Otto Rank (1993), Frederick Perls (1969), the main inspirer behind the Gestalt therapy approach, considered the experience of vulnerability, together with the experience of suffering that it entails, as an entirely unavoidable step in the path of human growth itself (Perls *et al.*, 1951/1994, p. 85 ff.). When the human being takes an "open" stance and even an attitude of abandonment towards vulnerability, that, in and of itself, promotes a healthy growth process, and leads us to overcome more rapidly the experience itself of fragility and pain (Perls *et al.*, 1951/1994, p. 133 ff.).

In contrast to this, a "closed" stance towards vulnerability, or the rejection of the suffering it entails and the spasmodic quest for "victory," for absolute control over reality, is the equivalent, for every human being, of shunning all vital growth processes and fuelling our neurotic aspects (Perls *et al.*, 1951/1994, p. 163 ff.). Thus, for Perls, it means forgoing forever the typical certitudes of "neurotic control" over reality, to acquire in their stead an adequate adaptive strategy to deal with the limits of the human condition, a mental well-being that comes solely from a "disinterested" relationship with the other, with the environment, and with life (Cavaleri, 2003).

In Perls' view, the only attitude able to foster a "healthy" adjustment to reality, even in the most difficult and problematic of conditions, is that of "creative disinterest" (Perls *et al.*, 1951/1994, p. 179 ff.). It is from disinterest, from an acceptance of the risk of losing, that creativity and mental well-being paradoxically emerge, and not from "victory" over oneself, over the other, and over reality in general. It is only such "disinterestedness" that brings us into full contact with the surrounding environment, sustaining our most authentic creativity and enhancing our capacity to grasp the strength, energy, and even vital eros that are hidden in vulnerability.

In the Gestalt therapy vision of the human condition, vulnerability always conceals within itself an unexpected and extraordinary "strength." It is only by opening up to the limit of vulnerability that such strength becomes accessible to us, enabling us to take possession of it and turn it into a driving element for growth, transformation, and life, even in such a dramatic and unsettling context as a pandemic. If interpreted and experienced creatively (Rank, 1993), the current pandemic crisis could turn into an opportunity to change the management of our planet. For example, economic growth could be harmonised with social inclusion and environmental protection in order to achieve sustainable development (Bellina, 2019). This integrated vision and sustainable development would also help to resolve the social and cultural contradictions that fuel racism today.

7.3 Human Potentiality

In recent years, the "liquid society" theorised by Bauman (2000) has been a highly authoritative conceptual paradigm of reference, helping us understand some of the disturbing aspects of globalisation, in particular individualism, social isolation, and relational fragility. During the pandemic, seeing the solidarity that emerged in many different forms, some were quick to pronounce the dawning of a new era and the "end of the liquid society" (De Giovanni, 2020). But unfortunately, this was not the case, and the way humans reacted to the pandemic proved to be very varied; in other words, "liquid". The reactions, quite naturally, have been many and vastly diverse, to the point of touching antitheses. There have been those who have sacrificed their own lives or have consciously given it to save others; those who have shut themselves away in their homes and in their solitude, like a "cocoon," remaining entirely indifferent to what was happening around them and desensitising themselves to the pain of others, or even seeing them simply as potential "spreaders of plague"; those who risked being infected by the virus to be at the service of others; and those who obsessively isolated themselves completely, behaving with irrational rationality and creating around themselves a sort of sanitary cordon giving them the illusion of controlling the virus and being invincible.

The diversity of reactions has characterised not only the behaviour of individuals but also entire local and national communities, trade union leaders, industrialists, and heads of state. How can it all be explained? What insights can the Gestalt therapy anthropological model offer to better understand the vast range of human reactions to the pandemic?

As we have seen before, the anthropological model developed by the founders of Gestalt therapy (Perls *et al.*, 1951/1994) highlights not only the positive aspects of the evolution of the human species but also the traps and dangers that it contains (p. 85 ff.). In their view, while initially our forebears were capable of fully merging the old and the new former ways of living, later, more evolved ways merged into an integrated whole. At a certain point in time, especially with the arrival of abstract thought and symbolic language, their mental capacity for integration was left significantly undermined by the excessive complexity their minds were then faced with.

For Perls *et al.* (1951/1994, p. 85 ff.) the inability to handle such extreme complexity in what is new brought about a "neurotic turn" in human evolution, a powerful urge to fall back on antiquated, though safer, forms of adaptation (Molinari, Cavaleri, 2015). So instead of continuing to merge the new with the old, the mind of our forebears learned to produce a "neurotic split" between the animal part and the human part of the self, learning to respond to the complexity of evolution with "regression" and "flight" back to forms of life that were more archaic but simpler and more tolerable. Confronted with the stress of having to integrate evermore complex aspects of reality, the human mind learned to activate two different adaptive strategies, one regressive and neurotic, the other creative and generative of new potentiality and new forms of integration between the old and the new (ibid.).

As Gestalt psychology has taught us (Wertheimer, 1945), the same reality can provoke different responses in the observer in both macro-systems and micro-systems. On the basis of how it is perceived, it can induce a return to the old or creative tension toward the new. As psychotherapists, we cannot intervene in political decisions, nor act on macro social systems. However, following in Perls' footsteps, we can, with every effort, support the vitality and creativity of our patients, the travail of their change, the novelty that is emerging in them.

8. Conclusion

To conclude, the pandemic has laid bare the extreme complexity and many contradictions of our globalised world. For human beings, it has meant not only dealing with the fear of death but also opening our eyes to a complex world that has suddenly become difficult to manage and control. Faced with this, some have responded with regression, seeing enemies everywhere, closing borders, and raising walls; others with creativity, conceiving "new things" and generating new forms of life, inclusion, and solidarity. In our pandemic-hit society, just like in the setting of a private practice, Gestalt therapists are called on to be agents of change, capable of promoting and supporting new potentiality and human forms – all those things that "can be" but "are not yet."

Notes

1 For a discussion of the "Great Unrest", see Cacciari (2016).
2 On the impact of the global economy on the community and on social relationships, see Bauman (2000). For a discussion of the issues of injustice, inequality, and the regression caused in Western countries by the global economy, see Atkinson (2015); Geiselberger (2017); Milanovic (2016); Piketty (2014); Saraceno (2015).
3 On the need to contextualise therapy work on the anthropological-cultural plane and connect it with developments in social sentiment, see Spagnuolo Lobb (2019).
4 On the gradual "regression" and on the growing "de-civilisation" of the contemporary world see Geiselberger (2017).
5 Alex Zanotelli (2003) uses the image of the "cocoon" to explain how Westerners insulate themselves and hide from the problems of poverty, social injustice, and human rights in the world, especially in the African continent.
6 *Competitive Individualism*, which is mentioned here, represents without a doubt the "dominant cultural model" that acted as a background to the election of Donald Trump in the United States.
7 On the evolutionary perspective in psychology see Buss (1998), Dawkins (1976), Pievani (2008), Pinker (2002), Tomasello (2005), Wilson (1975).
8 For more detailed studies on the subject see Cavaleri (2013a) and Spagnuolo Lobb (2013, p. 130).
9 For more detailed studies on the subjects in light of the most recent neuroscientific research, in particular of the "Polyvagal theory", see Porges (2011).
10 On the theory of the Self in Gestalt therapy see Spagnuolo Lobb (2013, 2016).
11 These considerations by Perls and Goodman, still very modern, find a strong validation in the most recent observations on the relationship between psyche and symbols by Galimberti (1999).
12 On the influence of Aristotelian thought on a few aspects of the development of Gestalt theory, see Cavaleri (2013b), Wheeler (1991).
13 Perls's and Goodman's idea of *creative adaptation* has been strongly influenced by Rank (1978). On this topic, see Cavaleri (2003, 2007).
14 On conflict as a space for recognition see Benjamin (2017); Honneth (1992); Ricoeur (2005).
15 On the "policy of recognition" see Bauman (2001). On recognition in "emotional bonds" see Benjamin (1988). On the "gift of recognition" see Molinari and Cavaleri (2015).

References

Anders, G. (1956). *Die Antiquiertheit des Menschen. Band I: Über die Seele im Zeitalter der zweiten industriellen Revolution* [The antiquity of man. Volume I: On the soul in the age of the second industrial revolution]. Munich: CH Beck.

Anders, G. (1964). *We, sons of Eichmann: An open letter to Klaus Eichmann*. Munich: CH Beck.

Aristotele. (1966). *Metaphysics*. Bloomington: Indiana University Press.

Atkinson, A. B. (2015). *Inequality: What can be done?* Cambridge: Harvard University Press.

Barbera, F., Gallerano, L., Nicoletti, A., & Raimondi, S. (2020). *Biodiversità a rischio* [Biodiversity under threat]. Roma: Legambiente.

Bauman, Z. (2000). *Liquid modernity*. Cambridge: Polity.

Bauman, Z. (2001). *Community. Seeking safety in an insecure world*. Cambridge: Polity.

Bauman, Z. (2013). La solidarietà ha un futuro? [Does solidarity have a future?]. In AA.VV., *Dono, dunque siamo. Otto buone ragioni per credere in una società più solidale*. Torino: UTET, 37–56.

Bellina, G. (2019). Modelli di sostenibilità per il terzo millennio [Sustainability models for the third millennium]. *Nuova Umanità, XLI*(4), 115–129.

Benjamin, J. (1988). *The bonds of love: Psychoanalysis, feminism, & the problem of domination*. New York: Pantheon Books.

Benjamin, J. (2017). *Beyond doer and done to: Recognition theory, intersubjectivity, and the third*. New York: Routledge.

Berger, P. L., & Luckmann, T. (1966). *The social construction of reality: A treatise in the sociology of knowledge*. New York: Doubleday & Company.

Braga, C., Calvo-Quiros, A. M., Contini, P., & Pellegrini, G. (2020). Migrazioni e inclusione [Migration and inclusion]. *Nuova Umanità, XLII*(2), 43–56.

Buss, D. M. (1998). *Evolutionary psychology: The new science of the mind*. Boston: Allyn & Bacon.

Cacciari, M. (2016). Il Grande Disordine. *L'Espresso, 30*, 14–17.

Capobianco, F., Perrelli, M. C., & Scarola, L. (2020). *Covid-19: Le lezioni (non) apprese della Fase 0* [Covid-19: Lessons (not) learned from Phase 0], www.vita.it/it/article/2020/04/20/covid-19-le-lezioni-non-apprese-dalla-fase-0/155092.

Cavaleri, P. A. (2003). *La profondità della superficie. Percorsi introduttivi alla psicoterapia della Gestalt* [The depth of the surface. Introductory paths to Gestalt psychotherapy]. Milano: FrancoAngeli.

Cavaleri, P. A. (2007). *Vivere con l'altro* [Living with the other]. Roma: Città Nuova.

Cavaleri, P. A. (Ed.). (2013a). *Psicoterapia della Gestalt e neuroscienze. Dall'isomorfismo alla simulazione incarnata* [Gestalt therapy and neuroscience. From isomorphism to embodied simulation]. Milano: FrancoAngeli.

Cavaleri, P. A. (2013b). Reich e Perls. Un confronto sempre attuale. *Quaderni di Gestalt, XXVI*(1), 81–89. DOI: 10.3280/GEST2013-001006.

Cavaleri, P. A. (2014), Il piacere della regressione. Gli stati di dipendenza e la funzione integrante del sé [The pleasure of regression. Dependency states and the integrating function of the self]. In G. Pintus & M. V. Crolle Santi (Eds.). *La relazione assoluta. Psicoterapia della Gestalt e dipendenze patologiche* (pp. 141–164). Ariccia, RM: Aracne.

Dawkins, R. (1976). *The selfish gene*. Oxford: Oxford University Press.

De Giovanni, B. (2020). *Il coronavirus è l'emblema della società liquida, tutto circola compresi i virus* [The coronavirus is the emblem of the liquid society, everything circulates including viruses], www.ilrifomista.it/il-coronavirus-e-l'emblema-della-società-liquida-tutto-circola-compresi-i-virus-58119/.

Erikson, E. (1968). *Identity, youth and crisis*. New York: W.W. Norton & Company.

Foucault, M. (2008). *The birth of biopolitics: Lectures at the Collège de France, 1978–1979*. New York: Palgrave MacMillan.

Freud, S. (1922). *Beyond the pleasure principle*. London, Wien: The International Psycho-Analytical Library.

Freud, S. (1930). *Civilisation and its discontents*. London: Hogarth Press.

Frewen, P., & Lanius, R. (2015). *Healing the traumatized self. Consciousness, neuroscience, treatment*. New York: W.W. Norton & Company.

Galimberti, U. (1999). *Psiche e techne. L'uomo nell'età della tecnica* [Psyche and techne. Man in the age of technology]. Milano: Feltrinelli.

Geiselberger, H. (Ed.). (2017). *The great regression*. Oxford: Polity Press.

Hobbes, T. (1983). *De Cive*. Oxford: Clarendon Press.

Hobbes, T. (1986). *Leviathan*. Oxford: Oxford University Press.

Honneth, A. (1992). *Kampf um Anerkennung. Grammatik sozialer Konflikte*. Frankfurt am Main: Suhrkamp Verlag.

Horney, K. (1937). *The neurotic personality of our time*. New York: W. W. Norton & Co. Inc.

Horton, R. (2020). *The COVID-19 catastrophe: What's gone wrong and how to stop it happening again*. Cambridge: Polity Press.

Köhler, W. (1925). *Psychological method for study of apes*. San Diego, CA: Harcourt, Brace & World.

Lasch, C. (1978). *The culture of narcissism: American life in an age of diminishing expectations*. New York: W.W. Norton & Co.

Lichtenberg, P. (1969). *Psychoanalysis radical and conservative*. New York: Springer Publishing Company.

Lichtenberg, P. (1990). *Community and confluence. Undoing the clinch of oppression*. Highland, NY: Gestalt Press.

Marcuse, H. (1970). *Reason and revolution: Hegel and the rise of social theory*. Boston: Beacon Press, or. ed. 1941.

Milanovic, B. (2016). *Global inequality: A new approach for the age of globalisation*. Cambridge, MA: Harvard University Press.

Molinari, E., & Cavaleri, P. A. (2015). *Il dono nel tempo della crisi. Per una psicologia del riconoscimento* [The gift in the time of crisis. For a psychology of recognition]. Milano: Raffaello Cortina.

Morris, D. (1967). *The naked ape: A zoologist's study of the human animal*. London: Jonathan Cape Publishing.

Panksepp, J., & Biven, L. (2012). *The archaeology of mind: Neuroevolutionary origins of human emotion*. New York: W.W. Norton& Company.

Perls, F. (1969). *Gestalt therapy verbatim*. Moab: Real people Press.

Perls, F., Hefferline, R. F., & Goodman, P. (1994). *Gestalt therapy: Excitement and growth in the human personality*. New York: The Gestalt Journal Press, ed.or. 1951.

Pievani, T. (Ed.). (2008). *L'evoluzione della mente. Le origini biologiche dell'intelligenza, della coscienza, del senso morale* [The evolution of the mind. The biological origins of intelligence, consciousness, and the moral sense]. Milano: Sperling & Kupfer.

Pievani, T. (2019). *La terra dopo di noi* [The earth after us]. Roma: Contrasto.

Piketty, T. (2014). *Capital in the twenty-first century*. Cambridge, MA: Harvard University Press.

Pinker, S. (2002). *The blank slate: The modern denial of human nature*. New York: Penguin Books.

Porges, S. W. (2011). *The polyvagal theory: Neurophysiological foundations of emotions, attachment, communication, and self-regulation.* New York: W.W. Norton & Co., Inc.

Porges, S. W. (2017). *The pocket guide to the polyvagal theory. The transformative power of feeling safe.* New York: W.W. Norton & Co., Inc.

Rank, O. (1978). *Truth and reality.* New York: W.W. Norton & Co Inc. (original published 1929).

Rank, O. (1993). *The trauma of birth.* New York: Dover Publications (original published 1924).

Ricoeur, P. (2005). *The course of recognition.* Cambridge: Harvard University Press.

Rifkin, J. (2014). *The zero marginal cost society: The internet of things, the collaborative commons, and the eclipse of capitalism.* New York: Palgrave Macmillan.

Rollo, M. (1950). *The meaning of anxiety.* New York: Ronald Press Co.

Rousseau, J.-J. (1968). *The social contract.* Harmondsworth: Penguin, or. ed. 1762.

Saraceno, C. (2015). *Il lavoro non basta. La povertà in Europa negli anni della crisi* [Work is not enough. Poverty in Europe in the years of crisis]. Milano: Feltrinelli.

Schütz, A. (1967). *Phenomenology of the social world.* Evanston, IL: Northwestern University Press, or. ed 1932.

Spagnuolo Lobb, M. (2013). *The now-for-next in psychotherapy. Gestalt therapy recounted in post-modern society.* Siracusa (Italy): Istituto di Gestalt HCC Italy Publ. Co.

Spagnuolo Lobb, M. (2016). Self as contact, contact as self. A contribution to ground experience in Gestalt therapy theory of self. In J.-M. Robine (Ed.). *Self. A polyphony of contemporary Gestalt therapists* (pp. 261–289). St. Romain la Virvée, France: L'Exprimerie.

Spagnuolo Lobb, M. (2019). La psicoterapia nella società post-moderna: uno strumento sociale a sostegno delle risorse umane del tempo [Psychotherapy in postmodern society: A social tool to support the human resources of the time]. In G. Fava Vizziello (Ed.). *Psicoterapie nella vertigine del cambiamento. Tra concepimenti senza sesso, migrazioni permanenti e sconosciuto potere tecnologico* (pp. 69–90). Padova: Cleup.

Straus, E. W. (1952). The upright posture. *The Psychiatric Quarterly, 26*, 529–561.

Taylor, M. (2014). *Trauma therapy and clinical practice: Neuroscience, Gestalt and the body.* Maidenhead, UK: Open University Press, McGraw-Hill Education.

Tomasello, M. (2005). *Le origini culturali della cognizione umana* [The cultural origins of human cognition]. Bologna: il Mulino.

Travaglio, M. (2020). *Tra inquinamento e mortalità per il Covid c'è un collegamento* [There is a link between pollution and Covid mortality], https://agi.it/cronaca/news//2020-04-30/particolato-inquinamento-coronavirus-covid-travaglio-8484721/.

Van Der Kolk, B. (2014). *The body keeps the score.* New York: Viking.

Wertheimer, M. (1945). *Productive thinking.* New York: Harper and Bros.

Wheeler, G. (1991). *Gestalt reconsidered.* New York: Gardner Press, Inc.

Wilson, E. O. (1975). *Sociobiology: The new synthesis.* Cambridge, MA: Harvard University Press.

Zanotelli, A. (2003). *Korogocho. Alla scuola dei poveri.* Milano: Feltrinelli.

The World Crisis and Gestalt Therapy

Response to Cavaleri

Comment by Gary Yontef

Gestalt therapy has always been a radically relational theory and practice. It seems to me that this age has a desperate need for a radically relational attitude by government leaders and ordinary citizens. The divisive tendencies of the human race have never been so dangerous as in this age of global business, politics, and military action. We need support for coming together for an emerging and creative sense of the possible.

We are living through a period of world crisis of hate, violence, and mass deprivation. The international and national social/political situations are marked by chaos and global suffering. Our governments and other agencies of regulation are frequently overwhelmed, incompetent, impotent, corrupt, or simply not concerned. At the same time, we are poisoning our air and water and driving many species into extinction. Many of us despair. In my practice I have not seen so many people bringing in their upset at general social and political situations since the era of the Vietnam War.

Is this sociological and political crisis the business of Gestalt therapy? Does the half century of Gestalt therapy theory and experience have anything to contribute? I think it is our business and we have some theory and experience to contribute. I caution though that while what we can contribute is worth explicating, we need some humility at extending our largely clinically derived perspective to the complex world of international political, diplomatic, and military processes.

There are core principles that apply to a variety of concerns, concerns of narrow or wide focus. They are principles of how to relate to others, how to gain clearer awareness, and how to think about the complexity of situations. In other words, our principles of dialogue, phenomenology, and field theory.

1. Dialogue

The kind of contact that Gestalt therapy theory and practice methodology calls for follows the principles of dialogue. Dialogue means meeting the other with recognition, respect, and acceptance rather than aiming to control the other and direct change or reform. This makes more likely a creative outcome that goes beyond any pre-established program. It makes possible the "together-with" that Cavaleri discusses.

The practice of inclusion is a specific principle that is key to understanding and practicing dialogue: Being open to, caring about, and attempting to facilitate experiencing the experience of the other so completely – as if one could feel it in your own body, while maintaining your own sense of self. In psychotherapy, the attempt to do this is a large part of the support the therapist brings to the development of the therapeutic relationship and progress in the patients' growth. This is the same regardless of the content of the situation and is especially relevant to working with someone from another culture. Caring about understanding the person from another culture, experiencing the world as the other person does, that is inclusion in practice. Even if true dialogue does not develop, being open to truly understanding the perspective of the other is necessary in order to be intelligent about relating to folk different than us.

Relating dialogically requires authentic presence. This means being fully present for the interaction; being emotionally involved, caring, congruent, appropriately self-disclosing, and radically open to the different experience of the other person.

Inclusion and presence and being open to what emerges from the dialogue is key to creative solutions. Commitment to the process of something emerging out of the dialogue means going beyond the either/or, win/lose reaction to differences that is often so destructive.

2. Phenomenology

The practice and skill at setting aside biases, preconceptions, so a clearer understanding can emerge is at the heart of the phenomenological method. In clinical practice, and in the rest of life, the phenomenological attitude helps identify biases so that we have a more accurate sense of the situation and our own process of observation, analysis, and emotional reaction.

The preconceptions that filter our understanding are even more magnified when one considers cross-cultural relationships. I am disheartened by how many ill-informed prejudicial beliefs seem to dominate the understanding, statements, and actions of our governments. For example, mischaracterisation of races, religions, ethnic groups, and so forth by some U.S. administration, like Trump, is quite alarming.

3. Field Theory

Simply trying to understand another person, or a family, or social situation involves multiple forces that combine to create the situation. There are always multiple forces interacting, with everything operating in the situation affecting everything else. And the situations are always changing, moving, becoming. The relatively simple linear causality model of Newtonian science is easier to understand and often misses the complexity that we absolutely need to understand and factor in to have a good chance of a creative outcome. Beware the ease and attraction of overly simple, polemical, and reductionistic analyses.

Obviously, the global situation is complex. This is true within nations, regions, and globally. We need to grasp historical and anthropological perspectives. It enhances our understanding of factors in the history of ethnic animosities, competition for resources, religious and cultural intensities, the organising principles of the powerful and the oppressed, and so forth that are at play in any given situation.

Overly simplistic ideas that reduce the complexity can be rhetorically satisfying and powerful but stand in the way of a more complex understanding. The profit motive and disregard for the needs of others that Cavaleri discussed are real and important. But is it only the profit motive of the Euro-American business people that cause the global unrest?

To me, it is obvious that while that is a potent variable, there are the other forces also operating.

4. Conclusion

Gestalt therapy as a radically relational theory and practice can contribute in an age that has a desperate need for a radically relational attitude by government leaders and ordinary citizens. In this age of global business, politics, and military action, the human capacity for hate, fear, and ignorance has never been as dangerous as it is now. We need to learn to come together for an emerging and creative future to be possible.

Chapter 4

Phenomenology and Gestalt Psychotherapy

New Challenges Under-the-Radar

Pietro Andrea Cavaleri

1. Phenomenology and Neurophenomenology

Phenomenology is born out of an attention towards "that which appears", towards "phenomenal reality", towards a world perceived and described "in the first person", with possibility of intuition of the "second person" perspective (Churchill, 2010). Interest in phenomenology, although in a different way, was already present in Kantian and Hegelian thought, but it was only with Brentano (1874) and Husserl (1910/1980) that it would give rise to a well-defined philosophical movement. Then, at the beginning of the 20th century, the phenomenological perspective would break into the world of psychology as well, almost simultaneously, with Jaspers (1913/1997) ushering in studies of psychopathology and "phenomenological psychiatry", and with Wertheimer (1912) giving birth to Gestalt psychology, specifically interested in how perceptive experience is organised and takes shape in the human mind.[1]

Lewin (1951) drew inspiration from the discoveries of Gestalt psychology for the development of his "field theory", as did Goldstein (1939), with respect to his research in the neurological and neuropsychological area. Laura Perls, for a substantial period of time, worked in Goldstein's laboratory, where brain-damaged veterans of the First World War were studied, and so did Frederick Perls for a shorter period. Subsequently, Goldstein's research would constitute the starting reference point for the "phenomenology of perception" theorised by Merleau-Ponty (1945/1962). Out of this rich and composite terrain would ultimately emerge the "phenomenology of the contact boundary" and the "phenomenology of the organism/environment field", developed by the founders of Gestalt therapy (Perls *et al.*, 1951).[2] We are dealing with a valuable legacy that to this day constitutes an indispensable reference for anyone who wishes to embark on a Gestalt clinical practice. It is however justified to wonder today, after seventy years, to what extent this phenomenological sensitivity, inherited from the founders, should be maintained intact or instead renewed, and further enriched by input from other sources.

In the last few years, an intense debate among Gestalt therapists has developed on how the field concept in particular might be revisited, still staying within a

DOI: 10.4324/9781003313335-6

coherent phenomenological perspective.[3] In Staemmler's view (2006), the field should be understood above all as the totality of subjective experience. Robine (2003) has expressed a similar stance. For him, the field constitutes in its essence a subjective phenomenon, negating the possibility of a shared field. Referring to the neo-phenomenology of Schmitz (1980), Francesetti (2015) describes the field as an atmosphere, as something ephemeral and fleeting, neither subjective nor objective.

Of a different opinion is Parlett (1991), who conceives of the field from a triadic perspective, composed of the field of one and that of the other, who, by interacting, co-create a third shared field, able to contain and influence the previous two. Very close to this position is that of Spagnuolo Lobb (2013, 2018). Conceiving the relationship between organism and environment on both the anthropological and socio-political levels, she affirms that the field perspective in Gestalt therapy encourages us to use non-dichotomous thinking (Spagnuolo Lobb, 2013, p. 79). It allows us to think of perception as a "relational product" strictly connected to the fullness of the concentration of the individuals involved at the contact boundary. In this way, they are able to grasp both what is internal and what is external. The fact that the self is considered in a medial position between organism and environment allows full subjectivity to coincide with full presence in objectivity. The more the individual is fully present in the "between", the more they take part in the field, the more their presence contributes to creating the conditions of the field (ibid., p. 80). It is from the phenomenological field created by the patient's modality of contact and by the therapist's response that the possibility emerges of supporting the spontaneous development of the patient's intentionality of contact (ibid., p. 118). "Perception is not an isolated process; it emerges and is cocreated together with the other and with the environment in general" (Spagnuolo Lobb, 2018, p. 58). Besides this, Wheeler (1991), McConville (2001), and Wollants (2012) have produced a thorough study on the epistemological plane. They have re-proposed with great consistency the need to re-evaluate the "phenomenological roots" that tie Gestalt psychotherapy to the Berlin school, in other words to Gestalt psychology.

This intense comparison on field phenomenology, which is of specific Gestalt interest, can be enhanced today by additional developments, which come from the most recent neurobiology of relational trauma and social engagement. A kind of maturity characterises our time because one can speak not only in terms of phenomenology, but also of neurophenomenology. In fact, if phenomenology describes phenomenal reality as such, neurophenomenology presumes to describe its neurobiological processes that make it possible, especially from the perspective of an embodied (cf. Kepner, 1995; Gallese, 2006) and a relational mind (cf. Siegel, 1999), from its origins (cf. Ammaniti and Ferrari, 2020). Of course, neurons are part of natural science, they are not a phenomenological reality. Nevertheless, there is a debate today between those who advocate the "naturalisation" of phenomenology (Gallagher, 2012) and those who oppose it (Giorgi, 1997). In this light, neurophenomenology could be conceived as an integral part of the same phenomenology, thus making a constant legitimate dialogue between "human sciences" and "natural sciences", between psychotherapy and neurosciences, outside of a dualism that might be obsolete (cf. Cozolino, 2020).

In the second half of the twentieth century, and in these two decades of the new century, there has emerged at breakneck speed a series of discoveries and new acquisitions, in the neuroscientific, psychological, and philosophical realms. They are an important challenge for us to deepen our Gestalt and phenomenological perspective. If we take up this challenge, we will immediately become aware of the fact that, in these last decades, a new "phenomenology of human relations" has arisen, almost "under the radar". Numerous researchers from multiple disciplines, clinicians from various approaches, and philosophers from diverse orientations have contributed in a different but significant way to this development. It is within this "under-the-radar phenomenology" that we are now trying to compare notes, in the conviction that we will find "nourishing" stimuli and "generative" pathways.

2. Beyond Every Dualism: Mind/Body Unity

What has always characterised the Gestalt therapy model is a phenomenological perspective contrary to every form of dualism, one which at times re-emerges in clinical practice. This represents a decisive rejection of both the organism/environment dualism and the mind/body dualism. Theorised by Descartes, mind/body dualism has heavily conditioned modern scientific thought and clinical practice right up until today. As we all know, Damasio (1994, 1999, 2010) exposed some time ago "Descartes' error". He gave rise to an authoritative field of research, which was able to show, on the neuroscientific level, how much the mind is rooted in the body, from which it emanates in a constant interaction with the world, thus describing a brain that "thinks the body" while it interacts with the environment. His research has substantively highlighted the relevance that emotions assume in decision-making processes, identifying the neuronal areas that are involved. Furthermore, by reasserting MacLean's triune brain theory in an original way, he has developed a theory of the self, identifying the different cerebral areas from whose interaction "the self comes to mind". Panksepp (2012), the father of "affective neurosciences", steered his research in a similar direction. He convincingly reconstructed a sort of "archaeology of the mind" capable of explaining the genesis and the neural mechanisms of the emotions, maintaining their absolute centrality in human relations. The discovery that "mirror neurons" play an important role in the shaping of a mind that is born out of a body in relation to the environment, is due to the work of Rizzolatti and Sinigaglia (2006) and Gallese (2006, 2011), and it is thanks to this that it has become possible to identify a neural system able to "simulate" the reality we perceive as external to us.

Thanks to this and to other numerous studies, "neurophenomenology"[4] has come into being today. It is able to provide support and neuroscientific cross-references to phenomenological observation. Unlike seventy years ago, today we can describe, from a phenomenological perspective, the field that is co-created by therapist and patient, and "in the first person" what "appears" while we expose ourselves to the median dimension of the "between", but in addition, we can also keep in mind those neurobiological and neurophysiological links involved in the "lived" experience. This "additional" level of consciousness, this "extra element", allows us to widen our understanding of what is happening "here and now", of the co-creation in progress, enabling us to express a more accurate observation of the field and of what flows into it, as well as to carry out a more insightful therapeutic intervention (Béjà, 2020).

Resorting to a metaphor can, even if only up to a certain point, help us to explain this passage better.[5] When we find ourselves in public, during a marionette performance, we are completely involved in what we are watching. We see colourful costumes, various characters moving from one side of the stage to the other. They speak and interact with each other. We are captured by their colours, by how they move, and by what they say. But if we leave the audience and go backstage, we become immediately aware of the existence of another perspective, different from the previous one. Reality which at first "appeared" to us in a given way is now revealed to be much more complex, and in some ways, even more fascinating. We meet the artists who, with their voice, their creativity, and their sense of beauty, have brought to life an absorbing performance, able to capture the attention and the fantasy of children and adults. Finally, we are able to better "understand" what we have "experienced" in all its particulars, an experience of which we have been co-protagonists.

Understanding in a phenomenological sense the multiple levels of complexity present in a co-created field allows the therapist to simultaneously have different perspectives and reading keys, to implement new tools, to make his/her interventions more insightful, and to demonstrate a better clinical ability. The phenomenological centrality of the experience described in the "first person", of the "lived" experience, can be supported by neurobiological and neurophysiological components underlying the "lived" ones, which patient and therapist explore in the co-creation of the shared field.

3. Trauma, Dissociation, and Polarity Conflict

Where the interaction between personal "life experiences" and neurophysiological processes emerges in all of its complexity is in the experience of trauma. Some neuroscientists have observed and analysed psychic suffering with much attention and sensitivity. For example, Van der Kolk (2014) provides an accurate description of the "experiences" linked to trauma and to the repercussions that these effectuate on the body, the brain, and on the entire nervous system.[6] Thanks to his research, it has been possible to grasp the proximity existing between the symptoms produced by war traumas and those caused by relational or affective traumas. Often, in both cases, those traumatised, in order to survive the triggering event, resort to the adaptive strategy of dissociation.

Fisher (2017), in referring to Van der Hart's "theory of structural dissocia-tion", recently described the adaptive dynamics of dissociation and has devel-oped a cogent psychotherapeutic model in support of the traumatised person. It is mainly Bromberg (2011) who has dwelled on dissociation as a "relational phenomenon". In order to articulate and advocate his data, he calls into play in a significant way the studies of Schore (1994) on the right hemisphere. Even though they start from different points of view, both Fisher and Bromberg pro-pose an interpretive and therapeutic model centred on the dissociation of parts of the self, one that is very close to the "polarity conflict" theorised by Gestalt psychotherapy through the contribution not only of Perls and Goodman but also other authoritative writers.[7]

The founders of the Gestalt approach conceive of mental suffering, that they refer to as "neurosis", as a "split" between two different parts or polarities, "one part is kept in unawareness, or it is coldly recognised but alienated from con-cern, or both parts are carefully isolated from each other and made to seem irrel-evant to each other, avoiding conflict and maintaining the status quo" (Perls *et al.*, 1951/1994, p. 16). Throughout history, human beings have learned how to defend themselves from their very complexity and from the conflicts that it inspires. We have learned to see in conflict not as an experience, in which different tightly con-nected polarities "dialogue" amongst each other (*et-et*), but as a painful wound that forces us to "choose" (*aut-aut*, either-or) between polarities that appear to be mutually exclusive (cf. Cavaleri, 2020). Out of this, according to the founders, comes the fragmenting of the personality, the "split" between spontaneity and deliberation, between body and mind, between the self and the outside world, between the personal and the social.

4. Neuroception Even Before Perception

Porges (2017) is an author of particular significance in the search for "under-the-radar phenomenology", which runs through contemporary neuroscientific research. Let us try to understand why. Since the beginning, the founders of the Gestalt approach have been interested in two principal themes: the "phenome-nology of intentionality" and the "phenomenology of perception" (cf. Cavaleri, 2003, 2013; Spagnuolo Lobb, 2013). With Porges' research on the vagus nerve and with his thoughts on "neuroception", a new challenge has emerged for the Gestalt approach. It entails having to confront a new and additional phe-nomenological perspective: the "phenomenology of neuroception". Porges maintains, in fact, that almost all of our behaviours are very much guided, before perceptive experience, by neuroceptive experience, which aggressively evades our consciousness, even though it passes through us and involves us completely.

Porges (2017) and Dana (2018) produced a first descriptive analysis of what we have called the "phenomenology of neuroception". What is revealed out of this is the important role that neuroceptive experience plays especially in social engagement. Neuroception, in fact, is defined as a process by which the nervous system evaluates a risk without resorting to conscious thought, automatically involving brain areas able to evaluate signs of security, but also of danger and threats to life. With these signs detected through neuroception, the physiological state of the organism is automatically modified for the purpose of guaranteeing its survival. However, a defective neuroception can reveal a risk where there isn't one, or instead, pinpoint elements of safety where risks may appear.

The system of social involvement, the system of fight-or-flight and freezing (collapse) depend on the neuroceptive experience and its automatisms. Other than with factors of a genetic nature, neuroceptive dysfunctionality can be linked, among other things, to abuse or neglect, to various kinds of traumas, and to experiences of inadequate co-regulation in childhood. In a Gestalt therapy context, the "aesthetic relational knowing", theorised by Spagnuolo Lobb (2018), can legitimately be considered an initial and significant contribution towards the development of a "phenomenology of neuroception" in the clinical field (cf. Cavaleri, chap. 7).

5. The Co-created Field and the Co-regulation of Reciprocal Recognition

Dissociation as an adaptive strategy to trauma, the interrelationship between neuroceptive dysfunctionality and dysregulated relational experiences constitute today issues of great clinical relevance. The topical nature of these themes directs us towards another field, which we first defined as "under-the-radar phenomenology". It represents a most recent branch of research and thought that concerns the centrality of recognition in human relations, in particular "reciprocal recognition" as a basic experience of human co-regulation and as an effective model of clinical intervention. Within the context of contemporary thought, Ricoeur and Honneth have studied this issue in depth.

In the tradition of phenomenology and with the intent to declare the dominance of reciprocity in relation to the other, Ricoeur (2005) highlights three different modalities with which to trigger pathways to recognition. The first, inspired by Husserl (1932/1988), could be defined as "analogic apperception" and consists of presuming that the other is analogous to me, that the other has a nature common to my own, and therefore I can recognise him through myself and my experience in life. The second, tracing back to Lévinas (1969), consists of giving precedence to the presence of the other and of exhibiting myself to their face, and to what it asks of me. In the third modality, suggested by the same Ricoeur, recognition occurs "between" the protagonists of the exchange; it is the result of the "between" that emerges from their mutuality, from the circularity of their reciprocal exchange. One is never the other. One always remains different from the other. But this does not prevent intimacy in the exchange, which is experienced in the making and the receiving of the gift of recognition. Thus, the mutuality, the reciprocity of the relationship does not become a fusional union, but can integrate the intimacy with respect, and always presents itself as the continuous exchange of a gift: the recognition of the difference of the other. From a different viewpoint, that of the Frankfurt School, Honneth (1992) claims that every human conflict is not generated so much by the predatory nature of the human being (*homo homini lupus*), but rather by an innate need for recognition, a need that is rooted in each of us. Human conflict, in all its forms, is interpreted not as a clash between antagonistic interests but rather as a "struggle for recognition", like an incessant request for one's own subjectivity, unique and one-of-a-kind, to be cognised and again re-cognised.

Benjamin (2017) proceeds along the same lines, but from the point of view of an intersubjective psychoanalytic context. In the wake of Beebe, Stern, and Tronick, she maintains that, just as in the mother/child dyad, in every significant bond as well, the relationship with the other is always marked by a sequence that is repeated: recognition-breakdown-restoration. After every initial "exchange of recognition", what follows is an inevitable and equally spontaneous "breakdown", that signals and causes everyone to experience the irreducible difference of the other, his/her distinct subjectivity. But after every breakdown, what ensues is always the need for "repair." At this point, however, the will to restore the relationship with the other can take on two opposite modalities. In the first, the overture towards the other is characterised by an affectively significant tension, aimed at re-cognising this other as a different subject than oneself, relinquishing every exercise of power or resistance over him/her and his/her diversity. In the second, on the other hand, what emerges is a marked intention to resist the other's difference and a strong desire to exercise over him/her every possible form of control, reducing this other to an object to subjugate, or to an object upon whom to exert one's power.

The first attitude opens a path towards "repair", towards realignment, towards reciprocal recognition as a co-created experience, towards the renewal of co-regulation after the deleterious breakdown. Instead, the second attitude fuels a misalignment, causes a failure of recognition, makes repair impossible, and condemns the relationship to dysregulation. Whereas in the first case each one fully experiences their own subjectivity, their own capacity to act and become compassionate, in the second case, the failure of recognition results in dissociation, and conceals to each one's consciousness significant parts of the self. Benjamin, in fact, declares that recognition and affective regulation determine each other. And so recognition of the effect on the part of the other promotes the integrative functioning within the self. Rereading within a Gestalt therapy context the co-creation of the field in the light of these stimulating ideas can certainly provide an extremely enriching opportunity. This is the attempt that Spagnuolo Lobb (2016, 2017a, 2017b) has made with her model of the "dance of reciprocity" (see Ch. 2), in which the recognition of the patient's (or child's) intentional movement and the therapist's (or caregiver's) reparative proposal of movement allow for the co-creation of a new field in which change to the relational dysregulations suffered by the patient is possible.

6. A Provisional Conclusion

We must keep in mind that phenomenology has always been a constituent feature of Gestalt psychotherapy (Amendt-Lyon, 2018). The model can continually regenerate and feed its own vitality, on the theoretical as well as the clinical level, to the extent that who practices it as a professional will know how to engage, not only with classical or academic phenomenology, but also with the various "phenomenological sensibilities", which, on many sides, materialise "under-the-radar" in many areas of learning, offering rich inspiration capable of revitalising and recontextualising the Gestalt therapy approach in the world of today and tomorrow.

Notes

1 See De Monticelli (2018) on the phenomenological perspective and on its current situation in the area of philosophy and psychology.
2 See, just as examples among many other writings, Cavaleri (2003, 2013), Bloom (2003) and the special issue of the journal *Gestalt Review* edited by Amendt-Lyon (2018), on the relationship between phenomenology and Gestalt psychotherapy
3 See Macaluso (2020) on this subject.
4 On the subject of neurophenomenology compare Varela (1996); Depraz *et al.* (2003); Lutz and Thompson (2003); Cappuccio (2006); Gallese (2006); Thompson and Zahavi (2007); Frewen and Lanius (2017); Stanghellini *et al.* (2019).
5 For an in-depth study of the metaphor proposed here compare Botto (2013).
6 In the Gestalt context, the experience of trauma is treated in depth by Kepner (1995) and Taylor (2014).
7 For an in-depth study of polarity conflict in Gestalt psychotherapy see Cavaleri (2003).

References

Amendt-Lyon, N. (Ed.). (2018). Special issue: Gestalt therapy and "new phenomenology". *Gestalt Review, 22*(3).
Ammaniti, M., & Ferrari, P. F. (2020). *Il corpo non dimentica. L'Io motorio e lo sviluppo della relazionalità*. Milano: Raffaello Cortina.
Béjà, V. (2020). Ways and means of the phenomenological attitude in a field perspective. The secret longing: A pragmatic clinical compass. *British Gestalt Journal, 29*(2), 33–39.
Benjamin, J. (2017). *Beyond doer and done to: Recognition theory, intersubjectivity, and the third*. New York: Routledge.
Bloom, D. J. (2003). "Tiger! Tiger! Burning Bright" – Aesthetic values as clinical values in Gestalt therapy. In M. Spagnuolo Lobb, & N. Amendt-Lyon (Eds.). *Creative license. The art of Gestalt therapy* (pp. 63–78). Wien, New York: Springer.
Botto, S. (2013). Le funzioni del sé, il loro substrato neurofisiologico e le interruzioni di contatto. Alcune ipotesi (The self functions, their neurophysiological substrate and interruptions of contact. A few assumptions). In P. A. Cavaleri (Ed.). *Psicoterapia della Gestalt e neuroscienze. Dall'isomorfismo alla simulazione incarnata* (pp. 136–146). Milano: FrancoAngeli.
Brentano, F. (1874). *Psychologie von empirischen standpunkt*. Lipsia: Lunker-Humblot.
Bromberg, P. M. (2011). *The shadow of the tsunami: And the growth of the relational mind*. London: Routledge.

Cappuccio, M. (Ed.) (2006). *Neurofenomenologia. Le scienze della mente e la sfida dell'esperienza cosciente* [Neurophenomenology. The sciences of the mind and the challenge of conscious experience]. Milano: Bruno Mondadori.

Cavaleri, P. A. (2003). *La profondità della superficie. Percorsi introduttivi alla psicoterapia della Gestalt* [The depth of the surface. Introductory paths to Gestalt psychotherapy]. Milano: FrancoAngeli.

Cavaleri, P. A. (Ed.). (2013). *Psicoterapia della Gestalt e neuroscienze. Dall'isomorfismo alla simulazione incarnata* [Gestalt therapy and neuroscience. From isomorphism to embodied simulation]. Milano: FrancoAngeli.

Cavaleri, P. A. (2020). A Gestalt therapy reading of the pandemic. *The Humanistic Psychologist*, *48*(4), 347–352. DOI: 10.1037/hum0000214.

Churchill, S. D. (2010). "Second person" perspectivity in observing and understanding emotional expression. In L. Embree, M. Barber, & T. J. Nenon (Eds.). *Phenomenology 2010, volume 5: Selected essays from North America, Part 2: Phenomenology beyond philosophy* (pp. 81–106). Bucharest: Zeta Books.

Cozolino, L. (2020). *The pocket guide to neuroscience for clinicians*. New York: W.W. Norton & Co Inc.

Damasio, A. (1994). *Descartes' error: Emotion, reason, and the human brain*. New York: Putnam.

Damasio, A. (1999). *The feeling of what happens: Body and emotion in the making of consciousness*. New York: Harcourt.

Damasio, A. (2010). *Self comes to mind: Constructing the conscious brain*. New York: Pantheon.

Dana, D. (2018). *The polyvagal theory in therapy: Engaging the rhythm of regulation*. New York: W.W. Norton & Co Inc.

De Monticelli, R. (2018). *Il dono dei vincoli* [The gift of bonds]. Milano: Garzanti.

Depraz, N., Varela, F. J., & Vermersch, P. (2003). *On becoming aware: A pragmatics of experiencing*. Amsterdam: John Benjamins.

Fisher, J. (2017). *Healing the fragmented selves of trauma survivors: Overcoming internal self-alienation*. New York: Routledge.

Francesetti, G. (2015). From individual symptoms to psychopathological fields. Towards a field perspective on clinical human suffering. *British Gestalt Journal*, *24*(1), 5–19.

Gallagher, S. (2012). On the possibility of naturalizing phenomenology. In D. Zahavi (Ed.). *Oxford handbook of contemporary phenomenology* (pp. 70–93). Oxford: Oxford University Press.

Gallese, V. (2006). Corpo vivo, simulazione incarnata e intersoggettività. Una prospettiva neuro-fenomenologica [Living body, embodied simulation, and intersubjectivity. A neuro-phenomenological perspective]. In M. Cappuccio (Ed.). *Neurofenomenologia. Le scienze della mente e la sfida dell'esperienza cosciente* (pp. 293–326). Milano: Bruno Mondadori.

Gallese, V. (2011). Neuroscience and phenomenology. *Phenomenology & Mind*, *1*, 33–48.

Giorgi, A. (1997). The theory, practice and evaluation of the phenomenological method as a qualitative research procedure. *Journal of Phenomenological Psychology*, *28*, 235–260. DOI: 10.1163/156916297X00103.

Goldstein, K. (1939). *The organism: A holistic approach to biology derived from pathological data in man*. New York: American Book Company.

Honneth, A. (1992). *Kampf um Anerkennung. Grammatik sozialer Konflikte*. Frankfurt am Main: Suhrkamp Verlag.

Husserl, E. (1980). *Ideas pertaining to a pure phenomenology and to a phenomenological philosophy – third book: Phenomenology and the foundations of the sciences*. Dordrecht: Kluwer (orig. ed. 1910).

Husserl, E. (1988). *Cartesian meditations. An introduction to phenomenology*. Dordrecht: Kluwer (orig. ed. 1932).

Jaspers, K. (1997). *General psychopathology – volumes 1 & 2*. Baltimore and London: Johns Hopkins University Press. (orig. ed. 1913).

Kepner, J. (1995). *Healing tasks: Psychotherapy with adult survivors of childhood abuse*. San Francisco: Jossey-Bass.

Lévinas, E. (1969). *Totality and infinity: An essay on exteriority*. Pittsburgh, PA: Duquesne University Press.

Lewin, K. (1951). *Field theory in social science*. New York: Harper & Brothers.

Lutz, A., & Thompson, E. (2003). Neurophenomenology: Integrating subjective experience and brain dynamics in the neuroscience of consciousness. *Journal of Consciousness Studies, 9–10*, 31–52.

Macaluso, M. A. (2020). Il concetto di "campo" in psicoterapia della Gestalt. Sviluppi e implicazioni [The concept of "field" in Gestalt therapy. Developments and implications]. *Quaderni di Gestalt, XXXIII*(1), 57–73. DOI: 10.3280/GEST2020-001005

McConville, M. (2001). Lewinian field theory. In M. McConville, & G. Wheeler (Eds.). *The heart of development, vol. 2: Adolescence* (pp. 26–53). Cambridge, MA: Gestalt Press.

Merleau-Ponty, M. (1962). *Phenomenology of perception*. London and New York: Routledge & Kegan Paul (orig. ed. 1945).

Panksepp, J., & Biven, L. (2012). *The archaeology of mind: Neuroevolutionary origins of human emotion*. New York: W.W. Norton & Company Inc.

Parlett, M. (1991). Reflections on field theory. *The British Gestalt Journal, 1*, 68–91.

Perls, F., Hefferline, R. F., & Goodman, P. (1994). *Gestalt therapy: Excitement and growth in the human personality*. New York: The Gestalt Journal Press, or.ed., 1951.

Porges, S. W. (2017). *The pocket guide to the polyvagal theory. The transformative power of feeling safe*. New York: W.W. Norton & Company, Inc.

Ricoeur, P. (2005). *The course of recognition*. Cambridge: Harvard University Press.

Rizzolatti, G., & Sinigaglia, C. (2006). *So quel che fai* [I know what you do]. Milano: Raffaello Cortina.

Robine, J-M. (2003). Intentionality in flesh and blood: Toward a psychopathology of fore-contacting. *International Gestalt Journal, XXVI*(2), 85–110.

Schore, A. N. (1994). *Affect regulation and the origin of the self: The neurobiology of emotional development*. Hove, UK: Psychology Press.

Schmitz, H. (1980). *New phenomenology. A brief introduction*. Bonn: Bouvier.

Siegel, D. J. (1999). *The developing mind: Toward a neurobiology of interpersonal experience*. New York: Guilford Press.

Spagnuolo Lobb, M. (2013). *The now-for-next in psychotherapy: Gestalt therapy recounted in post-modern society*. Siracusa: Istituto di Gestalt HCC Italy Publ. Co., www.gestalt italy.com.

Spagnuolo Lobb, M. (2016). Self as contact, contact as self. A contribution to ground experience in Gestalt therapy theory of self. In J-M. Robine (Ed.). *Self. A polyphony of contemporary Gestalt therapists* (pp. 261–289). St. Romain la Virvée, France: L'Exprimerie.

Spagnuolo Lobb, M. (2017a). From losses of ego functions to the dance steps between psychotherapist and client. Phenomenology and aesthetics of contact in the psychotherapeutic field. *British Gestalt Journal, 26*(1), 28–37.

Spagnuolo Lobb, M. (2017b). Phenomenology and aesthetic recognition of the dance between psychotherapist and client: A clinical example. *British Gestalt Journal*, *26*(2), 50–56.

Spagnuolo Lobb, M. (2018). Aesthetic relational knowledge of the field: A revised concept of awareness in Gestalt therapy and contemporary psychiatry. *Gestalt Review*, *22*(1), 50–68. DOI: 10.5325/gestalt review.22.1.0050.

Staemmler, F. M. (2006). A Babylonian confusion? On the uses and meanings of the term "field". *British Gestalt Journal*, *15*(2), 64–83.

Stanghellini, G., Raballo, A., Broome, M., Fernandez, A. V., Fusar-Poli, P., & Rosfort, R. (Eds.). (2019). *The Oxford handbook of phenomenological psychopathology*. Oxford: Oxford University Press.

Taylor, M. (2014). *Trauma therapy and clinical practice. Neuroscience, Gestalt and the body*. Maidenhead, UK: Open University Press, McGraw-Hill Education.

Thompson, E., & Zahavi, D. (2007). Philosofical issues: Phenomenology. In P. D. Zelazo, M. Moscovitch, & E. Thompson (Eds.). *Cambridge handbook of consciousness studies* (pp. 67–87). New York: Cambridge University Press.

Van Der Kolk, B. (2014). *The body keeps the score*. New York: Viking.

Varela, F. J. (1996). Neurophenomenology. *Journal of Consciousness Studies,* *3*(4), 230–349.

Wertheimer, M. (1912). Experimentelle Studien uber das Sehen von Begwegungen [Experimental studies on the vision of motion]. *Zeitschrift fur Psychologie*, *61*, 121–256.

Wheeler, G. (1991). *Gestalt reconsidered*. New York: Gardner Press, Inc.

Wollants, G. (2012). *Gestalt therapy. Therapy of the situation*. London: Sage.

Chapter 5

The Gestalt Clinical Data Sheet

A Phenomenological, Aesthetic, and Field Instrument for Gestalt Psychotherapy and Supervision

Margherita Spagnuolo Lobb, Elisabetta Conte, and Maria Mione

1. Introduction

We are presenting here a clinical tool based on what has been expressed in previous chapters. It consists of a data sheet capable of tracking the therapeutic situation beyond the patient's individual aspects: the patient's ground experience and the contextualisation of the distress that brought them into therapy, their self-actualisation within the therapeutic contact, and the phenomenological and aesthetic feeling of the therapist, that is the contact, the dance of reciprocity co-created between therapist and patient.

From a phenomenological, aesthetic, and field view, this instrument offers guidelines that orients the therapist towards comprehension of the *situation*, which is triggered with that particular patient, *and which includes the therapist*, and therefore towards a *relational* intervention, which takes into account the intentional reciprocal resonances and the "dance" of reciprocity between therapist and patient. The data sheet allows one to describe the therapeutic relationship and the patient's suffering while guiding the therapist's clinical thinking towards the coordinates of development within the relational key of Gestalt therapy. It allows for the systemisation of individual data and the designing of a therapeutic plan according to the situational Gestalt therapy model (see Wollants, 2012; Spagnuolo Lobb *et al.*, 2017).

The data sheet is useful in the therapeutic context and also in that of supervision and research. From a practical perspective, it can be used as a *guideline* for the therapist's diagnostic/clinical work, as a useful *teaching instrument* in student training, as a *record* of the practice of supervision, as well as a *tool for research* into individual cases.

Being a dynamic and not a static instrument, this clinical data sheet can be compiled in a short period with regards to the collecting of anamnestic data, while it demands, in its more procedural function, long-term reflection, and provides the possibility of updates during the evolution of the co-creation of the therapeutic relationship.

It includes the gathering of anamnestic data, of the patient's phenomenological descriptions of important events in his/her life, and of symptomology, as well as

DOI: 10.4324/9781003313335-7

a description of the therapist's perception both in relation to the functions of the patient's self and of the therapist's own participation in the treatment in relational terms. It also includes the therapist's description of the figure/ground dynamic in the co-creation of the contact with the patient, the consideration of the patient's intentionality, and its contextualisation in the experiential field generated within the specific therapeutic situation.

The Gestalt therapy data sheet presented here is a revised and expanded version of an already existing edition (Spagnuolo Lobb, 1997), utilised by all of the teaching staff of the Istituto di Gestalt HCC Italy. Compared to the previous data sheet, the current one takes into account some diagnostic and clinical aspects developed in recent years. They concern the evolutionary perspective (the "polyphonic development of domains", Spagnuolo Lobb, 2012, 2013), the presence of the therapist from the field point of view (Lewin, 1943; De Rivera, 1976) – that has been described as an aesthetic, relational way of knowing (Spagnuolo Lobb, 2018) – and the reciprocity of the therapeutic contact, namely what the therapist and patient do together kinesthetically in the creation of a "dance" (the "dance steps" model, Spagnuolo Lobb, 2016, 2017a, 2017b).

It encompasses different areas relative to the collecting of anamnestic data, to symptomatology information, to the analysis of the figure/ground relationship, to the formulation of diagnostic criteria, and to the identification of the contact intentionality to be supported during therapy. We will briefly summarise here the diagnostic and clinical areas taken into consideration and ultimately provide a practical application of the data sheet with a clinical case.

2. The Diagnostic and Clinical Areas

2.1. Significant Physiological Aspects

This area takes into consideration the visible physiological aspects in a first contact with the patient, on both the level of observable bodily structure and the level of information gathering on the primary physiological processes: ongoing diseases, the sleep/wake rhythm, eating habits, and pharmacotherapy, etc.

It also takes into consideration the potential intake of pharmaceuticals and if there are significant relationships with other specialists, including a psychiatrist. And lastly, we would want to know if the patient practices forms of alternative medicine (osteopathy, yoga, etc.).

2.2. Anamnesis

This area covers the family of origin, the current family, social adaptation, history of the symptom, and the attempts to resolve it.

Family of origin: what is highlighted here is the structure of the family of origin (the genogram, see Jolly *et al.*, 1980) and the description of the relationships within the family field (climate, relationships between siblings and between parents, see Minuchin, 1974; Satir, 1983), of important events that have marked the family history (deaths, relocations, accidents, separations of various kinds, hospitalisations, etc.), presence of myths, secrets, and taboos (Zuk and Boszor menyi-Nagy, 1971). It consists of an immersion together with the patient into their experiential ground, for the purpose of having a first picture of the relational ground in which they have been able to develop, with greater or lesser spontaneity, their own competencies and intentionalities of contact.

Current family: if it exists, what is described is: its structure, current experiences, and relevant events that characterise it.

Social adaptation: Here we analyse the patient's current overall social adaptation with respect to lifestyle, daily organisation, and work activity or study.

The symptom: In Gestalt therapy, the symptom is considered a creative adjustment in a difficult situation, the best way in which the organism has been able to tackle a particularly complex situation starting with the possibilities of self and hetero-support of which he/she can avail him/herself (Perls *et al.*, 1951/1994; Perls, 1992; Wollants, 2012). The symptom is viewed from a standpoint of (relational) contact, not an individual one, and is herein analysed from two perspectives.

Diachronic perspective: This comprises the history of the symptom and the suffering, paying close attention to the organism/environment relationship in the structuring of the symptom and in the evolution of the attempts to resolve it, as well as attention to the correlation between self-support and environmental support (see Thomae, 1968).

Synchronic perspective: Its aim is to analyse "how" the patient contacts the therapist in the telling of their symptom/suffering. It essentially consists of describing how the self unfolds in the here-and-now when the story of suffering is recounted to the therapist.

2. Figure/Ground Formation

The contact process in Gestalt psychotherapy is read as a progressive creation of emerging figures from an experiential ground (Wheeler, 1991).

> The self is in a continuous process in which creation and destructuration follow each other in the formation of figures and ground. . . . When we decide to make contact with the environment and then develop our self in the act of making contact and in the act of withdrawing from it, each moment of this process is a process of figure/ground that emerges from the contact.
>
> (Spagnuolo Lobb, 2015, pp. 33–34)

Ground:

> The ground experience . . . works as a support for the creation of perceptual figures, and is in its turn influenced by figure experiences. . . . I consider the ground as the acquired feeling of the body and of social roles; it is the given

situation in which the ego can deliberate on what to identify with and what to alienate from.

(Spagnuolo Lobb, 2016, p. 269)

What will be taken into consideration, in this section of the clinical data sheet, is the *id-functioning* – the ground experience from which the various possibilities emerge, the experience "beneath the skin", the place from where intentionalities of contact emerge – and the *personality-functioning* – the definition that the patient gives of themself starting with their own personal history (the "who I am"). We also consider the *polyphonic development of domains*. The different contact modalities, defined by Perls *et al.* (1951) as "losses of ego-functions" (introjection, projection, retroflection, confluence, egotism), acquired in previous contacts, can be seen in dimensional terms, along a continuum which goes from spontaneity to anxiety. In other words, one could have learned to introject (project, etc.) with greater or lesser anxiety. In this section of the clinical data sheet, the therapist will therefore observe how the patient actualises, during the therapeutic contact, habitual patterns of contact learned in his/her previous experiences throughout the entire evolutionary arc. It's like a relational "music" that the patient has learned to play in his/her previous contacts with the environment.

The concept of the polyphonic development of domains (Spagnuolo Lobb, 2012) is a way of looking, in the here-and-now of the session, at the client's development, in order to support the excitement for contact which has lost its spontaneity in development.

(Spagnuolo Lobb, 2016, p. 273)

Formation of the figure: From the ground of the patient's experiential possibilities, the current suffering and the intentionality of contact that the patient seeks to bring about (the now-for-soon to be) in therapy emerge in the figure. The therapist will observe whether the patient's resources "have kept their freshness or have become dormant" (Spagnuolo Lobb, 2016, p. 273). In this section of the clinical data sheet, the therapist will write about how the client is able to orient themself in the contact making with the therapist and spontaneously deliberate (ego-functioning).

The "dance steps" between therapist and patient: The interaction between therapist and patient can be described as a dance, considering the continuous adjustments happening between them, the desire and the pleasure of dancing together, what works, or in other words, the naturalness of their being-with. The focus of observation changes: from the patient to the phenomenological field in which they are inserted, to the reciprocal moving towards the other that characterises all of the interactions. The dance can be defined as the way they perceive each other, recognise each other, adapt to each other, take bold steps together, have fun with each other, connect with each other, and let themselves take care of each other (cf. Chapter 2).

3. Diagnosis

Descriptive diagnosis: The therapist formulates a diagnosis according to the criteria of a manual (for instance the DSM-5).

Gestalt diagnosis: He/she also formulates a Gestalt therapy diagnosis that does not just concern the single individual but also the relational phenomena co-created in the here-and-now of the therapeutic contact. In this section of the data sheet, the therapist will formulate a diagnosis in aesthetic, experiential, and field terms. The *aesthetic criteria* concern the quality of contact in the therapeutic field, for example the gracefulness (understood as *good form*), the rhythm (understood as *emotional regulation*), the fluidity (understood as *movement*). The first question that the therapist must answer on the clinical data sheet (external appearance of the person, immediate impression of the therapist, two/three adjectives) responds precisely to these aesthetic criteria and contributes to the formation of a diagnosis, which for us is a relational process. The experiential and field criteria concern the therapist's "vibration": in which movement of the patient does he/she feel a throbbing charge of energy that seeks to be recognised and accepted? These also include a description of the contact experience co-created by the patient and the therapist, for example a description of the "dance" on the part of both the therapist and the patient. The therapist's principal instrument in the formulation of this diagnosis will be their processes of resonance and attunement, that I have called *aesthetic relational knowing* (see Chapter 2). This aesthetic (sensory) and relational way of knowing is the instrument through which the therapist resonates with the client during the session, as well as the lens through which he/she looks at the client's vitality, the feeling the therapist experiences in the presence of the experiential field in which the client is immersed. This makes it possible for the therapist to understand in what situations of contact the patient manifests episodes of anxiety and the relative processes of de-sensitisation of the contact boundary.

Intentionality for contact to be supported in the therapy: In this part of the clinical data sheet, the therapist describes which contact intentionality is to be supported during the therapeutic process, and possible alternatives of therapeutic contact which could allow for the emergence of spontaneity and the re-sensitisation of the contact boundary.

4. Clinical Log

This last section of the data sheet allows the therapist to keep a clinical log of the sessions, report the evolution of the therapeutic process, and describe the prominent elements of each session.

5. A Clinical Example

We suggest that you consider the following clinical data sheet since it illustrates an example that has been filled out for the purpose of facilitating its comprehension and use.

===

Gestalt Therapy Clinical and Research Center of the Istituto di Gestalt HCC Italy

CLINICAL DATA SHEET[1]

- -

Date: . . . .
Patient: Paolo, 48 years, teacher.
Place and date of birth: . . . .
. . . .
Address: . . . .
. . . .
Telephone: . . . .
. . . .
Referred by: . . . .
. . . .

- -

Therapist's first impressions of the patient

- **Outer appearance**: description of what the therapist sees (2–3 immediate adjectives).

  Well-groomed, overweight, wary expression.

- **Relevant physiological aspects**: current diseases; breathing; posture and character armour (muscular stiffening due to retroflection); grounding, muscle tensions, direct or avoiding eye contact, facial expression; sleep/wake rhythm; eating habits; flexibility/adaptation abilities of bodily processes.

  Shallow breathing. A sufficiently fluid posture which however does not transmit a sense of bodily rootedness, the lower part of the body "slides" around the seat, he sits laterally, his gaze is rarely direct, he looks at me only fleetingly. Despite his excess weight, he seems to have little bodily consistency, little bodily ground in the lower part of his body. Sufficient flexibility of bodily processes.

  No current illness; regular sleep/wake rhythm; conflicted relationship with food: excessive and not very healthy consumption.

- **Medications**: Does the patient take medications? If so, what medication is he or she currently taking? Has he or she taken medications in the past?

  No medication being taken.

- **Other specialists?** Has the patient ever been in treatment with other specialists? If so, when?

  For two years the patient did psychotherapy with a therapist of psychodynamic orientation. The request for psychotherapy with me came after the termination of that process, which happened due to the relocation of said therapist, about three years ago.

6. Anamnesis

6.1. Family of Origin

- **Structure** (design the genogram of the family of origin)

  The patient is the eldest and first child, has a younger brother of 40, married with 3 children, another brother of 38, single, who has been living abroad for many years. Father, a retired corporate executive, comes from a very educated cultural environment. Mother has a degree in Literature. Both brothers are rather separated from the family of origin.

- **Atmosphere of the family** (description of the relationships inside the family): relaxed/tense; warm/cold; aggressive/avoiding conflict; accepting/dismissive.

  Tense climate, superficially warm but actually demeaning. Intense discord between the parents. Little expression of affection.

- **Relationship between siblings**

  Detached. Despite Paolo's requests to his brothers for a more regular relationship, his brothers show little willingness.

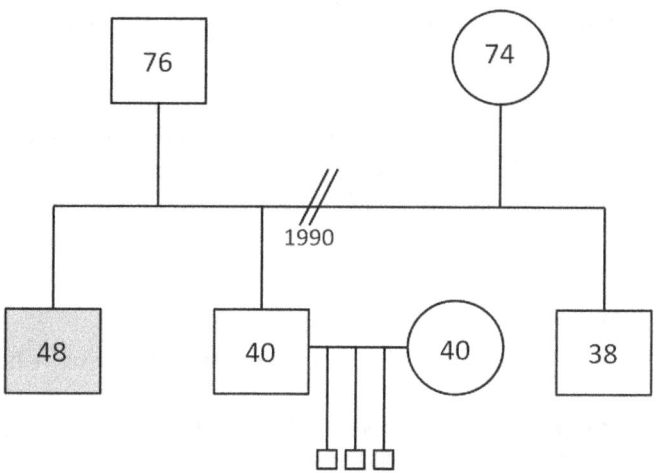

Figure 5.1 Genogram

- **Relationship between parents**: Avoiding conflicts? Aggressive and accusatory?

  *A very conflictual and completely accusatory relationship from the begin-
  ning. The parents separated when the patient was an adolescent. Afterwards both parents established other unstable affective relationships.*

- **Relationship between parent and children**: mention in particular: preferences/
  impartiality, respect of generational boundaries.

  *A very demanding and demeaning father with regard to Paolo and his sons
  in general, especially with respect to issues that concern social prestige.
  A very available and accessible mother but one who unloads all of her
  own anxieties, as well as a demand for exceptionality, onto the patient.*

- **Relevant events in the life-cycle of the family**: deaths, relocations, abortions and miscarriages, accidents, hospitalisations, separations, traumas of
  various types, etc.

  Separation of the parents, happened when the patient was 18 years old.

- **Myths, secrets, taboos of the family of origin**.

  Myth: socio-cultural prestige relative to the family history.

6.2. Current Experience

- **Current family**: if existing, describe its structure, atmosphere and relevant events.

  *He is single. He has had two important relationships, the last one ended
  slightly before the start of therapy. At present he begins relationships
  with women in a desensitised and compulsive way. Joins chat rooms and
  has very superficial relationships.*

- **Social adaptation**: describe life style, daily organisation, relationships, work,
  or study.

  *Poor network of friendships, he feels alone. Very much desires a relationship
  with others and at the same time is very centred on himself and on his
  need to be admired by others.*
  *The day-to-day routine essentially revolves around work where he has expe-
  rienced conflicts with colleagues.*

6.3. Symptom

What kind of suffering does the patient bring and what kind of narrative do they offer?

- **Diachronic perspective**: history of the symptom (or suffering): when did
  it begin, what was going on in the patient's life? How did he or she or they

attempt to cope with it? Have they had the feeling of being able to cope or one of failure? How have they experienced the organism/environment relationship in these attempts to address their suffering? In what critical moment of the personal and transgenerational life-cycle did the breakdown take place? What kind of environmental and personal support was lacking? It is important to highlight the close correlation between environmental support and personal support.

The patient remembers a pervasive and great sense of suffering since he was a child, with an intense sense of loneliness and lack of support on the part of his parents. He learned to react by withdrawing from contact with others as well as from his own body, and trying to achieve brilliant results in all fields. All of this was experienced in considerable solitude. He has never felt seen or supported on an environmental level. Since he was a boy, he has developed a great propensity towards obsessive thought and fantasies of an imagined future for himself, filled with grandiose and satisfying situations which, precisely for this reason, frighten him by feeding his sense of inadequacy. He is aware of having created little in his life on the affective level and of being very alone.

- **Synchronic perspective**: description of current symptom (or suffering). How does the patient speak about it? Describe the id-functioning and the personality-functioning with respect to the description of the symptom: the "here-and-now of the narrative", the way the self is constituted here-and-now in the words that the patient chooses.

Paolo comes with a great ability to analyse and a great awareness of his situation; he is very intelligent but unable to connect with his emotions. Initially, in telling me about his suffering (inadequacy and loneliness alternating with a sense of self as being a slightly special person, obsessive traits) he doesn't seem to perceive me at the contact boundary, telling stories rich in particulars and details, and interesting as well, but in a monologue completely disconnected from my presence. He lacks breath support and there is no full bodily ground (bodily desensitisation) because of which, in the story of his symptoms, he seems to shrink and become more "plaintive", with little embodied presence. He attempts some spurts of energy by appealing to his personality-function (he knows he is a good teacher, a very intelligent person, capable of awareness of what is happening, he knows he can be witty and can joke in an ironic and refined way); his voice is then raised, and he becomes apparently more energetic in providing preconceived solutions, in saying what he might need, or how he should act, or in carrying out extensive self-criticism.

7. Figure/Ground Formation

7.1. Ground

Description of what we grasp of the ground of the patient, of how he or she fits into their world.

- **Id-Functioning**: describe how the patient makes contact by means of his or her body, how he or she moves in their environment, how he or she breathes, the ground.

  The ground is charged with fear: the creative adaptations attempted up until now are no longer effective in curtailing his fear of failure, and the fear of not being able to cope. Not being able to count on the ground of the id-functioning to carry out his excitement for contact (shallow breathing, little embodied presence), when an emotion arises during therapeutic contact, it becomes desensitised, veering towards intellectualisation or complaining. His body stays quite static in the lower part, like a useless "encumbrance", his feet never stick to the ground, while the upper half is very mobile and participatory.

- **Personality-Functioning**: verbal copy of the self, how does the patient describe him or herself.

  He defines himself as a complex person with antithetical features. He knows he is a man with good assets, intelligent, sensitive, curious, and a lover of new things, but also a man who feels lost, alienated, disoriented, and discouraged, with a huge sense of failure. His biggest fears relate to the fact that others may not see his value and to his loneliness.

- **Polyphonic development of domains**: in the here-and-now of the session, look at the development of the patient. When do we feel him or her to be fluid, spontaneous, and present at the senses, or when do we sense him or her to be not fully present and we feel the boundary is desensitised? How does the patient integrate introjecting, projecting, retroflecting, and confluence in the contact with the therapist? Describe what the patient has learned in his or her life in terms of domains; his or her "habitual" ways of fitting into the world; what "protective resistances" has he or she learned over time. For example, how has he or she learned to introject in the past?

  The suffering, as a result of childhood experiences, of not feeling sufficiently seen in terms of his needs or recognised in his intentionality to connect with his parents, and trying to be like they wished him to be, has left a ground of loneliness and the fear of not having any worth. The domains that have been mostly acquired with anxiety seem to be projection (the impetus and the courage to connect with another have been replaced by control, by over thinking, by avoidance, by procrastination) and retroflection (the ability to stay with his own energy and his own reflections has grown into a sense of being special, and caused a certain grandiosity which has not facilitated the search for reciprocity).

What especially stands out in the first period of therapy: long meticulous stories, rich in detail, in which the patient is often consumed by excessive doubt, hoping that I may understand all of his good reasoning (his sense of worth) without ever fully seeing me (doing things by himself). At present he has made progress in staying in contact with me but, if a situation of greater closeness is created, he will easily retroflect, going back to doing everything by himself and excluding the other.

He retains a certain freshness in knowing how to show his attractiveness (healthy charm) in the narration of some events (trips, work episodes) (domain of retroflection), just as he still has the curiosity to learn and understand (domain of introjection) when he allows himself to learn, in therapy, something on the relational level that he feels touches him, and, in such a case, the excitement of learning is maintained and he can truly assimilate the novelty. Despite many negative paternal introjections, he is beginning to be able to introject good things from therapy.

7.2. Formation of the Figure

- **Ego-functioning**: the patient's capacity to orient him- or herself in the contact and to make choices. Describe of the patient's modality of contact with the therapist.

  Presently Paolo is realising that he is better able to perceive his needs. In therapy, he can break some old rigid pattern without fear, such as looking me intensely in the eye for a few seconds, or saying to me that I mean a lot to him, or becoming critical (but in a healthy way, not whining) of me, thus exercising in a fuller way his ego-functioning. The rigidity of the figure (the fixed figure of the obsessive) still often prevents his choices from being spontaneous and fully experienced. He is very focussed on himself and the goals that he thinks he must fulfill (self-consciousness) but at the same time he realises that the work on the therapeutic relationship is indispensable for him.

- **"Dance steps" between therapist and patient**: they express the unique reciprocity between psychotherapist and patient.

  After a year of therapy, Paolo and I have achieved a comfortable connection at the beginning of a session; we can count on a shared language, on having a certain reciprocal familiarity with respect to our way of encountering each other (the ground building). Getting started with our senses requires work and concentration on our part (the perception of each other), and even if he knows how to recognise my moving towards him (recognition of contact intentionality) he cannot yet fully welcome it inside himself. I feel interested in him and I am trying to recognise and sustain our contact intentionality, reminding him of some moments of our past therapeutic history (the ground building). Thanks to this, Paolo is able to take a bold step together with me, telling me that in that moment he is trying to bring me with him by not avoiding my gaze, and sitting for a moment in silence (taking bold steps together). In that moment, I have the sensation that we are connecting, although I am aware that instant will dissipate quickly. I point this moment out to him, a moment in which we have "touched" each other so that it might reinforce our relational ground (ground building – connecting with each other). In that moment, I see from the softening in his eyes, which immediately avoid mine, that he has grasped our closeness (giving himself up to a small moment of intimacy). It is all he is able to do towards entrusting himself to me, and already he is slipping away and, perhaps, one day we will be able to smile about this together (having fun). I say good-bye with the faith that this small thread that has united us may feed the hope for the possibility of a stronger future connection, even if we are both aware that it will take a lot longer to build it.

8. Diagnosis

8.1. Descriptive Diagnosis

- **DSM-5 criteria**.

    Narcissistic disorder with obsessive-compulsive traits.

8.2. Gestalt Therapy Diagnosis: Implemented by Means of the Aesthetic Relational Knowing of the Therapist (Attunement and Resonance)

- **Aesthetic Criterion**: grace (*good form*), rhythm (*emotional regulation*), fluidity (*movement*) + vibration of the therapist (in which of the patient's expressions does the therapist feel the vibrant drama?).

    I feel the patient's experience as dramatic in the session any time that the awareness of his desperate need for the presence of the other (of the therapist) beside him to calm his fears intertwines with his actual retreat from the other (from the therapist). The other's presence is only contemplated on a level of desire but never embodied, never reached through a feeling that is also emotional/corporeal. Since the other was never there when he needed it, and not having been able to experience such closeness, he continues to act as if the other is not there. Contact intentionality is always in the search for the other but can never spontaneously evolve.

- **Phenomenological and field criterion**: description of the experience of the field and of movements. How does the therapist describe his/her own experience of making contact with the patient? How does the patient describe his/her own experience of making contact with the therapist? What feeling does the therapist get from the field that is created during the session?

  Sometimes a deep sense of solitude circulates between us, and I also feel it inside me, even if we are with each other and the other person is dear to us. Thus, it is easy to get lost and look for security in analysing and explaining things (Paolo explicitly requests this from me) and in making connections with his childhood experiences, but in the end no explanation can bring that rootedness, which can act as a dam against fears, and the sense of having done little for him persists inside me. And so I have to breathe and feel my weight and my feet that touch the earth, remind myself that Paolo and I have a work history together that has lasted for more than three years and a bond, which, because it is so delicate, is precious and important for me (and also for him? How frightening it is sometimes not to be sure of this!) and I can be with Paolo and feel strong in this sensation. In this way, I can make contact again with my body, my interest in us, and the sense of tenderness I feel for Paolo, for this struggling between anxieties and fears, understanding everything but not being able to find a way to quieten him down in anything. I renew contact with my desire to be able to help him and to feel that we can connect with each other, and that he can "carry me deep within himself" (finally feelings, bodies, and not only words!), to savour a real closeness by taking my affection without me asking anything in return. This inner listening reactivates my presence on the contact boundary, in our therapeutic encounter, and allows me to formulate welcoming but firm interventions, sometimes ones that are also guiding, in order to provide containment to his ruminating without losing the sense of my availability and his being dear to me.

- **The anxiety comes mainly from . . .** (What situation triggers the anxiety)?

  The thinking that he has lost so many possibilities in the past by pursuing patterns of avoidance, and at the same time, being afraid to give up these patterns. Never finding relational rootedness that could help him face up to his fear. The fear of being poorly judged and the shame.

8.3. Intentionality of Contact to Be Supported in the Therapy (Therapeutic Now-for-Next)

- **In order to calm the anxiety** and allow the spontaneity of the psychophysical and relational processes to emergence, it is advisable to . . .

  To help him to experience that being with the other gives him support against loneliness.

To help him develop body awareness.
To support the passage from self-consciousness to awareness.

• **On the individual level**: messages that should be encouraged or avoided

Use messages that:
  • *give value to the perception of his own emotions;*
  • *support experiences in which the patient perceives his own value with-*
    out needing to be perfect or impressive and in which he demonstrates
    authentic interest in the other, without manipulations;
  • *help the patient to grasp the nuances of his own feelings.*

• **On the group level**: encourage activities . . . and avoid . . . (social life and/or group therapy)

To learn to show his need and desire of the other without any superfluous ele-
    ments, to make the first step towards the other.
To avoid confrontational attitudes.
To give greater value to the affective acknowledgements of others for him.

===

9. Clinical Diary[2]

Describe the relevant features of each session.

_ _

10. Conclusions

We hope that readers may find this clinical data sheet to be a tool that helps them adequately set down their therapeutic observations of their patients, that clinical trainers may find it to be a useful teaching and supervising support for their students and that researchers may be able to use it for the clinical dimensions upon which they do their research.

Ultimately, we like to think that in using this implement, psychotherapists may not see this technique as an end in itself but as a way in which they "implement themselves" in a clinical situation, with all of their professional abilities and life experiences that they have accumulated and integrated.

The chapters that follow will always contain one or more clinical cases, described by means of this data sheet (sometimes explicitly shown, and other times left implicit).

Notes

1 Elisabetta Conte is the therapist of this patient, whose personal data have been changed for privacy purposes.
2 A blank clinical data sheet is published as an appendix in this book.

References

De Rivera, J. (1976). *Field theory as human-science: Contributions of Lewin's Berlin Group*. New York: Halsted Press.

Jolly, W., Froom, J., & Rosen, M. G. (1980). The genogram. *The Journal of Family Practice, 10*(2), 251–255.

Lewin, K. (1943). Defining the "Field at a Given Time". *Psychological Review, 50*, 292–310.

Minuchin, S. (1974). *Families and family therapy*. Cambridge, MA: Harvard University Press.

Perls, F., Hefferline, R. F., & Goodman, P. (1994). *Gestalt therapy: Excitement and growth in the human personality*. New York, NY: The Gestalt Journal Press, or.ed., 1951.

Perls, L. (1992). *Living at the boundary*. New York: Gestalt Therapy Press.

Satir, V. (1983). *Conjoint family therapy*. Palo Alto, CA: Science and Behavior Books.

Spagnuolo Lobb, M. (1997). Linee programmatiche di un modello gestaltico nelle comunità terapeutiche [Programmatic lines of a Gestalt therapy model in therapeutic communities]. *Quaderni di Gestalt, 24/25*, 19–38.

Spagnuolo Lobb, M. (2012). Toward a developmental perspective in Gestalt therapy, theory and practice: The polyphonic development of domains. *Gestalt Review, 16*(3), 222–244.

Spagnuolo Lobb, M. (2013). Developmental perspective in Gestalt therapy. The poliphonic development of domains. In G. Francesetti, M. Gecele, & J. Roubal (Eds.). *Gestalt therapy in clinical practice. From psychopathology to the aesthetics of contact* (pp. 109–130). Siracusa, Italy: Istituto di Gestalt HCC Italy Publ. Co., www.gestaltitaly.com.

Spagnuolo Lobb, M. (2015). The body as a "vehicle" of our being in the world. Somatic experience in Gestalt therapy. *British Gestalt Journal, 24*(2), 21–31.

Spagnuolo Lobb, M. (2016). Self as contact, contact as self. A contribution to ground experience in Gestalt Therapy theory of self. In J.-M. Robine (Ed.). *Self. A poliphony of contemporary Gestalt therapists* (pp. 261–289). St. Romain la Virvée, France: L'Exprimerie.

Spagnuolo Lobb, M. (2017a). From losses of ego functions to the dance steps between psychotherapist and client. Phenomenology and aesthetics of contact in the psychotherapeutic field. *British Gestalt Journal, 26*(1), 28–37.

Spagnuolo Lobb, M. (2017b). Phenomenology and aesthetic recognition of the dance between psychotherapist and client: A clinical example. *British Gestalt Journal, 26*(2), 50–56.

Spagnuolo Lobb, M. (2018). Aesthetic relational knowledge of the field: A revised concept of awareness in Gestalt therapy and contemporary psychiatry. *Gestalt Review, 22*(1), 50–68. DOI: 10.5325/gestalt review.22.1.0050.

Spagnuolo Lobb, M., Conte, E., & Mione, M. (2017). La scheda clinica gestaltica: presentazione di uno strumento di lavoro [The Gestalt clinical data sheet: Presentation of a working tool]. *Quaderni di Gestalt, XXX*(2): 67–82. DOI: 10.3280/GEST2017–002005.

Thomae, H. (1968). *Das individuum und seine welt* [The individual and his world]. Göttingen: Hogrefe.

Wheeler, G. (1991). *Gestalt reconsidered. A new approach to contact and resistance*. New York: Gardner Press Inc.

Wollants, G. (2012). *Gestalt therapy. Therapy of the situation*. London: Sage.

Zuk, G. H., & Boszormenyi-Nagy, I. K. (1971). *Family therapy and disturbed families*. Palo Alto, CA: Science and Behavior Books.

Psychopathological Situations in the Clinical Fields of Human Relations

Chapter 6

Ring-a-Ring O' Roses, a Pocket Full of Posies[1]

Gestalt Psychotherapy and Childhood Suffering

Silvia Tosi and Elisabetta Conte

1. The Condition of Children in Today's World

Children born today in the western world live in conditions of greater well-being with respect to their peers a few decades ago. The infant mortality rate has considerably decreased; there is excellent healthcare and better nutrition; the educational cycle is guaranteed from early childhood. Despite these very positive conditions, those who work with children and their families are witnessing an increase in distress: many parents are experiencing difficulties in their relationship with their youngsters, and many children are expressing aggressiveness and hyperactivity. Their outbursts are becoming harder and harder to contain, or they are manifesting problems on the physiological level (sleep, nutrition, somatisation). The job of parenting is a very difficult one today: due to lack of time, heavy work schedules, personal problems, and the fast pace of our lives, parents are often unable to spend time with their children and so delegate care to the school, babysitters, grandparents, and tablets. The act of caring for and protecting does not always coincide with being together, with supporting with one's presence, with one's body, with one's time. The child needs to be able to share his/her feelings, not only the positive ones, and to feel that his/her parents can handle them. The possibility of being recognised even through fatigue, through sadness, and pain allows children to express themselves, live through, and overcome even difficult emotions. The health emergency caused by Covid-19 has forced parents into sharing time/space with their children in an entirely new way, one which requires a considerable creative adjustment. It consists of co-constructing together that presence, that being-there in which new possibilities are created. The complexity of current society (globalisation, migratory movements, work insecurity, climate change, terrorism, environmental disasters, pandemics) has certainly created a ground characterised by insecurity, anxiety, destabilisation, danger, and loss that cannot *not* have an impact on individuals and families.

The process of perceptive and emotional desensitisation[2] that is so widespread today is an attempt to feel less, to anaesthetise all these lived experiences. As Gestalt therapists, we are interested in the organism's relationship with the environment and in the way in which the organism and the environment co-create

DOI: 10.4324/9781003313335-9

their contact (Perls *et al.*, 1994; Robine, 2006; Cavaleri, 2003; Macaluso, 2015; Spagnuolo Lobb, 2013a, 2016a).

In the face of the complexity of our present world and its stresses, some relational disorders of children seem to be increasing: a sensory apathy, which generates desensitisation and indifference, as well as the phenomenon of dissociation (Conte and Tosi, 2016; Spagnuolo Lobb, 2016b). We do not yet know to what extent the current pandemic will aggravate (or not aggravate) these processes. Many children seem to have developed greater anxiety over these months of the pandemic (Andolfi, 2021; Dalla Ragione *et al.*, 2021); many of them express fears and angst over death. We can define desensitisation as the impossibility of feeling completely, through one's senses, the contact boundary with the other (Spagnuolo Lobb, 2013a; Spagnuolo Lobb and Rubino, 2015). An aesthesia,[3] the not-feeling, reduces the possibility of defining oneself through the process of co-creation and of being able to grasp all of the possibilities of the field (Francesetti, 2015; Sampognaro, 2016; Spagnuolo Lobb, 2016b).

The Gestalt approach to children is a phenomenological, field, and an aesthetic one (Arfelli Galli, 2013; Spagnuolo Lobb, 2016b). Aesthetic knowing, "sensitive knowledge", brings us back to our condition of embodied beings since it is a corporeal knowing, embodied in the senses, and in the resonating of the body. One of the main risk factors in childhood development comes directly from bodily desensitisation (Spagnuolo Lobb *et al.*, 2016). The key role of the bodily exchange between child and caregiver has been confirmed by the neurosciences[4]; in addition to many experts of the world of childhood, we herein cite Stern (1985, 2010), Ammaniti and Gallese (2014), Frank (2001, 2016a, 2016b), Frank and La Barre (2011), and Maggio and Tosi (2020). This embodied suffering, present at the contact boundary, can assume many forms and many levels of severity along the spontaneity/desensitisation continuum depending on its scope and on how early was the onset (Conte and Tosi, 2016).

In order to combat the afflictions of today's world, ones which we encounter in our clinical work as well as in our social life, as Gestalt therapists we are interested in recovering the ability to co-create the experience of the encounter with the other in a creative and spontaneous way. Spontaneity is a quality of the contact process that is characterised by being fully and consciously at the contact boundary. This enables a re-sensitisation of the boundary itself. In the work with children and their families, it is very important to be present with one's senses open, to be sensitive enough to grasp the harmony and vitality present in their being in contact, otherwise we can have desensitisation, loss of spontaneity, and blocking of the intentionality for contacting (Tosi, 2016; Conte and Tosi, 2016). "A primary task of psychotherapy with children is to foster the processes of secure attachment which, in our language, translates as supporting the self-regulation between caregivers and child, that is the spontaneity of creative adaptation, in full awareness" (the fullness of the oneself-with-the other sensation, as opposed to emotional and bodily desensitisation) "and with the parents' spontaneous acceptance of a healing role" (Spagnuolo Lobb, 2016b, p. 30).

We will present hereafter some theoretical concepts that have guided our reading of childhood pathology in a phenomenological and field view, first considering the suffering of the child as a being-with type of suffering. We will then describe the case of a young patient by means of a Gestalt clinical data sheet in which the child's malaise as well as the therapeutic relationship will be analysed, following some phenomenological, aesthetic, and field coordinates.

2. Psychopathology

2.1 The Suffering of Being-With

Paolo, 6 years-old, in the first grade, passes his time in class making baby noises; Marco, 8 years-old, almost every night hits his head repeatedly against the wall of his bedroom; Nadine, 11 years-old, doesn't talk, almost as if she were mute, she cries and has a hard time going to school. What is happening to these children? What is depriving them of their serenity, of their spontaneity, of their "earnestness" (Perls *et al.*, 1994, p. 80)? The symptoms displayed by a child represent a creative adaptation, a vital act that signals the presence of a difficult relational field. The suffering expressed by a child, in Gestalt psychotherapy, is not read as an individual malaise but is viewed from a relational perspective: a suffering of the "between", which is born at the contact boundary with the environment that is significant for him,[5] and which limits the possibilities for the growth of the child, a highly sensitive receptor. The child, a messenger of suffering (Levi, 2016), expresses malaise in the first person, but the central hub is the phenomenological field into which he is placed and the reciprocal moving towards each other of the child and the caregivers. The place where this process occurs is the contact boundary. The way in which the child and the caregiver co-create the contact boundary gives rise to a greater or lesser rich experience, depending on whether there is the presence of harmony and vitality or desensitisation.

2.2. The Loss of the Ground

The suffering of being-with undermines the formation of that ground of basic relational experiences upon which the child can develop the ability to advance his/her own intentionalities for contacting, his/her own sense of self, and the ability to differentiate him/herself: it "is the flow of the dance with the caregivers, with the significant adults; the child learns, knows him/herself and grows at the contact boundary with the other, experiencing the mutual attunement and resonance between him/herself and the adult" (Spagnuolo Lobb, 2016b, p. 31). Neuroscience confirms this thesis. Porges (2017) points out how, from a polyvagal perspective, deficits in the feeling of safety are closely related to the onset of physical and mental illness and how relational grounding is of fundamental importance. A sense of security is founded on the basic support that the caregiver is able to give to the child by making him perceive love, recognition, the receiving of adequate care, the attention to his needs, and respect for roles as taken for granted (Spagnuolo Lobb, 2016b). When the child cannot draw on these presumed securities, the excitement for novelty has no support and is felt not as a possibility for growth but as a loss of ground, an ' "indescribable' (Spagnuolo Lobb, 2003) experience of existential vulnerability, coupled with unbearable pain" (Levi, 2013, p. 278).

Every symptom of a child is therefore a suffering to do with contact, a "mortification of the tension towards contact" (Spagnuolo Lobb, 2016a, p. 29), an unrecognised, or interrupted, or incomplete intentionality to connect with the caregivers. The bond of recognition is an "essential social act" (Robine, 2015; Molinari and Cavaleri, 2015; Honneth, 1992) which, on the one hand, determines the structuring of subjectivity, and on the other, the building of a social network. Those intentionalities that are recognised and supported can develop into clear experiences, rich in vitality; those that are ignored become blocked and their development can produce confusion and pain (Conte and Tosi, 2016; Kedrova, 2016; Spagnuolo Lobb, 2016b).

2.3 The Importance of the Ground: Diagnostic Overview

The ability to fully be at the contact boundary (achieving the integrity of the experience) and the ability to assimilate new contacts, together with the results of previous growth, allows one to maintain and update one's own emplacement in the face of continuous changes (perceiving the continuity of experience) (Conte and Mione, 2008), so that what is co-created at the contact boundary is integrated within the child with the previous acquisitions and with the intentional impetus to connect with the caregivers. Reading this process according to the theory of the self (Perls *et al.*, 1994; Spagnuolo Lobb, 2001, 2016b; Robine, 2015), the here-and-now experienced by the child is a creative *Gestalt* that summarises in a diachronic sense the contacts which gradually become acquired over the course of his/her development and which will constitute the experiential ground of the self from the being-with through the body (the id-function) and through the social definition of the self (personality function). In a synchronic sense, such a *Gestalt* summarises the present intentionalities which support the on-going contact between the self and the caregivers (ego function). Spagnuolo Lobb suggests the concept of "the polyphonic development of domains"[6] to denote the co-created ground experience, which comprises the contacts and the acquired contact modalities, and the concept of the "dance steps"[7] to indicate the figure provided by the current process of the co-creation of the contact experience between child and caregiver, but also between child and therapist. In this figure/ground relationship, so that the figure may emerge with clarity and light, the ground of the domains provided by the experience of the relationships with the caregivers must be relaxed, rich with inferred securities and full of closed *gestalten*, so that it can support the emerging of excitement at the contact boundary. When the ground is characterised by anxious experiences, the ego function cannot be easily determined.

3. The Gestalt Clinical Data Sheet

The Gestalt clinical data sheet (Spagnuolo Lobb *et al.*, 2017; see also Chapter 5) is a work tool developed by the Istituto di Gestalt HCC Italy, displayed in this chapter. We use it here to present a case of childhood malaise. The data sheet allows one to describe the therapeutic relationship and the child's suffering from a Gestalt viewpoint, directing the use of anamnestic data and clinical thought towards phenomenological, aesthetic, and field coordinates.

Istituto di Gestalt HCC Italy – Centro Clinico e di Ricerca HCC Italy
CLINICAL DATA SHEET

Date . . . .

Patient: Nino, 8 years old
Place of birth:
Date of birth:
Referral: colleague
Reason for referral: aggressive and oppositional behaviour

First impressions of the therapist

- **External features of the child:**

  Smiling, red hair, blue eyes.

- **Relevant physiological features:**

  No on-going illnesses; regular sleep/wake rhythm; reasonable relationship with food; direct gaze, expressive facial countenance, moves in a pronounced way; bodily processes: straight posture, accentuated stiffness, movement is not fluid, high muscle tone, and mostly tense, difficulty approaching, little flexibility and capacity to adapt.

- **Daily life:**

  Regularly goes to school, plays sports and engages in extracurricular activities: talks with pleasure about his extracurricular and sports activities while he tends not to talk about school, which he seems to attend with difficulty.

- **Pharmacotherapy:** *No intake of pharmaceuticals*
- **Other specialists:** *A year ago, Nino was taken by his doctor father to a psychologist who works in his hospital. The father discontinued the process not having had the answers he was looking for. He was not available to provide the name of the colleague for possible contact.*

4. Anamnesis

4.1 Family of Origin (Figure 6.1)

- **Structure**

    The eldest. He has a seven-year-old sister, very introverted, who, as a baby, was diagnosed with autistic spectrum syndrome, afterwards revealed to be incorrect. The girl exhibits relational problems with friends and her brother. She speaks little, and uses physical means to a great extent to express herself. Since January she is in therapy with a colleague with whom we are collaborating.

    Mother: 44 years of age, only child. She works for a large company in the fashion industry.

    Maternal grandparents: both 68 years of age, retired, living outside Milan.

    Father: 50 years of age, second child, has an older sister. Pulmonologist in an important public hospital in Milan.

    Paternal grandparents: Grandfather, 80, suffers from senile dementia. Grandmother, 75, ex-teacher, lives in her house in Milan and takes care of her grandchildren a few afternoons a week.

- **Family atmosphere**

    The relationships within the family are very tense and disparaging. Considerable verbal aggressiveness is noticeable between all the members of the family ("everyone against everyone")

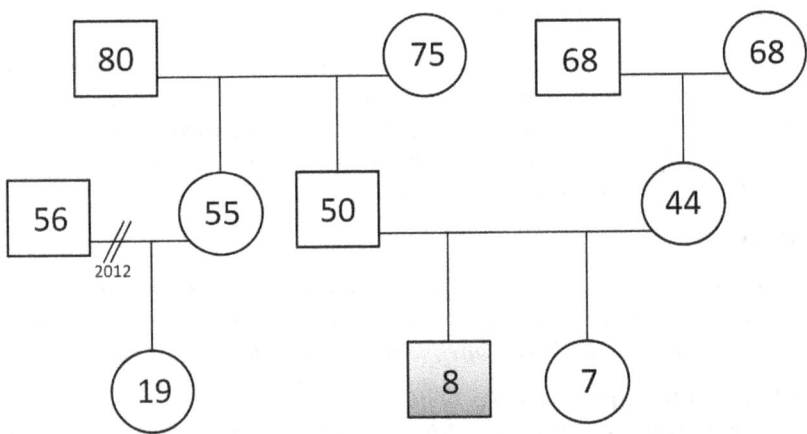

Figure 6.1 Genogram

- **Relationships between siblings**

  There are relationship problems between the two siblings, who often fight in a violent manner both verbally and physically. In talking about it, the parents seem to be overwhelmed by their children's aggressiveness.

- **Relationship between parents**

  The two parents have relationship problems and conflicts, and exhibit aggressive and accusatory modalities.

- **Parent/children relationships:** *Mother/Nino relationship: very negative, aggressiveness and tension are present. The relationship between the mother and the sister seems less conflictual but equally non affective. The mother seems to be emotionally and physically distant from her children, not very present both qualitatively and quantitatively. Nino is very angry with her.*

  Father/Nino relationship: a good relationship, warm and affectionate, structured around play but there is role confusion. The relationship between the father and the sister is always based on play, but there is more distance. The father, more present, spends a lot of time with the children, especially with Nino, but he tends to put himself on the same level as them, not providing containment. Nino is very attached to his father.
  Both parents attest to having difficulty with their children, whom they define as unmanageable and who "always do whatever they want".

- **Relationships with the parents' family of origin**

  Problems emerge with both families of origin, in which the parents feel judged as inadequate. The maternal grandparents are considered by both parents to be closed off and anxious. The paternal grandparents are considered by the mother as "always over the top" and by both parents as clowns.

- **Relevant events in the family life cycle**

  In 2019, when the therapy started, many important events in Nino's life occurred: the parents decided to change Nino's school due to socialisation difficulties with classmates and in June the child began his therapy process; during the summer the mother was operated on her knee and for a few months was not very mobile; in September the mother changed work and that meant being closer to home and a greater presence in her children's lives; Nino began the school year in his new school; towards the end of the year the senile dementia of the paternal grandfather worsened until a definitive admission to an Assisted Living Residence (Residenza Sanitaria Assistenziale, RSA) was required.

- **Myths, secrets, taboos of the family of origin**

  No specific myths, secrets, or taboos revealed.

4.2 Present Experience

- **Social adaptation**

  Nino is not "well-adapted"; his behaviour is often strange and unsuitable in contexts such as school, family, peer groups. In school he has relationship difficulties and often manifests aggressive behaviours (especially verbal) with his classmates who tend to isolate him. He talks back to teachers who complain that they cannot contain him (with one teacher who makes him feel recognised and who, he, in turn, recognises, things go a bit better). Nino's aggressive reaction is closely tied to his not feeling seen or recognised. In the family, with his parents and sister, he is very aggressive, just as he is with his grandparents, who however contain him and do not let him overwhelm them. In the session he appears reasonable. He enters easily into a relationship, even though with initially provocative modalities, and he is capable of accepting limits.

4.3 Symptom

The child's suffering is expressed through great rage and aggressive behaviours both in relation to his friends and family members, while that of his parents is highlighted in their difficulty handling their children. The suffering at the contact boundary is manifested in the impossibility of the family members to give recognition to the intentionalities for contacting of the various members. The parents seem particularly immersed in a sort of "desensitisation" which prevents them from seeing their children's attempts at reaching out to them.

- **Diachronic perspective**

  The parents recall that Nino's temperament has always had these characteristics; they describe him as a child who has always engaged them a great deal. Nino has "hated" his little sister from the beginning. Starting elementary school has increased his relational difficulties.

- **Synchronic perspective**

  Nino is a very sensitive and intelligent boy and appears to be aware of his suffering. At the beginning of our meeting, as he does with everyone, he tries to test me in order to understand if I see him, if I am there for him, revealing, with his modalities of being in a relationship, his need to be seen and reached out to. He lacks breath support and there is no full bodily ground: he moves quickly and in an agitated way as if there is no possibility of finding a rhythm with which he can rely on someone, relax, and rest. When he speaks about music, movies, computer games, what emerges is great competence and capacity to stop and devote his attention to these things. In these moments I feel that he has connected with me.

5. Figure/Ground Formation

5.1 Ground

- **The ground experience in neurotic, psychotic, borderline, post traumatic (due to abuse or sudden loss) perception[8]:**

    The ground is filled with anxiety. There are few securities taken for granted, so that the basic ground is not secure on either the bodily or the relational level. Nino's entire self is in danger. It is not possible for him to feel his own body and find a definition of self since there is little differentiation between the organism and the environment, and therefore there is no experience of feeling a self in contact. The figures that emerge are linked to the anxiety of the ground rather than co-created at the contact boundary (psychotic perception).

- **Id function:**

    The ground lacks rootedness: Nino constantly moves around a great deal. He does not remain seated. His eyes are wide open. He goes from activity to activity very quickly. Not being able to count on the ground provided by the id function to direct his excitement, and to contain it in such a way as to be able to perceive his own solidity, the excitement becomes "liquid", giving the image of a spinning top that cannot stop.

- **Personality function:**

    Nino defines himself as an aggressive naughty child, who wants to hit others.

- **Polyphonic development of domains:**

    Nino does not seem to have ever been heard, seen, and contained by his parents, especially the mother. This leaves him feeling a constant need to get the other's attention at all costs. Some of the domains seem to have been acquired, up to this point, with anxiety:

- *Confluence: Nino's body is always very tense, eyes wide open, limbs rigid, as if it has never been possible to "lose himself in an embrace"*
- *Projection: the energy to reach out to the other is explosive and overblown, so much so as to engulf the other without seeing him and feeling seen.*
- *Introjection: the stiff position of vigilance and defence seems to prevent him from receiving nurturing from the other and from the environment. Nino rejects school, his teachers, and his classmates.*

5.2 Figure Formation

• **Ego function**

> *He enters into contact with the therapist in a direct and disruptive way. He asks. He is well-disposed towards relating, accepts limits if they are clear and circumscribed. In the beginning he appeared tense and anxious. Now he laughs and easily lets himself go.*

Dance steps between therapist and patient: Experience of the Movements and Kinesthetic Resonance[9]

*At the start of the session, even after a month that we have been meeting, Nino enters the room with a lot of energy, quite stiff, and with high muscle tone. He moves within the surroundings without perceiving my presence. I sense his tense body. He moves jerkily and struggles to stay still and relax. My body, too, stiffens and tends to move around him. I have to raise my voice to be heard. We move around the room without a clear direction and without meeting one another. Only when I re-concentrate on my breathing, and on the placement of my feet on the floor and stop, can I relax and be with him. He always seems to be on the alert in the relationship. He looks at me wide-eyed. His posture is straight and stiff; the more I root myself to the ground, the more he begins to see me and move towards me. Sitting on the floor on the cushions or on the big balls allows us to relax, to lower our voices, to find our shared ground (**construction of the ground**), to be able to count on reciprocal modalities of encountering one another, familiar to us, as we begin to perceive each other with our senses open to our relationship (**perceiving each other**). After some questions about how his week went, starting with what emerges from our being at the contact boundary, we begin to play.*

*I see that he is alert to my presence. I am still. I feel solid with him. I feel that I am able to oppose and hold his driving force. Sensing that I am here for him allows us to connect. The body tone of each of us is lowered. Our gazes meet and our movement becomes more fluid. Our gestures are directed towards the other. We recognise each other in our contact intentionality. He squints his eyes, looks at me, and smiles. I feel my breathing becoming more regular and slower. My muscles relax. I feel that I can move closer and we can sit next to each other, play a game, and find a new equilibrium together. Nino knows and feels that I am there for him. He recognises me in my intentionality and I recognise him in his reaching out to me with all that energy, which I felt could overwhelm me on the first occasions, and which now instead I feel to be warm and full of resources (**recognising one another**). (Nino takes the sponge ball and throws it very forcefully against the wall from which it then bounces off and it is not possible to stop it. I look at him and the ball and I say to him that I like his energetic toss of the ball). During play, we adapt to each other gradually, receiving each other's movements and feelings, and transforming them in order to be able to find a good rhythm* between us *(adapting to each other)*. *(Nino's tosses of the ball become more and more focussed and the intensity more modulated in keeping with my tosses and vice versa). For Nino, reaching out and being reached, being able to "grab" onto the other is something difficult and new; he seems to enjoy it and vigorously request it: he suggests a game where we have to "take each other" with the ball. I perceive in my body that it relaxes and in my breathing that it becomes fluid, that when I am able to make him feel my presence he can feel that I am there, that I see him and contain him. We are ready to do something new together: we lower the intensity and the game with the ball becomes a way to be in contact, fluctuating with a gentle rhythm* **(taking bold steps together)**. *We have fun. It is a new way for us to be together, to nurture each other in a shared rhythm* **(having fun)**. *I feel that we have connected, we have let ourselves go. We have found our rhythm* **(connecting and letting oneself go towards the other)**. *For Nino, it is still difficult to be able to consolidate the me-with-you experience without anxiety, to be able to assimilate such an experience and make it his own in a subsequent exploration. Nino can only relax with the other for a short space of time: after a little while, during which we are interacting in a fluid way, something gets interrupted and I sense that my heart and my breathing are accelerating again. I lose my ground, while Nino leaves again with his stiff movement and without direction, with his breathing blocked in his upper body.*

6. Diagnosis

6.1 Descriptive Diagnosis

– **Criteria according to the DSM-5**

   Oppositional defiant disorder

6.2 Gestalt Diagnosis Made by Means of Aesthetic Relational Knowing (Attunement and Resonance)[10]

– **Aesthetic criterion:** *Through his agitation and inability to stay still, what is transmitted to me is his great need to be seen and acknowledged as a child who is still small, alone, and needy, just as is also transmitted his huge appeal to be stopped, contained, and embraced. I feel tenderness for all the energy that he will not give up in order to execute this intentionality of his.*

• **Phenomenological and field criterion:**

   Nino's agitation confuses me. I feel overwhelmed by his movement. I feel as if I am being carried along, and so I begin to move, to talk, to raise my voice in order to be heard. I feel as if I cannot lean on anything. I feel like a butterfly constantly crashing into the light. When I meet his gaze, he often appears frightened. Sensing this emotion of his makes me feel more in contact with him and it allows me to find a foothold from which to take off. We can stay in the fear, in the sadness, and in the anger. I can contain him.

Anxiety principally caused by . . . *Anxiety is manifested whenever Nino does not feel seen and recognised in his desire to connect with the other person who is important to him, or when he does not feel helped in his need to be contained and held.*

6.3 Intentionality for Contacting to Be Supported in Therapy (the Therapeutic Now-for-Next)

• **In order to calm the anxiety:**

One must help him to experience the feeling of being contained and held by the other so that this novelty once experimented with on the contact boundary can modify the old patterns of perception.

In the session: One must prioritise those games and messages that help him to feel seen and recognised, for example the game of charades. Games of attunement (dance, musical instruments). Shared drawing. Shared story-telling, for instance by using illustrated cards and "story cubes".[11]

In school: One must avoid ignoring him when he exhibits aggressive behaviour, and encourage a better attitude to listening.

In the family: one must be more fully with him, foster shared games recognising his abilities. One must seek dialogue that replaces continuous chastisement.

7. A Work Model With the Child, His Parents, and His Environment: The Setting and the Therapeutic Process

Our model (Conte and Tosi, 2016) of the developmental phase envisages work with the child and the environment. Psychotherapy with the child takes place only after a first phone contact with the person who formulated the request for help (activation of the co-created field), followed by at least one session with the parents (exploring the ground), a meeting with the entire family (intentionality for contacting during growth) and possibly a meeting with the teachers, and, lastly, individual psychotherapy with the child (recuperating the spontaneity).

We maintain that it is important to involve, through structured encounters (interviews, family sessions, meetings), the educational figures of reference (parents, teachers) in accordance with the role of each, since they constitute the ground that supports the therapist/child care relationship. During the entire duration of therapy, the parents are involved in the treatment process by means of monthly or bi-monthly meetings of feedback and engagement (every situation is difficult and therefore the best form of their involvement in the therapeutic process will be evaluated and agreed upon with the parents).

We will illustrate hereafter the individual work with the child[12] through the experience with Nino.

Nino's father phones me in June, 2019, after the end of school. Nino's parents are seeking help because they are worried about their son's aggressiveness, which they do not understand. Nino is always very angry, in school, with his classmates and the teachers, at home, with his sister and especially with his mother. The anger is manifested with physical and verbal violence. What emerges is an aggressive family field that is neither caring nor supportive.

8. The Individual Setting: Restoring Spontaneity

8.1. Consultation

Initially we suggest a consultation in order to understand together how to help the child and the parents to feel better. The consultation is already structured as a therapeutic intervention whose objective it is to help the parents better comprehend the child's difficulty, and to support and mobilise parental, family, and social resources. If the consultation process allows the child to be recognised in his intentionality for contacting and if there is no deep suffering in the field, the child can often overcome his distress and continue on his path to growth. If instead the consultation process reveals a deeper sense of suffering, depending on the need which arises, on the age of the child, on the needs of the family, we suggest individual or group psychotherapy for the child, family therapy, or a caregiver-child therapy, or parental support. The outcome of the consultation could also conclude with a referral to another service or professional (e.g. child neuropsychiatry).

The consultation involves: two meetings with the parents (an initial one and a final one of feedback), a family meeting, and 3-5 meetings with the child. During the meetings with the child, we suggest a path towards getting to know each other through drawing, storytelling, and play. Sometimes, if necessary or requested, we also administer assessment tests (e.g., the WISC-IV, *Wechler Intelligence Scale for Children-IV*) and/or projective tests (e.g., the Duess Fables, the *Children's Apperception Test*, etc.). Both during and after the completion of the drawings, we always ask the child to tell us what he/she is drawing and if he/she wishes, to tell a story starting from what is on the piece of paper. During these inquiries, the therapist is active and interacts based on the material co-created in the session.

From the Duess Fables (1940) Nino's experiences clearly emerge:

The bigger lamb attacks the smaller one in order to get all of the mother's milk because he doesn't like eating grass. The smaller lamb goes to the mother to complain. The mother yells at the bigger one, and so he gets angry and kills everyone and is left all alone.

The consultation process ends with giving feedback to the child and the parents of what has emerged from the meetings.

In the feedback meetings with Nino and his parents, I tell and show what has emerged from the sessions and I suggest psychotherapy for the child along with sessions of support and engagement with the parents.

8.2. Psychotherapy

Once the consultation phase is concluded, psychotherapy begins. Whatever the choice of setting, the parents are always part of the therapeutic process and will be helped to find keys to the reading and concrete tools to support their intentionality for contact with their children, and to give strength to the ground upon which the sense of family security rests (Tosi *et al.*, 2013).

Psychotherapy is the moment in which the child/therapist relationship and the co-construction of their encounter, as well as the therapist's ability to give support to the "between" become fundamental, thus facilitating within the child the possibility of experimenting with new creative adaptations.

In the individual sessions, the therapist works with the child by keeping in mind certain therapeutic questions: What is happening between us? What is emerging from our meeting one another? How does the pain emerge on our contact boundary? In what way can we build a good adult-child encounter? How do our bodies meet each other? What is the incomplete gesture of this child in his relationship with me? How can I be the calm and secure ground that supports the excitement for contact of this child in order to restore his spontaneity?

Example of a session (October 2019):

Nino comes into the room and begins to play by himself with the ball. He throws the ball forcefully and higher and higher. He doesn't look at me. I try to speak to him but he doesn't respond. I stand up and approach him but I can't become part of his game. I feel my body stiffen more and more and I realise that I have no desire to play ball. I sit down and look at him. My body relaxes. I sense that I want to stop him, stop his moving around without direction. I ask him how he is. He stops. With the ball still in his hands, he tells me that he is angry. At school his teacher yelled at him because he hit another boy. The more I ask him questions, the closer he comes towards me. He puts down the ball and sits beside me. He tells me that this boy was making fun of him for something and that his only friend in class also began to make fun of him, and then another boy joined them. He was about to cry, but then, instead of crying, he stopped being sad and hit the boy. He tells me through his tears that he was very happy to get angry. Instead of crying, he defended himself. My breathing is blocked and I feel sad. I ask him how it is now that he is crying with me. He says it's good because I don't tell him that he mustn't cry. At home, when he is about to cry, his father laughs and his mother, if she's there, tells him to stop. I start breathing normally again. We look at each other and we smile. Nino picks up the story cubes (a game he often uses), we throw them, and we invent a story based on the images, each of us recounting a small part – the story of the boy that seemed angry at everyone and instead was sad. He asks me to re-read to him the story and asks if he can take it home. He wants to read it to his mother and father.

At the end of the entire process, we suggest a feedback moment devoted to the child and one of his parents. We ultimately suggest a family session in order to discuss together all that has emerged from the work and as a way to end the intervention. Sometimes, as a conclusion to therapy, the therapist writes a story for the child (Finn, 2007) based on what happened during the sessions. We use this technique as a means to facilitate the assimilation of the therapeutic process and as a way to "savour" the importance of the experience of having built together a good relational ground.

8.3 Therapy with Nino During the Lockdown

When the first lockdown began, therapy with Nino was abruptly halted due to the restrictions.

During the health emergency period, the therapeutic question was: How do we keep the therapeutic process alive and give Nino an experience of continuity in such a complicated moment in time? We know that the relationship between the psychotherapist and the child during particularly stressful periods is of fundamental importance, the work of psychotherapy being an occasion to strengthen and expand a safe and secure base: therefore it was necessary to continue to communicate and be in contact, using all the available technology.

Initially, when we still thought that we would come out of the lockdown in a short space of time, I kept up contact with Nino and his parents through phone calls. The aim was not to do telephone therapy but to maintain connection and continuity. When Nino, during one of these calls, asks me when we would see each other again, and not being able to give him a face-to-face appointment, I suggest a video call. Nino and his parents accept the proposal with enthusiasm. From that moment on, Nino and I regularly meet on a video call once per week. Therapy is still ongoing and proceeds remotely according to this setting:

- *Same day and schedule as the face-to-face therapy*
- *Once a week*
- *5 minutes at the beginning and at the end together with the caregiver*
- *Space for himself (his bedroom).*

The particular nature of therapy with children is that it takes place through play, through the co-creating of stories, through bodies and being present. How is it possible to maintain these special elements through remote therapy? The aesthetic relational knowing (Spagnuolo Lobb, 2018) is the tool with which we resonate with our little patient during the meeting through the screen. By working on the contact boundary with our little patient, we see what emerges in the encounter, and we work on the "between". Children, unlike us, are "digital natives". Video calls can become relational and play material, just like the house, the objects, and possible pets.

We use Nino's space (his room and other corners of the house, his toys and puppets (stuffed animals), his dog) as resources; in addition, the video call and all the potential offered by technology become part of the therapeutic relationship (e.g. short videos, photos, emoticons, chats).

The parents then become more greatly involved. This is surely a new process that forces us to face limits and resources, which we can only approach with curiosity and humility.

9. Conclusion

We have wanted, in this chapter, to highlight some important aspects for dealing with childhood malaise (the pathology). We have considered the symptom as an expression of not an individual but as a relational suffering, one which brings to the surface the importance for the child of the recognition of his own intentionality to connect with his parents, the importance of a ground that allows a sufficient corporeal and relational rootedness, with a view to counteracting the processes of desensitisation. We have tried, by means of Nino's clinical case, to give body and voice to the theoretical concepts expressed here.

During the pandemic, in the frequent lockdown periods, children were forced to live 24 hours a day with their parents. On the one hand, especially for the youngest and in reasonably good families, this was reassuring and was able to facilitate the building of a solid ground provided by rootedness and a sense of belonging. On the other hand, the parents, like all of us, felt that they did not have any kind of certainty to give to their children. They felt fragile, fearful of the virus, of economic collapse, and the lack of nurturing social relationships. The risk was in teaching children the opposite of what one previously advocated: use the internet, watch videos, keep your distance from people we love, stay locked in the house.

As we set these conclusions down, we are still in the midst of the pandemic, children are taking their classes at home, and by now we know that they are, together with adolescents, one of the most penalised groups. The atmosphere of hope and change experienced in the first lockdown is no longer here, and the novelty of distance learning, at first welcomed enthusiastically, has given way to an alienating routine. We hope that the ideas presented in this chapter can spark discussions around thinking about how to help these youngsters, in post-pandemic times, to find once more new and exciting ways to make contact with the other, ways in which to integrate this pandemic experience, and to renew contact with their own bodies, enjoying again all the possibilities (affective, recreational, athletic) which they can provide.

Notes

1 These are the first words of a nursery rhyme known around the world. Children sing it while holding hands, and finally falling down laughing. The nursery rhyme, originally from England, and born, according to some, in order to exorcise the Great Plague of 1665, boasts a secular tradition: *Ring-a-ring o'roses, A pocket full of posies, A-tishoo! A-tishoo! We all fall down.*

2 We mean that process in which "when the environment is perceived as threatening or confusing, or the contact experience becomes painful and unsustainable, the contact occurs anyway, but loses the quality of awareness and spontaneity, the contact experience is characterised by anxiety. This implies desensitisation of the contact boundary: it is necessary to put part of the sensitivity to sleep in the here-and-now of the contact with the environment" (Spagnuolo Lobb and Rubino, 2015, p. 35).

3 From the Greek *anaisthēsía* "insensitivity", derived from *aisthēsis* "sensation", with the prefix *an*-privative.

4 For the concept of embodied empathy compare Gallese *et al.* (2006).

5 For the concept of psychopathology as the pathology of between-ness, of the interaction of the individual with the environment compare: Yontef (2001), Spagnuolo Lobb (2013a), Francesetti (2015), Francesetti *et al.* (2013), Salonia (2013), Sampognaro (2016).

6 For the concept of "polyphonic development of domains" cf. Spagnuolo Lobb (2012, 2013b, 2016a).

7 For the concept of "dance steps" cf. Spagnuolo Lobb (2016a)

8 We wish to reiterate that we are describing a ground experience and not making a diagnosis.

9 In the reading of the dance steps, the close correlation between environmental support and personal/body support is also highlighted here in the reading of the relational movements of Frank (2001, 2016a, 2016b), Frank and La Barre (2011).

10 For the concept of "aesthetic relational knowing" cf. Spagnuolo Lobb (2018).

11 We are referring to commonly used games that can be found on the market.

12 For a detailed illustration of the other phases compare Conte and Tosi, 2016.

References

Ammaniti, M., & Gallese, V. (2014). *La nascita dell'intersoggettività. Lo sviluppo del sé tra psicodinamica e neurobiologia* [The birth of intersubjectivity. The development of the self between psychodynamics and neurobiology]. Milano: Raffaello Cortina Editore.

Andolfi, M. (2021). Il bambino e la pandemia [The child and the pandemic]. In *Conference on line. La psicoterapia al tempo della pandemia*, www.cptf.it/it/la-psicoterapia-al-tempo-della-pandemia/.

Arfelli Galli, A. (2013). *La psicologia evolutiva nella scuola della Gestalt. Le ricerche in area tedesca nel periodo 1921–1975 [Developmental psychology in the Gestalt school. The researches in the German area in the period 1921–1975].* Università di Macerata: Eum Edizioni.

Cavaleri, P. A. (2003). *La profondità della superficie. Percorsi introduttivi alla psicoterapia della Gestalt* [The depth of the surface. Introductory paths to Gestalt psychotherapy]. Milano: FrancoAngeli.

Conte, E., & Mione, M. (2008). La relazione educativa nella postmodernità: l'età della fanciullezza [The educational relationship in postmodernity: The age of childhood]. In A. Ferrara & M. Spagnuolo Lobb (Eds.). *Le voci della Gestalt. Sviluppi e innovazioni di una psicoterapia* (pp. 174–179). Milano: FrancoAngeli.

Conte, E., & Tosi, S. (2016). Between Spontaneity and Intentionality of Growth: Gestalt therapy and children. In M. Spagnuolo Lobb, N. Levi, & A. Williams (Eds.). *Gestalt therapy with children. From epistemology to clinical practice* (pp. 101–122). Siracusa: Istituto di Gestalt HCC Italy.

Dalla Ragione, L., Medde, P., & Stallone, T. (2021). *I disturbi e i disordini alimentari all'epoca della pandemia* [Eating disorders and disturbances in the pandemic era], www.enpap.it/news/2021/01/webinar-disturbi-e-disordini-alimentari-allepoca-della-pandemia/.

Düss, L. (1940). La méthode des fables en psychoanalyse [The method of fables in psychoanalysis]. *Archives Psychologie Geneva, 28*, 1–51.

Finn, S. E. (2007). *In our clients' shoes: Theory and techniques of therapeutic assessment*. Mah, NJ: Earlbaum.

Francesetti, G. (2015). From individual symptoms to psychopathological fields. Towards a field perspective on clinical human suffering. *British Gestalt Journal, 24*(1), 5–19.

Francesetti, G., Gecele, M., & Roubal, J. (Eds.). (2013). *Gestalt therapy in clinical practice. From psychopathology to the aesthetics of contact*. Siracusa, Italy: Istituto di Gestalt HCC Italy Publ. Co., www.gestaltitaly.com.

Frank, R. (2001). *Body of awareness. A somatic and developmental approach to psychotherapy*. Highland, NY: Gestalt Press.

Frank, R. (2016a). L'esperienza del movimento: la risonanza cinestesica come sentimento relazionale. Intervista a Ruella Frank a cura di F. Maggio e S. Tosi [The experience of movement: kinesthetic resonance as a relational feeling. Interview with Ruella Frank by F. Maggio and S. Tosi]. *Quaderni di Gestalt, XXIX*(1), 9–24. DOI: 10.3280/GEST2016-001002.

Frank, R. (2016b). Moving experience: Kinaesthetic resonance as relational feel. In M. Spagnuolo Lobb, N. Levi, & A. Williams (Eds.). *Gestalt therapy with children. From epistemology to clinical practice* (pp. 87–99). Siracusa: Istituto di Gestalt HCC Italy Publ. Co., www.gestaltitaly.com.

Frank, R., & La Barre, F. (2011). *The first year and the rest of your life. Movement, development and psychotherapeutic change*. New York: Routledge.

Gallese, V., Migone, P., & Eagle, M. N. (2006). La simulazione incarnata: i neuroni specchio, le basi neurofisiologiche dell'intersoggettività e alcune implicazioni per la psicoanalisi. *Psicoterapia e Scienze Umane, XL*(3), 543–580.

Honneth, A. (1992). *Kampf um Anerkennung. Grammatik sozialer Konflikte* [Struggle for recognition. Grammar of social conflict]. Frankfurt am Main: Suhrkamp Verlag.

Kedrova, N. (2016). Restoring the melody of contact. In M. Spagnuolo Lobb, N. Levi, & A. Williams (Eds.). *Gestalt therapy with children. From epistemology to clinical practice* (pp. 157–168). Siracusa: Istituto di Gestalt HCC Italy.

Levi, N. (2013). The gilded cage of creative adjustment: A Gestalt approach to psychotherapy with children and adolescents. In G. Francesetti, M. Gecele, & J. Roubal (Eds.). *Gestalt therapy in clinical practice: From psychopathology to the aesthetics of contact* (pp. 265–280). Siracusa: Istituto di Gestalt HCC Italy Publ. Co.

Levi, N. (2016). Between caring and respect. Ethical aspects of Gestalt psychotherapy with children. In M. Spagnuolo Lobb, N. Levi, & A. Williams (Eds.). *Gestalt therapy with children. From epistemology to clinical practice* (pp. 63–86). Siracusa: Istituto di Gestalt HCC Italy.

Macaluso, M. A. (2015). Beyond the Perls-goodman model: From the organism-environment field to the relational field. *Gestalt Review, 19*(3), 233–250. DOI: 10.5325/gestaltreview.19.3.0233.

Maggio, F., & Tosi, S. (2020). *Il domani in movimento. Sostenere l'intenzionalità di contatto dei bambini* [Tomorrow in motion. Supporting children's contact intentionality]. Lecture presented at the International Seminar: Il domani dei bambini, tra relazioni intime e istituzioni. Mondello, Palermo: Istituto di Gestalt HCC Italy, 7/8 febbraio.

Molinari, E., & Cavaleri, P. A. (2015). *Il dono nel tempo della crisi. Per una psicologia del riconoscimento* [The gift in the time of crisis. For a psychology of recognition]. Milano: Raffaello Cortina Editore.

Perls, F., Hefferline, R. F., & Goodman, P. (1994). *Gestalt therapy: Excitement and growth in the human personality*. New York, NY: The Gestalt Journal Press, or.ed., 1951.

Porges, S. W. (2017). *The pocket guide to the polyvagal theory. The transformative power of feeling safe*. New York: W.W. Norton & Company, Inc.

Robine, J.-M. (2006). *La psychotherapie comme esthetique*. Bordeaux: L'Exprimerie.

Robine, J.-M. (2015). Il campo e la situazione, il self e l'atto sociale essenziale. Intervista a cura di Maria Mione. Commenti di M. Spagnuolo Lobb, G. Francesetti, P.A. Cavaleri [The field and the situation, the self and the essential social act. Interview by Maria Mione. Comments by M. Spagnuolo Lobb, G. Francesetti, P.A. Cavaleri]. *Quaderni di Gestalt, XXVIII*(2), 9–24. DOI: 10.3280/GEST2015-002002.

Salonia, G. (2013). Gestalt therapy and developmental theories. In G. Francesetti, M. Gecele, & J. Roubal (Eds.). *Gestalt therapy in clinical practice: From psychopathology to the aesthetics of contact* (pp. 235–250). Siracusa: Istituto di Gestalt HCC Italy Publ. Co.

Sampognaro, G. (2016). Working with the developmental age in Gestalt therapy. In M. Spagnuolo Lobb, N. Levi, & A. Williams (Eds.). *Gestalt therapy with children. From epistemology to clinical practice* (pp. 169–190). Siracusa: Istituto di Gestalt HCC Italy.

Spagnuolo Lobb, M. (2001). The theory of self in Gestalt therapy. A restatement of some aspects. *Gestalt Review, 5*, 276–288. DOI: 10.5325/gestaltreview.5.4.0276.

Spagnuolo Lobb, M. (2003). Therapeutic meeting as improvisational co-creation. In M. Spagnuolo Lobb & N. Amendt-Lyon (Eds.). *Creative license. The art of Gestalt therapy* (pp. 37–50). Wien, NY: Springer.

Spagnuolo Lobb, M. (2012). Toward a developmental perspective in Gestalt therapy, theory and practice: The polyphonic development of domains. *Gestalt Review, 16*(3), 222–244.

Spagnuolo Lobb, M. (2013a). *The Now-for-Next in psychotherapy: Gestalt therapy recounted in post-modern society*. Siracusa: Istituto di Gestalt HCC Italy Publ. Co., www.gestaltitaly.com.

Spagnuolo Lobb, M. (2013b). Developmental perspective in Gestalt therapy. The poliphonic development of domains. In G. Francesetti, M. Gecele, & J. Roubal (Eds.). *Gestalt therapy in clinical practice. From psychopathology to the aesthetics of contact* (pp. 109–130). Siracusa, Italy: Istituto di Gestalt HCC Italy Publ. Co., www.gestalt italy.com.

Spagnuolo Lobb, M. (2016a). Self as contact, contact as self. A contribution to ground experience in Gestalt therapy theory of self. In J.-M. Robine (Ed.). *Self. A poliphony of contemporary Gestalt therapists* (pp. 261–289). St. Romain la Virvée, France: L'Exprimerie.

Spagnuolo Lobb, M. (2016b). Gestalt therapy with children. Supporting the polyphonic development of domains in a field of contacts. In M. Spagnuolo Lobb, N. Levi, & A. Williams (Eds.). *Gestalt therapy with children. From epistemology to clinical practice* (pp. 25–62). Siracusa: Istituto di Gestalt HCC Italy, www.gestaltitaly.com.

Spagnuolo Lobb, M. (2018). Aesthetic relational knowledge of the field: A revised concept of awareness in Gestalt therapy and contemporary psychiatry. *Gestalt Review*, *22*(1), 50–68. DOI: 10.5325/gestalt review.22.1.0050.

Spagnuolo Lobb, M., Levi, N., & Williams, A. (2016). Introduction: From dental aggression to suffering of the "between". In M. Spagnuolo Lobb, N. Levi, & A. Williams (Eds.). *Gestalt therapy with children. From epistemology to clinical practice* (pp. 13–20). Siracusa: Istituto di Gestalt HCC Italy Publ. Co., www.gestaltitaly.com.

Spagnuolo Lobb, M., Conte, E., & Mione, M. (2017). La scheda clinica gestaltica: presentazione di uno strumento di lavoro [The Gestalt clinical data sheet: Presentation of a working tool]. *Quaderni di Gestalt*, *XXX*(2), 67–82. DOI: 10.3280/GEST2017-002005.

Spagnuolo Lobb, M., & Rubino, V. (2015). Le esperienze dissociative in psicoterapia della Gestalt [Dissociative experiences in Gestalt therapy.]. *Quaderni di Gestalt*, *XXVIII*(1), 27–48. DOI: 10.3280/GEST2015-001003.

Stern, D. N. (1985). *The interpersonal world of the infant: A view from psychoanalysis and developmental psychology*. New York: Basic Books.

Stern, D. N. (2010). *Forms of vitality. Exploring dynamic experience in psychology and the arts*. Oxford: Oxford University Press.

Tosi, S. (2016). Psicoterapia della Gestalt con i bambini: un modello di lavoro di gruppo [Gestalt psychotherapy with children: A model of group work]. *Quaderni di Gestalt*, *XXIX*(1), 91–100. DOI: 10.3280/GEST2016-001007.

Tosi, S., Cucchiani, A., & Vitali, R. (2013). "Grazie e a rivederci". Tra identificazioni e autonomia: forme di intervento terapeutico nel Servizio Pubblico ["Thank you and see you again". Between identifications and autonomy: Forms of therapeutic intervention in the Public Service]. *Quaderno dell'Istituto di Psicoterapia del Bambino e dell'Adolescente*, *37*, 53–65.

Yontef, G. M. (2001). Relational Gestalt therapy. In J.-M. Robine (Ed.). *Contact and relationship in a field perspective* (pp. 79–94). Bordeaux: L'Exprimerie.

Chapter 7

Children of "Broken" Relationships

Repairing the Ground of the Parental Experience

Paola Canna and Manuela Partinico

1. Introduction

The radical changes that have characterised the socio-cultural reality of the last fifty years have inevitably affected couples and families. The decade between 1970 and 1980 in Italy was especially plentiful in terms of reforms, among which the divorce law that represented a momentous turning-point and a civil conquest was one of the most important. Besides opening a path to a revision of family law, it established equal responsibility for both spouses and a greater balance in the rights and duties between parents, liberating generations of women and children once forced to remain in violent situations.

With respect to the past few decades, today we are witnessing a complexity dictated by the instability of couple relationships and by the ever-growing number of separations, outcomes produced by a type of society that generates precariousness and uncertainty, the "liquid" society (Bauman, 2005). In a context where the speed of change sweeps away every expected security and all long-established notions, the social trauma of the Covid-19 pandemic has become an amplifier and an emblem of an already present vulnerability (Spagnuolo Lobb, 2020). The speed at which the virus spreads and its dangerousness have blatantly highlighted the fragility of humans; what is even more obvious is just how slim that thread is that binds intimate relationships together. The forced togetherness, the co-management of daily life, the constrained spaces, the social isolation, and the restrictions imposed on us have determined the drastic and sudden collapse of a safe ground, upon which the organisation of family, work, and relationship life relied. This unexpected change exposed the weakness of certain relationships, that were already difficult, increasing their distresses, and in many cases, making pre-existent or buried couple crises explode.

The fragility of couple relationships, according to Spagnuolo Lobb (2013a), has stood out not so much due to the difficulty of "staying in the relationship" but more for the difficulty of "feeling in the relationship". The issues that are documented, already from the first year of shared life, highlight different degrees of "bodily desensitisation": from feeling how emotionally involved with and attracted one is to one's partner, to the development of disorders related to the

DOI: 10.4324/9781003313335-10

sexual sphere. The more or less complete ability to stay spontaneously in a relationship with the other is also a relevant diagnostic indicator in the identification of dysfunctionality, which concerns the experience of parenthood. Examples of this are found in cases of "premature parenthood", in which young couples who have had children before having carried out a choice as a couple, delegate the primary care to their families of origin, abdicating their parental role, in order to keep their own individual spaces. In other cases, what is illustrated is a "split parenting", where the role of parent is often borne by a single hyper-responsible and legal spouse, while the other, running away from his/her duty, stimulates in the partner the same nurturing attitudes addressed towards the children. Ultimately, "separated parenthood" can also be transformed into a dysfunctional experience, when the conjugal break-up, accompanied by intense conflict, becomes a fixed figure, such that it prevents the "seeing" and "hearing" of the children, left alone to self-manage their emotional experiences. The inability of the parent to provide relational and bodily containment to the children's suffering, in turn, leads to their corporeal and emotional desensitisation, the only outcome to the painful lived ordeal of the family. These family experiences, which are sometimes traumatic, can impact young generations with various – some less, some more – serious forms of vulnerability like, for instance, new dependencies, current forms of anxiety disorders, social withdrawal, and different maladaptive behaviours.

Every separation is a rupture of the ground of the family relationships: it causes an experience of fragmentation and uncertainty in children, something that aggravates the sense of social precariousness in which they are immersed. What is needed are new preventative and mental health care measures that can respond in a more contemporary way to the malaise which the children in today's society are living through.

2. Mediation as a Means Towards a Good Separation

It was around the Seventies, as a response to the social and cultural changes that were hitting relationships and the family, that mediation, as an extra-judicial measure for couples, facing the difficult transition of separation, was born.

The first form of mediation was introduced, legally speaking, by means of matrimonial rules applied to divorce. Subsequently, negotiation was developed, with which, through management techniques of conflicts coming from the context of organisations, some sort of support was offered to the parties in order to identify common interests and be able to satisfy shared advantages (Haynes and Buzzi, 2012).

Thanks to the contribution of some psychotherapy and social science approaches another stream of mediation made headway, one in which the work emphasis was placed more on relational and family type issues rather than on the negotiation of the parties involved (Cigoli, 1991; Chianura et al., 2011).

The goal that brings together all mediation is to create "a space for communication" between the parents in order to build a stable collaboration agreement for the benefit of the children. Mediation, generally speaking, takes place in the presence of the single parental couple and envisages three distinct moments: the pre-mediation phase, eventually finalised to evaluate the level of conflict between the parties and the feasibility of the path forward; the actual mediation, during which the topics of contention within the couple are dealt with; the drawing up of the shared agreements on all the problematic points brought to the mediation table. Only a few models include one or more sessions with the children, whether for the purpose of explaining to them what is happening to their parents or of evaluating the level of distress and maladaptation caused by their experience (Mastropaolo, 2010).

Gestalt mediation, utilised here, places attention on the reciprocity between parents and children and between the children, drawing on recent developments in the Gestalt field approach (Spagnuolo Lobb, 2013b, 2018) and therefore considering the separation situation as an experiential field to take care of. It is not possible to deal with the suffering of the children without addressing the contribution brought by the parents' suffering in the separation situation.

From the Gestalt perspective, separation is not considered a personal or couple failure; rather, it is analysed from a procedural perspective as an expression of a present suffering in the "here-and-now" of the couple relationship that is applying pressure towards a new form or *gestalt*.

Starting from the assumption that the separation experience divides the couple but not the parenting, or, in other words, they are always "parents together" (Spagnuolo Lobb, 2013a), Gestalt mediation has as a specific focus the safeguarding and the recovery of the parental relationship, so that the children may be able to continue to count on the security of the experiential ground at the root of the relationship between the father and mother. With the break-up of the conjugal relationship what becomes prioritised is guaranteeing the "ground of the parental experience",[1] the secure support for the children.

A first fundamental step concerns the distinction between the couple bond, which is about to end, and the parental bond, which will last forever. The possibility of keeping the two levels of personal identity ("partner of" and "parent of") distinct is reached through the emergence of the Spontaneous Parental Personality Function (SPPF). In Gestalt psychotherapy, the personality-function is the ability to establish a relationship with the other through the social definition of the self (Spagnuolo Lobb, 2013b, p. 107). In Gestalt Mediation, we speak of the SPPF to indicate the way to be fully and spontaneously in a relationship through one's own parental self.

In the following, we wish to illustrate how the Gestalt mediatory process results in an intervention especially suitable for the prevention and treatment of the suffering of the children and of the intimate relationships in current familial and social scenarios.

3. The Suffering of Children in the Separation Experience

Conflict is a "normal" element in the life of two people. It is the indispensable space in which to experience the difference between the self and the other (Cavaleri, 2017). If the differences that have surfaced are so deep that the relationship is rendered irreparable, the partners are obliged to acknowledge the inevitability of the break-up. The separation, therefore, is configured as a resolution to the unbearable tension within the family's phenomenological field[2] and as the closure of a gestalt.

How does a familial field, imbued with aggressiveness, manifest or coerced, influence the experience of the children? What contact intentionality underlies the destructive clashes between the parents that are separating?

In the following cases, two different situations of conflictual separation will be presented along with their relative influence on the family field. Gestalt mediation, when possible, envisages some sessions devoted to the children, in which the mediators "resonate" with their suffering and offer an emotional containment. In this sense, as emerges in case no.1, the Gestalt mediation may also be considered a therapeutic tool for the children.

Case no. 1   A Mediation Situation: The mediation setting is composed of two Gestalt mediators with the parental couple and, in a designated session, of the co-mediators with the children

Luisa and Marco attend a consultation due to a serious conjugal crisis that seems to have arrived "like lightning out of the blue". She is 40 years old and since childhood has cultivated a passion for music that she has set aside to devote herself to the family – but with a growing sense of dissatisfaction.

Marco is 52 years old and works as a surveyor for the municipal offices where they reside. He has always played a very responsible role, directly managing his children and wife and undervaluing the need for Luisa to fulfil herself as a musician. The couple has two children: Edoardo, 18 years old, a student at an Arts Secondary School, and Laura, 16 years old, registered at a professional institute, learning to be a chef. In the last few weeks, Luisa has been living in another city, about thirty kilometres from the family home, together with a musician with whom she says she is in love. In the face of this event, the husband "has barricaded" himself in the house with his children and his profound pain.

The youngsters are invited to the meeting. They talk about suffering as they watch their father close in on himself and be preoccupied by financial matters, while confessing to feeling "abandoned" by their mother who has left the home so suddenly.

Edoardo feels that he is the "caretaker" of the torment and anger permeating their father; this situation shifts the father/son relationship onto an almost symmetrical axis, increasing the son's sense of responsibility and his subsequent emotional burden. Laura, on the other hand, has become the "substitute" for the mother in all the domestic chores and in the family organisation; the assumption of a strictly managerial role increases her emotional distance from her father, dismantling the parent/daughter relationship.

The youngsters speak about having known of their mother's move to the home of her new partner only when it was a *fait accompli*. Every time that Laura meets with her, she consumes her mother's emotional confidences as if she were her intimate friend and keeps her secrets. Edoardo describes himself as the one observing from afar, feeling overlooked and kept at a distance by his mother. Laura participates with excitement in her mother's falling in love, in her transgression, in the impulsiveness with which she has acted, and thus living the experience of adolescence denied to her. For Edoardo, on the other hand, his mother deprived him of this experience, reserving for him the only role left open: that of the responsible and independent adult.

We learn from their stories that the suffering experienced by each of them, and the weight of the parents' separation, up until this point, has never been the subject of shared discussion. Edoardo and Laura have endured their pain alone, propping themselves up in silence.

In the phenomenological-experiential field of the session, what circulates is a sense of loss and profound solitude that forcefully sweeps over us, the mediators, affecting us quite deeply. Within the suffering that permeates the context, the beauty of Edoardo and Laura is striking, and it takes on a distinct character: their strength, their dignity, and their ability to persevere even autonomously are most touching. The two young siblings, in this desolate wasteland, have learned to move with delicate fluidity and grace. The pain derived from the physical and relational absence of both parents wanders freely and directionless and awakens in us the instinct to rescue them and respond to their need for relational rootedness. We communicate the desire to be of help to them so that they may be able to feel that someone is there to whom they can entrust their lived experiences, their emotions, and what is stirring in their bodies.

During the meeting, we listen to the pain of Edoardo, unable to manifest his distress in the relationship with both parents: with his mother who is too distant, with his father because he is too full of his own grief as an abandoned husband. Laura expresses at length and in tears her great sense of emptiness due to her mother's absence and the lack of the tranquil atmosphere that used to exist "when I set the table and pulled out 4 forks!" Her body is motionless, trapped in a subtle but continuous shiver. She would like to spend more time with her mother, but cannot confide this to her father, fearing she would hurt him and cause a negative reaction. Gradually, as the words flow, their bodies begin to loosen up. For the first time, Edoardo and Laura open up in a touching and personal account that makes them aware of how much they share in common, and of how much they have kept secret from each other until this moment. What strikes us is the bodily energy that can be found in the two siblings. It is not expressed through emotions of anger, which could give rise to a conflict with regards to their parents. On a symptomatological level, their suffering, which has not had a relational containment in the parental couple, comes to light in specific risky behaviours: the boy has developed an intense dependency on smoking, and has admitted to abusing light drugs, while the girl is committing acts of self-harm, methodically making cuts to her wrists.

In the family gestalt, they appear uprooted and their emotions, without containment, are the cause for a desensitisation of their bodies. These dysfunctional behaviours appear to us as attempts to control the de-anchoring that they have suffered, the sudden loss of ground security, splintered by the abrupt break-up between their parents, and the attempt to reconnect with their own body and feel it to be alive once again.

Case no. 2   Support Situation for Separated Parenting:
The mediation setting is composed of one Gestalt mediator and the separated parent

Agnese, Pietro, Federico, and Davide are the four children of Giancarlo, a banking agent, a fifty-year-old, divorced from Susanna 4 years ago. The children, 18, 16, 14, and 10 years old respectively, live with their mother and spend some days with their father according to the separation agreement. From the moment of leaving Giancarlo's house, the mother accentuated her disparaging attitude towards the father, something already underway during their married life, leading to an obvious annihilation of the fatherly figure and to a progressive estrangement from the children. At the time of separation, Agnese, the eldest, was completely withdrawn from the relationship with her father and was refusing to go to dinner to his house together with her brothers. Pietro occasionally complied with the obligations to visit when it was convenient for him. Federico was collaborating with his mother's control strategy, letting her know how his father was managing his little brother. Davide, the youngest, let himself be guided by his mother's agenda, never making a request for an alternative, even when at his father's house.

The separation between Giancarlo and his ex-wife perpetuates and aggravates the conflictual and power dynamic already present in the conjugal relationship. The hostility of the children and the conflicts that are generated represent the fixed figure of the field of family relations, which heavily influences the way in which the children relate which each other and with each of their parents. The children's suffering is explained through their intentionality of contact, unexpressed and suffocated by the urgency of the conflict between the parties. From the stories of the father, what is striking is the obvious contrast on generational lines: while the parents are constantly occupied with their fight, animated by the strong emotions of anger and mutual hostility, the children are not expressing any demand for support, and their emotional component seems "frozen" behind attitudes of apparent indifference. The sons, in different ways, manifest behaviours of closure and withdrawal while the daughter is plagued by a pervasive dermatitis, and has developed an eating disorder of the bulimic kind that is gradually becoming more evident. Amongst them there is no sense of complicity or alliance. They seem like distant islands in a turbulent sea. They do not demonstrate any kind of affection or sadness for their father, or any rebellious reaction with regards to their mother, who imposes coercive rules even on the older children.

Giancarlo, after the first four years of separation, begins a process of support for separated parenting and it is here that he conveys the massive grief of his failure: an unwanted marital break-up, the physical detachment and the emotional loss of his four children, the lack of recognition and the impossibility of expressing his role as a father.

What is striking about Giancarlo is his imposing, tall, and robust physique, his deep voice and firm tone, and how he moves through space with large and generous gestures. His elegant attire, in accordance with his role, is attenuated by his relaxed bearing, which is not formal in the least. Right from the first sessions, he proves to be a sociable man, confident and authentic, open to expressing his personal emotions, to the point of allowing himself to burst into tears.

In the shared field, one perceives the drama of having lost not only a united family but also the relationship with his four children, to whom he is much attached. His pain of loss provokes an empathic reaction of suffering in me for his sense of failure which he conveys, but at the same time, I also feel a certain annoyance for his difficulty to react like a "grown man" to the injustices and intrusions of his ex-wife, even in terms of the separation. In the relational field, what hovers in the air is his fear in relation to the mother of his children and the anxiety around making a mistake, all of which generates frequent and urgent requests for help from the mediator for relational and communication issues to do with her.

These perceptions of the relational field allows the Gestalt mediator to create a therapeutic relationship by means of which Giancarlo may be able to have an experience of recognition and self-esteem, achieving a personal "renewal". To the pressing demands dictated by fear and insecurity, the Gestalt mediator supports the capacity to listen to himself and find his own strength, beginning with his body and role and ability as a father (Spontaneous Parental Personality Function).

The process of separated parenting support is healing Giancarlo's wound, caused by the devaluation of his identity, and restores recognition and space for the expression of his assets, boldly put on view with each of his children and with their mother.

Agnese, the firstborn, is beginning to turn to her father to ask for advice and concrete help. During a period of intense conflict with her mother, Giancarlo is encouraging Agnese to re-establish a dialogue with her. And thus, she is unexpectedly beginning to resume her visits to her father's house, and to spend summer vacation with all of her brothers. Giancarlo not only recognises his own relational abilities but also the importance of being father to his adolescent sons. He approaches Pietro and Federico with more confidence, using their passion for basketball, and bravely asks them for help in the management of his house. New spaces of communication and fun are being opened up between Giancarlo and his sons, and this moves them to participate in their visits to their father with greater interest and motivation. Thanks to a more assertive attitude and one that conforms to his role as a father, Giancarlo is able to express himself more firmly in relation to his ex-wife, asking to be able to share in the educational guidance and decisions regarding Davide, the youngest son.

4. Treating the Children's Suffering Through Supporting the Ground of the Parental Experience

Infant Research has provided a broad contribution to the observation of primary relationships, documenting the wealth of the communicative and affective exchanges in the mother-child dyad (Ainsworth *et al.*, 1978; Emde, 1991; Trevarthen, 1998; Tronick, 1989). The intersubjective viewpoint and in particular the studies of Stern *et al.* (1998), on the concept of "implicit relational knowledge", have offered up a description of how the primary interactions are modelled on a dyadic rhythm through the internalisation of mutual expectations (Stern, 1985). In addition, based on the consideration that the father-mother-child triad represents a unified system right from the first months of life, Fivaz-Depeursinge has demonstrated that the relationships are always structured according to a triadic model (Fivaz-Depeursinge and Corboz-Warnery, 1999). In line with previous contributions, the Gestalt perspective considers the complex experiential field which emerges in the relationships between parents and children, in which the different relational threads get woven and unwoven. The experience of separation is considered a boundary event within a single field of perceptions, where every member is present and exists in relation to each other. The suffering at the boundary between the father and the mother contributes to the formation of the figure at the boundary between the child and each parent. What happens at the contact boundary between child-father and between child-mother also influences the exchange between the two parents.

In accepting this reference map, the Gestalt paradigm goes beyond the concept of duality and introduces the logic of the field (Spagnuolo, 2013a, p. 171) as a fundamental element that contributes to the experience of embodied pain through the bodies, the looks, the gestures, the silences, and the breathing. The experiences and malaise of the children are included in the relational viewpoint and are part of the shared situation. Edoardo and Laura, in case no.1, participate in the dynamic between the parents, one, by taking care of the father, and the other, by taking care of the mother, sacrificing the sharing and the closeness between siblings. Giancarlo's children, in case no. 2, react to the game of power and conflictuality that exists between the mother and the father, depriving themselves of a relationship with him and of relationships with each other. The field perspective represents the specific map which guides the Gestalt procedural work. It goes beyond the approach of psychoanalysis and more recent psychotherapies, based on the task of making explicit what is implicit. The treatment consists of supporting the emergence of *spontaneity*, thus facilitating the implementation of the contact intentionality that has not been completed successfully and the re-sensitisation of the boundary (Spagnuolo Lobb, 2013a, p. 171, 2015, p. 30). In the cases addressed here, the valorisation of parenting facilitates a healthy rebalancing in the relationship with the children. For example, the assumption of maternal responsibility on the part of Luisa allows the daughter to distance herself from the role of friend/confidante. Marco, being able to count on the collaboration with Luisa, can enjoy more light-hearted and fun spaces with his adolescent children. Giancarlo's children rediscover and regain the affection and the authoritativeness of the father by counterbalancing the relationship with their mother.

In Gestalt mediation, we can identify four steps that represent the basic procedures of the work.

The *first step* of the mediation process consists of the *phenomenological observation of the co-created relational field*. The phenomenological reality of the here-and-now of the mediation session is a diagnostic tool that allows one to distinguish separations of low conflictuality (case no. 1) and separations of high conflictuality (case no. 2). The orientation and the subsequent choice of the type of intervention to undertake arise out of this preliminary analysis: mediation with the parental couple (case no.1) or mediation with a single parent (case no.2). Separations of low conflictuality are those that are suited to classically defined mediation work. In these cases, the negative emotions resulting from the conflict belong to the ground and enable the emergence of the parents' motivation to participate in confrontation and dialogue in order to protect the children from the trauma of the marital break-up. In separations of high conflictuality, which are almost universally considered unresponsive to mediation (Chianura *et al.*, 2011), the Gestalt mediation process, thanks to its field epistemology, operates with a single parent, working on the system of relationships. By means of this methodology, which we have called *Support for separated parenting*, the mediator "substitutes" for the absent parent in open conflict, taking on the role of collaborating co-parent.

The fundamental objective of the *second step* of the mediation process is the *restoration of the ground of the parental experience*. How does one reach this goal? In the *separated parenting of low conflictuality*, it is attained by making the Spontaneous Parental Personality Function emerge (SPPF), and it is based on the recovery of those strengths that gave rise to the couple's initial falling-in-love phase. In case no.1, Marco's sense of responsibility, reliability, and security, and Luisa's creativity, light-heartedness, and sociability, having become an obstacle in the couple's relationship, gain a new value and meaning if transferred and seen in the relationship with the children. The emergence of the SPPF modifies the familial field of the relationships. This work, in fact, concerns not only the specific competencies, which everyone possesses in the relationship with one's children, but allows for the mutual recognition of the parental identity, namely how each parent has become "that father or that mother that I appreciate", once again making possible the experience of being valued and *connecting* with the other. The relational good that has developed in the previous experience of marital and family life in this way is renewed through the parental relationship (Molinari and Cavaleri, 2015; Partinico and Canna, 2020) and alleviates the pain of the break-up of the couple relationship. This restructuring of the field eases the conflictual climate that one usually experiences during a separation process, promoting a more peaceful ground where the child may be able to become rooted in a more secure way. In *the separated parenting of high conflictuality*, which entails only one parent present in the mediation setting, the mediator, immersed in the situational field, by means of aesthetic relational knowing,[3] uses his/her own perception for looking together with the patient at that specific child as if he/she were the co-parent. In this process, as in clinical example no. 2, the mediator perceives Giancarlo's life force, reflecting his full identity as adult and father. The work on the SPPF frees the parent from the couple conflict in which he feels entangled, thus allowing the sensitisation of the contact boundary with each of his children.

The *third stage* of the mediation process consists of looking at the *now-for-next of the separated parenting*, supporting the contact intentionality of the individuals. This passage represents the cornerstone of Gestalt mediation, the key element, which allows for the emergence of new figures. In case no.1, Luisa, who in married life was only able to express herself in the role of wife and mother, withdraws from the family to realise her dream of becoming a musician; the support to intentionality has enabled the integration of the dimension of personal realisation with the parental one, facilitating the renewal of the personality-function. Working with Marco has brought about the recovery of a lifestyle that is less burdensome and more committed to sociability, for many long years suffocated by the hyper-responsible assumption of the role as head of the family. In case no.2, Giancarlo's ability to take care of his children and a greater sense of self-esteem have been the bridge towards the fulfilment of a new family and couple experience – the first made possible by the decision of the older boys to go and live permanently in their father's home, the second by the experience of a couple relationship of equals, where he can also express the strong and protective side of his character towards the female figure.

The *fourth and last step* concerns the stage of formalization and *closure* of the mediation process. After the work of support in order to facilitate the emergence of the *now-for-next* (in other words, the tension over the change in the partners), implicit in the separation experience, one proceeds to the drafting of the shared and long-term agreements, which will be included in the act of legal separation to which is entrusted the division of assets and the calculation for maintenance payments to which the children are entitled. The agreements include the decisions which the parental couple has made relative to potentially problematic or conflictual issues brought to the mediation table. An example of this could concern aspects of communication between the parents, educational choices, the management of health problems, the time for spending with the children, as well as the introduction of a new emotional relationship, etc. These are integral to the reorganisation of the family field and the rearrangement of the relationships, an inherent component of the rehabilitation of the *ground of parental experience*.

To sum up, the Gestalt mediation process is structured within an experiential field, according to four steps:

1. *Phenomenological observation of the field*, from which the orientation towards the type of mediatory intervention arises, on the basis of the separations of high or low conflictuality;
2. renewal of the ground of the parental experience through the recovery of the SPPF, as a specific work methodology on conflict in Gestalt psychotherapy;
3. focussing on the now-for-next of the separated parenting, supporting the contact intentionality of the individuals;
4. *drafting of the agreements*, shared and long-term, often experimented with over the course of time.

4. Conclusions

Gestalt psychotherapy, availing itself of a phenomenological, aesthetic, and field perspective, sees the separation experience as a boundary event, out of which a new relational process can originate. It is an expression of the evolutionary impetus that achieves new intentionalities, which encourage a reorganisation of the field of family relationships. Within this perspective, the couple break-up and the collapse of the ground of familial security can be transformed into an evolutionary change that influences not only individual identities but also the experience itself of parenthood, by rejuvenating it.

Separation can be seen, however, as one of the possible evolutionary stages of the family life cycle.[4] Nevertheless, such a process is not exempt from suffering, for both the couple and the children, who, as previously explained, are not generally considered during the course of mediation. The conjugal break-up, the inevitable consequence of the no longer productive conflict, never divides parenting. The work of restoring the ground of the parental experience, substantially compromised by separation, becomes the specific treatment that helps the children get through the ordeal of the change.

In conclusion, Gestalt mediation can be considered a treatment method of the "broken" relationships of the familial field. Appreciation of the differences as well as the recovery of the Spontaneous Parental Personality Function release the parents from their couple's conflict and allow for the emergence of new figures: the children within the separation experience. The contact boundary between parents and children becomes re-sensitised, allowing these latter the experience of being seen in their pain and of finding an emotional containment and a more secure rootedness in their primary bonds.

Repairing the disconnected ground of the familial relationships thus allows the children to spontaneously access both parents and to move more securely in the world because they are free to live the experiences and responsibilities appropriate to their age group.

Notes

1   For the ground of the parental experience we are referring to the sensorial and corporeal ground that orients the meanings and the actions undertaken in the parental role and guides the contact intentionality within the parents/children relationship. It is the being-present in the here-and-now, with the perception of one's own parental self and the field perception.
2   For the definition of phenomenological field we refer the reader to Chapter 4.
3   By aesthetic relational knowing we mean "the instrument through which the therapist resonates with the client during the session, and as well the lens through which s/he looks at the client's vitality, the feeling the therapist experiences in the presence of the experiential field in which the client is immersed" (Spagnuolo Lobb, 2018, pp. 17–63).
4   Separation, seen as a further evolutionary stage of parenting, deserves to be inserted into the Gestalt model of parenting of Spagnuolo Lobb (2016) with the designation of *Shared parenting in the separation situation*.

References

Ainsworth, M. D. S., Blehar, M., Waters, E., & Wall, S. (1978). *Patterns of attachment: Assessed in the strange situation and at home*. Hillsdale: Erlbaum.
Bauman, Z. (2005). *Liquid life*. Cambridge: Polity.
Cavaleri, P. A. (2017). Il riconoscimento reciproco, anche nella coppia, attraversa il conflitto [Mutual recognition runs through conflict, even in the couple]. *Conflitto e Mediazione, Etica per le professioni, 3*, 13–19.
Chianura, P., Chianura, L., Fuxa, E., & Mazzoni, S. (Eds.). (2011). *Manuale clinico di terapia familiare. Volume II: le buone prassi nella terapia sistemico-relazionale* [Clinical handbook of family therapy. Volume II: Best practices in systemic-relational therapy]. Milano: FrancoAngeli.
Cigoli, V. (1991). Dalla parte delle famiglia. Come procedere alla sua tutela nei casi di pseudo scisma coniugale e di divisione dei figli [On the side of the family. How to proceed to family protection in cases of pseudo marital schism and child division]. In C. Saraceno & M. Pradi (Eds.). *I figli contesi*. Milano: Unicopli.
Emde, R. N. (1991). Positive emotions for psychoanalytic theory: Surprises from infancy research and new direction. *Journal of the American Psychoanalytic Association, 29*(Suppl. 1), 5–44.
Fivaz-Depeursinge, E., & Corboz-Warnery, A. (1999). *The primary triangle. A developmental systems view of mothers, fathers, and infants*. New York: Basic Books.
Haynes, J. M., & Buzzi, I. (2012). *Introduzione alla mediazione familiare. Principi fondamentali e sua applicazione* [Introduction to family mediation. Basic principles and its application]. Milano: Giuffré.
Mastropaolo, L. (2010). Crisi e conflitto: mediazione familiare, "intervento per il cambiamento". Percorsi differenti della Scuola Genovese [Crisis and conflict: Family mediation, "intervention for change". Different paths of the genovese school]. In L. Chianura,

P. Chianura, S. Mazzoni, & E. Fuxa. *Manuale Clinico di Terapia Familiare*. Milano: FrancoAngeli.

Molinari, E., & Cavaleri, P. A. (2015). *Il dono nel tempo della crisi. Per una psicologia del riconoscimento* [The gift in the time of crisis. For a psychology of recognition]. Milano: Raffaello Cortina.

Partinico, M., & Canna, P. (2020). Il processo mediativo secondo la prospettiva gestaltica. Il caso di Elena e Giovanni [The mediation process according to the Gestalt perspective. The case of Elena and Giovanni]. *Quaderni di Gestalt, XXXIII*(1), 85–97. DOI: 10.3280/GEST2020-001007.

Spagnuolo Lobb, M. (2013a). *The now-for-next in psychotherapy: Gestalt therapy recounted in post-modern society*. Siracusa: Istituto di Gestalt HCC Italy Publ. Co., www.gestaltitaly.com.

Spagnuolo Lobb, M. (2013b). Developmental perspective in Gestalt therapy. The poliphonic development of domains. In G. Francesetti, M. Gecele, & J. Roubal (Eds.). *Gestalt Therapy in clinical practice. From psychopathology to the aesthetics of contact* (pp. 109–130). Siracusa, Italy: Istituto di Gestalt HCC Italy Publ. Co., www.gestaltitaly.com.

Spagnuolo Lobb, M. (2015). The body as a "vehicle" of our being in the world. Somatic experience in Gestalt therapy. *British Gestalt Journal, 24*(2), 21–31.

Spagnuolo Lobb, M. (2016). Lasciarsi trasformare dai figli. Proposta di un modello estetico di genitorialità [Letting children transform us. Proposal for an aesthetic model of parenting]. *Quaderni di Gestalt, XXIX*(1), 25–39. DOI: 10.3280/GEST2016-001003.

Spagnuolo Lobb, M. (2018). Aesthetic relational knowledge of the field: A revised concept of awareness in Gestalt therapy and contemporary psychiatry. *Gestalt Review, 22*(1), 50–68. DOI: 10.5325/gestalt review.22.1.0050.

Spagnuolo Lobb, M. (2020). Gestalt therapy during coronavirus: Sensing the experiential ground and "dancing" with reciprocity. *The Humanistic Psychologist, 48*(4), 397–409. DOI: 10.1037/hum0000228.

Stern, D. N. (1985). *The interpersonal world of the infant: A view from psychoanalysis and developmental psychology*. New York: Basic Books.

Stern, D. N., Bruschweiler-Stern, N., Harrison, A., Lyons-Ruth, K., Morgan, A., Nahum, J., Sander, L., & Tronick, E. (1998). The process of therapeutic change involving implicit knowledge: Some implications of developmental observations for adult psychotherapy. *Infant Mental Journal, 19*(3), 300–308.

Trevarthen, C. (1998). *Empatia e biologia. Psicologia, cultura e neuroscienze* [Empathy and biology. Psychology, culture, and neuroscience]. Milano: Cortina.

Tronick, E. Z. (1989). Emotions and emotional communication in infants. *American Psychologist, 44*(2), 112–119.

Chapter 8

Gestalt Psychotherapy and Complex Trauma in Preadolescence

How to Support the Integration of the Body, Emotions, and Words

Rosanna Militello

1. An Encounter "Without Words"

Lidia comes into the therapist's office with a worried expression, following the care facility coordinator with hesitant steps. First, she hesitates to sit down, clearly implying that she is not at all enthusiastic about being here. She looks perplexedly around, holding herself tight within her jean jacket, and keeps on mumbling incomprehensible words under her breath while the coordinator, in a spirited manner, invites her to introduce herself with the clear intent of getting a smile out of her. Lidia is a pretty girl of eleven years old, even though she seems to be a little younger. Her body is wiry and lean. Her blonde and smooth hair frames a gaunt, freckled, and sharp-edged face, while a rebellious lock extends over her big eyes, of an intense blue colour, which stay hidden from the gaze of the other. Neat in appearance, she sits down with a bewildered look. Maintaining her worried countenance, she whispers in a small voice her name. Shyly, she immediately acknowledges, speaking clear and unequivocal words, her apprehension and embarrassment ("I don't like it here at all!!"). For the entire time of the encounter, Lidia, short of breath, continues to look around and pull down the sleeves of her jacket until she completely hides her hands. She makes herself as small as possible, pulls her legs up to her chest, and shrivels up inside her shoulders, while her downcast eyes keep trying to avoid mine and settle on what is outside the window. I listen to her silence; I observe her movements: awkward, uncertain, anxious; I see her shame in her continuous avoidance of my eyes, her embarrassment; I feel a mess of intense emotions on my skin: a mixture of impotence, tenderness, uneasiness, and fear.

It is exactly from this phenomenological field (in which, just as it happens to Lidia, every word of mine also seems "senseless and so dies in my throat") that the therapeutic process is initiated; an arduous and delicate "journey", characterised by deviations, halts, and regressions; a torturous path in which staying in the relationship becomes a difficult commitment to build and maintain. But Gestalt psychotherapy, insofar as it is an *aesthetic model*, teaches us to look at that beauty that belongs to the human and to every contact born out of an encounter. It helps us to recognise how the violated youngster has made a masterpiece out of his/her

DOI: 10.4324/9781003313335-11

life, despite the humiliations and degradations which his/her *self-in-development* has experienced. The relational strategy, which the child brings into therapy, is the fruit of his/her *creative adaptation*, the best response possible in the face of the situations experienced. The diagnostic model, based on the co-creation at the contact boundary (cf. Spagnuolo Lobb, 2013, 2015, 2016a, 2016b), is the map that orients the observation and reading of what happens in the "between" of the treatment setting. The phenomenological lenses of observation allow the therapist, although remaining concentrated on the "here-and-now", to grasp the complexity of the being-there on the part of the young patient.

They allow the therapist to give voice to those silent embodied words, which contain a trace of the stifled and sometimes frozen intentionalities of contact. The aim is to grasp and bring to light the small seeds of the *now for next*, despite the severe scars and the outrage endured (cf. Militello, 2011). The Gestalt gaze must focus on the dance that the therapist and patient co-construct (cf. Spagnuolo Lobb, 2017) – a unique synchronicity, where the therapist's competent and human interest meets the young patient's attempt to entrust him/herself to the therapist. A dance made up of continuous adjustments, in which there is no "right" therapeutic move, but a continuous monitoring, curious and receptive, made up of attunement, recognition, and emotional synchronicity. In this co-created space-time, the steps, at first uncertain and barely fluid, become, through the process of the therapeutic work, bolder and bolder and more and more harmonious. The Gestalt therapist uses his/her own aesthetic competence, namely his/her own sensoriality, as an instrument for attunement and resonance. This feeling, which Spagnuolo Lobb (2016b, 2018) defines as *aesthetic relational knowing*,[1] becomes an elective Gestalt tool, because it allows one to contextualise the therapist's aesthetic emotions in the phenomenological field activated by the patient and grasp the non-explicit intentionalities of contact. A compass, therefore, which helps to orient oneself, without distortions or manipulations, in the phenomenological field, out of which emerges the wounded child's experience, thus allowing one to identify the right direction for a more effective and suitable intervention, in absolute antithesis to the malicious relationships the child has experienced. Attention is concentrated on the process, on *how* the therapist/patient encounter takes place, prioritising the perspective of the perceptive experience. What is created is a new meeting, a third reality in which it becomes fundamental to support and provide the young patient the possibility of being in a relationship with greater presence and spontaneity, overcoming those habitual obstructions enacted in previous experiences, which suppressed the possibilities of connecting with the other in the fullness of a self that is still fragile and in the process of formation (*ibidem*). In this process (a delicate one, fraught with difficulty), the therapist helps the child, who has been harmed, to focus attention on the present moment. It is only by being in the "here-and-now", in the free, safe, and clean therapy space that it becomes possible to help the child patient in the search for a vocabulary based on feeling; to guide the youngster in listening to his/her sensations and emotions that surface out of the background; to bring out the corporeal embodied experience as a figure that has become intrinsic to the relational process. Therapeutic treatment and change are possible by means of the work of stitching together the body, emotions, and words, precisely because the working through of the trauma cannot be separated from a deep experiential integration of the *young-wounded-self*. Gestalt therapists look at how the child positions him/herself before them, what physiology the child expresses, how the youngster narrates his/her story, how the patient moves, and how the patient's trauma has taken shape in his/her body. Besides looking at the *figure*, the therapist moves his gaze over the *ground*. The ground is precisely the terrain which the trauma has pervaded, where confusing sensations and unexpressed emotions, which have been introjected undigested, have become entangled.

2. The Thick Blanket of the Unspeakable: Lidia – A Tale Waiting to Be Told

When Lidia arrives at the child-care facility, she seems to be a difficult child to treat. Intolerant of the idea of living in that setting, she exhibits a total mistrust towards adults. Repeatedly, she attests to being capable of taking care of herself and also of her brother, and wanting to go home. The first months after her placement are delicate, characterised by a marked sense of immobility and stagnation in which she shows all of her opposition. She has little patience with the rules and is confrontational. She often takes on the role of leader, demonstrating improper and almost delinquent behaviours and modalities. Her relationships are regulated by the law of the strongest and the most cunning. She raises her hands to the smaller children. She challenges the decisions of the care workers with contempt. Relationships with the adults are characterised by manipulation, alternating with seductive and aggressive attitudes. She seems to be wearing a protective sheath, a rigid suit of armour that never lets her show her fragile side. Never a tear, an emotion that might have something to do with tenderness; never a gentle word, a request for closeness and help. Her ground is full of fear; her ways of doing things and being with others are wary and oriented towards substantial reactivity. It is as if Lidia is always on the alert, at the mercy of an extreme and non-regulated neuro-vegetative activation. Her senses are concentrated and focussed on grasping every small signal of danger, even of the most innocuous and non-dangerous kind.

What is known about Lidia when she arrives at the facility is truly very little. She is defined by the manager of the care community as a "tsunami, a complicated and intensely problematic subject", capable of disrupting, in a matter of weeks, the difficult relational equilibrium of the host facility. Lidia's case reaches the attention of the judicial authority when the school informs Juvenile Court of the confidences of Paolo, Lidia's only younger brother, who tells his teacher in class of the scenes of violence, which it seems he has been witnessing together with his sister. In fact, he reports that his father, who has a precarious job, usually lingers in the tavern and there, together with his friends, plays cards and drinks "heavily".

Then, late at night, drunk, and exuding a nauseating smell of wine, comes home, angry, nervous, and beats his mother and breaks everything. Paolo is eight years old and in the third grade of elementary school. Lidia has begun the first year of middle school. Following the intervention of Social Services, it is discovered that the family is very neglectful and abusive.

The extended family network, well-known to local services for sensitive incidents of family abuse and maltreatment, cannot guarantee any support because it is deemed to be devoid of trust, respect, and resources. Juvenile Court, judging the parents incapable of fulfilling their responsibilities, entrusts the children to social services. Lidia and Paolo are placed in care – two different residences but ones which are part of the same facility. The parents have the right to a weekly visit.

3. The Evolution of the Therapeutic Journey: The Post-Traumatic Reaction as the Creative Adaptation of the Self

The weeks flow by one after another while the meetings seem to repeat the same *clichés* over and over. Lidia, slumped in the armchair, goes from a deafening silence, in which everything in the room seems heavy and oppressive, to moments of energetic excitement in which she begins to weave foul-mouthed gibberish whose objective is to "contaminate", not only the space and time which we struggle to create, but also the effort of the person patiently endeavouring to give her the possibility of "creating a home" in a reassuring place that provides an atmosphere of "protection and care". The clinical work with a minor, who lives in a care home, cannot be thought of as a "closed door" therapy. Although combating, in fact, the protective treatment space from abusive invasions, and always keeping the therapeutic aim abundantly clear, the therapist has to keep in mind the reality of the surroundings – a reality made up of anxieties and delicate moments, in which there is an interplay of different figures: police, judges, neuro-psychiatrists, social workers, but also families of origin and foster families. A psychotherapist knows that it is not possible to be an active part of this process but keeps informed of the facts and the delicate moments in the legal process, not only because in these moments the support to provide the child becomes more important, but also because in these stages, the traumatic memories, which the child has dissociated in order to continue to survive, very often are exacerbated and reactivated by means of symptoms and disturbances of various kinds. These are moments that must be managed "by more than one set of hands", with a knowledgeable and skilled network, in order to allow the child or the "injured" adolescent to be able to benefit from the emotional compensation and make sense of the experience suffered. Complex trauma, namely the set of symptoms that results from cumulative interpersonal traumas and which is experienced over the course of development, undermines the basis itself of existence, compromising self-image, trust, and relationships. The clinical framework becomes more articulated and complex in the work with children since, if repeated abuse in adult life threatens the securities of a personality already formed, in childhood, a traumatic experience has the potential to deform the developing personality, which is also vulnerable from a physiological viewpoint. In this regard, Spagnuolo Lobb (2016a, p. 38) states: "The foundation of security that a mother provides the child is the "given" ground with which the child faces the world". For Gestalt psychotherapy, the child builds the experience of the self thanks to the "dance" with the significant figures: he/she learns, knows him/herself, and grows at the contact boundary with the other, experiencing mutual attunement and resonance between him/herself and the adult (compare Spagnuolo Lobb, 2018). In Gestalt psychotherapy, the self is considered the experience of the world (cf. Spagnuolo Lobb, 2016b). The contacts acquired contribute to the building of the experiential ground of the self and this explains how early relational traumas can interfere with the normal development of the person in various areas, giving rise to pervasive damage and complex psycho-pathological situations. I am touched by Lidia's wariness and at the same time by her curiosity. I grasp her intentionality, suffocated by ambivalent emotions: on the one hand, I feel her desire and her curiosity to want to meet me; on the other hand, I sense her fear of this contact, in which I strongly discern her blocking of trust. In addition, the abused child lives hidden between the desperate need to be seen, recognised, and the need to put up extremely high walls, to avoid leaking anything that could expose the distressing experience. After around three months from our first meeting, Lidia asks the care-workers for the first time if she can move the session forward. I accept her proposal without hesitation; I feel that it represents a good possible opening. Lidia is beginning to experience that maybe the "time together" (a time that never seems to flow but just to stand still), despite her constant attacks, does not get shaken up, but is stable and ready to embrace her. Her words are striking when she turns up for the appointment. She asks me: "How long do I have to spend in this room?" "As long as you like", I answer her. "Tell me, how long would you like to be here?" "Not more than fifteen minutes," she answers, "I have nothing to say to you!" I look at the clock on the wall: it's 4:15 P.M. "Then we have only fifteen minutes. At 4:30, we'll say good-by, and if you want, we will meet again, but only if you want." Lidia looks at me and agrees. She tells me, with few but essential words, and only at my instigation, about her "new school". Then, she asks me when she can go to the other care centre to see her brother, to help him with his homework. Time passes quickly, but I have not forgotten our pact. I interrupt her and point to the clock. It is 4:30. Lidia looks at me surprised. She does not say anything. Perhaps she would have liked to continue. I ask her if she is willing to come again. She nods. Then, when she reaches the door, she wants me to know that she will only come if she hasn't already gone home. Her sly look, her mumbling reply, her holding back and taking her time represent her creative adaptation; the best possible solution, the cleverest, for creating and generating a semblance of security, which can help her to withstand the tough situations into which she has been forced. She leaves the room, her body still stiff. She turns around, looks at me, raises her hand, a slight gesture, a farewell, a small sign.

I feel that something is changing. In terms of the process, what strikes me and touches me, in this wish of hers to keep her distance, is the spurt of courage and her cautious audacity. I read it as a positive possibility – the cocoon of a nascent desire to open up. I would like to pass on this feeling of mine to her, but I feel that the way I proceed must be prudent, in order to give her the opportunity to experiment with a "right time" to feel comfortable, secure, at home. I await, with confidence, her step, her sign.

My feelings, unfiltered by any interpretation, my *Aesthetic Relational Knowledge* (Spagnuolo Lobb, 2016a, 2018), becomes the compass that allows me to intuit the intentionalities of contact not made explicit by Lidia. Our relationship is slowly becoming the topsoil in which small seedlings, which are involved with new processes of a transformative kind, are beginning to take root. My way of being, together with Lidia's small responses, creates "that something more" capable of modifying and enriching our perceptions. Other elements of novelty are added to our way of encountering each other. The therapeutic change, made up of small and brave steps, is born out of an implicit shared relationship, comprised of those *now moments* (cf. Stern, 1985, 2004) that destabilise the present. These are the precise small elements of novelty that, if they are taken advantage of in an opportune manner, make change and the building of our relational ground possible.

And it is in this way that the encounters, week after week, become more anticipated by Lidia. The time for "being together" gets longer and longer even if often, a sheet of silence suddenly seems to envelop her, as she becomes shorter of breath. It is precisely at such times that the need to move, to wander about the room, and escape contact seems strong. Step by step, the continuity of the space and of "patient time", which little by little we are able to co-create, is configured like a fundamental therapeutic action. We are learning to know each other, to "make small things together", to weave the mesh of a new way of meeting one another, to experience that nascent security capable of breaking down the wall of mistrust and worry, behind which Lidia has remained cornered. In the meantime, the care-workers observe and then report on the weekly meetings made with the parents. These are moments of confidences whispered in the ear, of winks and promises made allusively, which make Lidia nervous. After the visits, she appears more irritated and uncontrollable. The workers in the centre in which Paolo, the brother, resides, are beginning to observe highly sexualised behaviours and language in the boy. Once in a while, Paolo makes small and confused revelations in which he speaks of family scenes mixed with physical and sexual violence, revelations which later are invariably retracted after having spent time playing with his sister Lidia in the common garden of the two residences. Following these warning signs, Juvenile Court interrupts the parents' weekly visits and the meetings between the siblings begin to be monitored. After a few weeks, Paolo and Lidia are summoned to the Office of the Prosecutor. Before the Prosecutor and the appointed expert, Paolo says nothing. Lidia leaves the Courthouse very angry and annoyed: "You have to leave my brother alone. . . . You only need me, and there's nothing to say anyway!" We well know that very often you cannot superimpose the timing of the court over that of the minor, and therefore, in compliance with the Public Prosecutor, in order to avoid impositions and pressures which could be configured as abuse within abuse, or rather "institutional abuse", the meetings in the legal framework are suspended to give Lidia the time necessary to soften her rigid contact modalities, imprinted onto her control of herself and the situation. After this hearing, Lidia begins to have bad dreams. In the middle of the night, she screams in terror, waking up her roommates. She often wets the bed. It is clear that the signs, symptoms, and behaviours are small pieces, which have to be read and recomposed in order to be able to reveal their full complexity and the totality of the picture. Even during the day, Lidia is becoming more aggressive; this is what the care-workers are writing in the log book. She reacts with kicks, punches, and threatening language. She approaches others looking for a physical confrontation. In our meetings, too, Lidia exceeds the window of emotional tolerance: Her body stiffens, she clenches her jaw, she grinds her teeth, and once again she goes back to attacking with gestures and tough and overbearing attitudes, unaccompanied by speech.

The holistic perspective of Gestalt psychotherapy, in highlighting that "the whole is always greater than the sum of its parts", has always emphasised the central role of the body, fundamental in the creation of emotion and meaning. Contemporary neural science, through the clinical evidence of *neuro images*, has confirmed the intuitions of the Gestalt psychotherapy founders, underscoring that the mind has an innate tendency towards integration, while traumatic situations, by creating stiffness and fractures, block this natural tendency.

The Gestalt therapist's eyes are focussed on the somatic narrative in order to be able to observe phenomenologically the process more than the content. Attention only to thoughts and only to words, in fact, can keep the therapy at a superficial level in that, very often, in abusive situations, words are absent, while everything is hidden beneath a thick blanket of the unspeakable.

What therefore becomes important – together with the building of the ground – is that skilled work of emotional regulation, necessary to begin to put together, in a delicate task of stitching, sensations, emotions, and words (compare Siegel, 1999; Dana, 2018). Staying emotionally regulated, attentive, and accepting towards a defensive adolescent is fundamental for building trust.

I watch Lidia, her outburst, her nervous posture, and her agitated gestures. After remaining steadfast with my senses open and attuning myself to her emotional states, I use my firm and reassuring voice to bring her back into the space of the here-and-now, where one can give voice to pain and the unspeakable.

4. The Here-and-Now: The Vitality of Contact and the Development of the Relationship

One day, I give her a present of a binder with coloured pages and I invite her to put down her thoughts, fears, and desires. I explain to her that this is a technique

I use with other children to enable me to know them better and to help them feel better. They are small and simple instruments that enrich my "tool kit": exercises, drawings, and stories that vary on the basis of age and aim, not only to create the foundation for meticulous and difficult clinical work but also to make that terrain fertile. This is to bring to light small seedlings of awareness that concern sensations and emotions that have been buried inside serious and painful memories.

As Spagnuolo Lobb states (2016a, p. 33), we can say that a child psychotherapist who deals with relational traumas must possess skills capable of being harmoniously integrated with each other. One must know how to read the complexity of the relational, emotional, and social components of which the injured child is the carrier. One must know how to recognise the signals and the modalities with which the young victim expresses malaise. What is needed is to integrate Gestalt clinical work on children and adolescents with models of development and of child psychopathology, with the neurobiology of complex trauma and with the traumatic experiences (cf. Finkelhor and Browne, 1985) of the different forms of maltreatment, without forgetting the experiential ground and the pathological dynamics of the abusive families. Moreover, the therapist is also required to have the *know-how*, that is, to have a large "tool kit" to use in the various and challenging phases of therapy, precisely when it is very difficult for words to take shape and find their voice. Ultimately, the psychotherapist is called upon to *know how to be*, namely to possess that important emotional preparation, the result of meticulous work on his/her own grey areas.

It is necessary, when faced with the ambivalent experiences of the child, for the therapist to avoid having "smudged glasses", which could prevent the recognition of aesthetic emotions that are activated in the phenomenological field. This failure of recognition could undermine the delicate process of taking charge and the complicated therapeutic process as well.

For Lidia, too, the pages, pens, and coloured pencils become the bridge for creating contact exactly where words struggle to come out. Lidia looks at me perplexed, takes the package, and with surprise in her eyes, while she scrutinises everything, adds in a faint voice: "But I don't know how to draw, I just can't, I'm all thumbs, I really suck at this, too!" As often happens to victimised children, Lidia, suffocated by a fierce sense of self-contempt and lack of value, says the same words over and over. She is almost embarrassed in front of this gift which she accepts with surprise, but for which she is convinced of being undeserving. "But can I really keep it? Is it really mine?" Having grown up in an uncertain unpredictable environment, and not having been seen in her childhood needs, Lidia has gone forward with the clear-cut perception of "not being worth anything", of "not measuring up". She drags with difficulty the heavy weight of this stigma, which becomes even more exacerbated when she finds herself facing her peers.

Living the experience first-hand that relationships, even those that are certain and taken for granted, are not a source of security and trust, has created a stagnant and muddy ground, from which it is difficult to get free.

Her reticent ways and the need to hide herself, to withdraw from contact seem to be the only expedient for not being swallowed up in that flurry of sensations that make her feel inadequate, bad, and impotent. Uneasy and awkward, both in words and movement, Lidia, surprised and excited by the unexpected gift, sketches an uncertain heart on the first pink page, the one "of pretty things". Inside the heart she writes her name and mine, too: "Diary of Lidia and Rosanna". She smiles shyly as she is intent on colouring. The she looks up "to see" where I am, if I'm looking at her, if my attention is on her. I am right there – still, solid, accepting. Lidia smiles again, her body more relaxed. With pride, she puts the pink sheet back into the binder. Small and proud gestures that give the *sense of us*, of our growing relationship made up of effort, courage, and a great commitment to be able to dismantle the introjections necessary for the re-construction of the Self. It is thanks to the use of creative techniques and tools, invented from time to time, that Lidia is beginning to give voice to the unspeakable nature of her feelings and emotions, and to give order to her thoughts that have been disrupted by that warped view of life, unfortunately penetrating her in an overwhelming way. Through the game of "let's crack the ugly secrets", Lidia outlines in her notebook, in clear and precise words, the vanquished borders of her self, made small and fragile by malevolent relational intrusions. After having written entire pages of "I can't say it, I don't know how to say it", in which she lets the threat and injunction to keep silent emerge, always telegraphically, she abandons resistance and begins to give voice to the fear and the need to find someone who may be ready to believe her and accept her painful story ("and if then they don't believe me? What could happen? If no one will believe what I say?"). The revelation proceeds in fits and starts, but we well know, as the literature abundantly confirms[2] that the divulging is not made of one single event; it does not follow the logic of all or nothing. Revealing is a process, an uneven and torturous path, difficult to traverse. Lidia, suffocated by fear, by shame, trapped by and adapted to an ignoble vision of life, goes from wanting to vomit to holding back. It is difficult to give voice to what she has lived through. In the face of the surfacing of her memories, still too fresh, she tends to run away, to become estranged, enacting attitudes of distancing and flight. It is difficult to name the obscenity and the inner upheaval. If, on the one hand, the pain seems to soften and melt; on the other, in an abrupt and overbearing way, she often returns to poisoning, making it physically difficult for her to be in the "here-and-now". The oval of her face becomes tough, is transformed into a mask of pain and struggle; her eyes go back to eluding, as she seems to chew on bitter words, and suffocate her sobs, and hold her fear inside.

The involvement of Claudia, a member of the care staff, into our meeting space becomes fundamental for working better, for reinforcing Lidia's courage, for acknowledging those small flashes in which her ability to move and take action is glimpsed, and for finally dismantling the veil of secrecy. The work in collaboration with the Prosecutor's Office – which is waiting for the "right moment" to meet Lidia – also becomes important, as well as with local services which, unfortunately, continue to tell a story of an absolutely incompetent parental couple, who ignore every appointment and show no sign whatsoever of being open to discussion. Eventually we learn that the mother has moved to northern Italy because she has a new partner.

5. The Work on Shame

The relational ground, that sense of security that is born out of our encounter, becomes a more and more solid one, helping Lidia to get to know herself a little more, and to become more mistress of herself, of her feelings and emotions. She is learning to find, within the therapeutic space, and through the hard work of stabilisation, mirroring, and connection, alternative strategies to her explosive anger. She is learning to feel that "right heat" and that confidence that will carry her beyond the therapy space, and allow her to make more significant relationships with her peers and with the other child-care workers, to ask for advice, to begin to confide in others, and to live an "almost normal" adolescence. It is within this new openness that it becomes crucial to work on shame – a very real barrier to emotions, making the therapeutic process difficult, and risking condemning to isolation the still fragile young victim, whose borders are blurred. Shame, in trauma work, even more so if the trauma is complex, plays a central role because it is the result of a pervasive sense of inadequacy, vulnerability, and self-hatred, continually aggravated by the beliefs and meanings that the victims have attributed to the experiences of humiliation and fear.

Lidia, like a slow and heavy snail, bears on her very own shoulders a cumbersome burden, of which her body conserves the memory.

Shame is an absolutely destabilising emotion, which requires a gradual and modulated approach. Confronting it means venturing into a world of great pain, in which it is easy to become dysregulated, by losing one's anchor in the present and one's connection to the therapist. The heart of the intervention has as its aim to work through, one step at a time, the pain tied to the traumatic experiences of the past, in order to dissolve the rigid *gestalts* of the malevolent relationships previously experienced, without however generating overwhelming emotions and without re-traumatising the patient during the therapeutic process itself. Often, in trauma work, the ability or the wish to remember is mixed up with the terrifying fear of reliving the experience one has endured. For this reason, it becomes important to guide the patient, with compassion and empathy, to achieve small steps, in order to experience and feel, without any forcing, just "a granule at a time of that serious malaise that immobilises and swallows him/her, pulling along the mind and the body from the "here-and-now" into the "there-and-then" (cf. Kepner, 1993; Taylor, 2014, 2015).

Lidia is being supported, by means of small exercises, to be in the present, to trust in the safe space that we have created together, thus being able to give voice, in unhurried fashion, to a burning sense of unease that runs right through her.

Finally, she can explore that compassion towards herself as it becomes a health-giving ray of light, at first faint and then more and more radiant. It has now become possible for her to accept that sense of vulnerability tied to her inability to fight back – that unbearable fallibility for not having been a mindful and caring sister with regard to Paolo. For the purposes of giving adequate voice to shame, we draw a mountain together. The goal is to be well-equipped before the climb, in order to be able to reach the top, learning, step by step, to observe ourselves and the world from a different perspective. Every "climbing" movement, even if laborious and full of pain, is a small step that allows one to go forward and loosen the tight grip of humiliation. Every step towards the summit becomes a small and important conquest, able to help Lidia to have a new awareness, necessary to give her the strength to return once again to the notebook and recount what is too hard to put into words.

6. An Experiential Field Which Enables the Integration of the Body, Emotions, and Words

And so it is like this that her feelings, imbued with disgust, impotence, and horror, leak out in tiny droplets. Evermore a participant and a trusting one, she is able to reveal in her notebook the important fragments linked to the sad events ("My father kissed me in the mouth, in the bed, the big bed, he said to me, I love you too much . . . what can I do?") the story becomes clearer and clearer, vivid and all too raw, a story of inappropriate touching, of being forced onto the big bed to watch pornographic videos, the better to learn and then satisfy the instincts of that perverted adult. He, stripped in every sense of the word of his protective role, disrupted and rendered Lidia's self-in-the-making even weaker, confusing the grammar of the affective register with that of the distinctly sexual ("you're really good! You're better than your mother"). The written words, in a trembling script, make palpable the immediate attack on the self and on the functions of the ground. The body, profaned in its integrity, has been the theatre where the sad experiences were consummated. The indignity is unspeakable. Unutterable is the pain of a body not only objectified, but humiliated and seized in its subjectivity literally by the one who was supposed to protect it. The attack undermines the personality function of the Self at its foundations ("are you better than your mother?"). Lidia doesn't know who she is (Is she the daughter? Has she been the partner? Has she stolen the place of her mother?). She has endured a pervasive outrage so severe as to make the ground, acquired through identity certainties, collapse.

Clinical work is hard and taxing. But Lidia, recognised by now in her daring for having shattered the violation and the preoccupation with not being believed, confirmed in her value as a person, is also able to give voice to the trauma-inducing experiences (Finkelhor and Brown, 1985) of which abuse is the ultimate carrier. Tears finally trickle down onto the blue pages of the notebook, now managing to tell the story of impotence and deceit ("what could I do? He said it would be the last time"), but also the sense of guilt for not having protected her little brother ("I haven't been a good sister . . . my brother has suffered for everything that he has seen, but I didn't know how to defend him") and once again the sense of betrayal, the indignation towards her mother and the adults in the family, who, though knowing, did not do anything to stop the obscenity ("my mother has always been weak, and then she got engaged to someone else, she was no longer interested in us; my uncle, my father's brother, knew everything. He told my father off when I tracked him down, but then everything always went back to the way it was before.") The therapeutic journey with Lidia continues on a weekly basis. Much work has been done, but much remains to be done. However, we have reached the time to take on the stress of the pre-trial hearing, in which the presence of the psychotherapist is required as psychological support. Lidia knows that I cannot enter the room, but she also knows that I am there, that I will be there. During the course of the interrogation, conducted by the auxiliary of Justice, she manages, in a heartfelt way, and with a statement, to be absolutely consistent and congruent with her words, to not only make clear and unambiguous the story of the reprehensible events, but she is also able to finally release the tears and that host of sensations that she has learned to feel in her body, to recognise in her emotions, and to tell with the right words.

Notes

1 Aesthetic relational knowing can be considered as a tool by means of which the therapist resonates with the patient during the course of the session, a sort of lens through which he looks at the patient's life situation. It moreover allows the therapist to grasp the implicit intentionality of contact with which the patient experiences the contact boundary (cf. Spagnuolo Lobb, 2013, pp. 35–36, 2018).
2 Compare Carini et al., 2001; Roccia, 2001; Malacrea and Lorenzini, 2002; Foti, 2001, 2007; Fergusson and Mullen, 1999; Luberti and Pedrocco Biancardi, 2005; Castellazzi, 2007; Dettore and Fuligni, 2008; D'Ambrosio, 2010; Cartei and Grosso, 2016; Onofri and La Rosa, 2017.

References

Carini, A., Pedrocco Biancardi, M. T., & Soavi, G. (2001). L'abuso sessuale intrafamiliare [Intrafamilial sexual abuse]. Milano: Raffaello Cortina Editore.

Cartei, V., & Grosso, F. (2016). Oltre il silenzio. Come elaborare e superare il trauma dell'abuso subito nell'infanzia [Beyond the silence. How to process and overcome the trauma of childhood abuse]. Milano: FrancoAngeli.

Castellazzi, V. L. (2007). L'Abuso Sessuale all'Infanzia [Childhood Sexual Abuse]. Roma: LAS.

D'Ambrosio, C. (2010). L'abuso infantile. Tutela del minore in ambito terapeutico giuridico e sociale [Child abuse. Protection of the child in the therapeutic legal and social context]. Trento: Erickson.

Dana, D. (2018). The polyvagal theory in therapy: Engaging the rhythm of regulation. New York: W.W. Norton & Co Inc.

Dettore, D., & Fuligni, C. (2008). L'abuso sessuale sui minori. Valutazione e terapia delle vittime e dei responsabili [Child sexual abuse. Assessment and treatment of victims and perpetrators]. New York, NY: McGraw-Hill.

Fergusson, D. M., & Mullen, P. E. (1999). *Childhood sexual abuse: An evidence based perspective*. Thousand Oaks: Sage.

Finkelhor, D., & Browne, A. (1985). The traumatic impact of child sexual abuse: A conceptualization. *American Journal of Orthopsychiatry*, *55*(4), 530–541. DOI: 10.1111/j.1939-0025.1985.tb02703.x.

Foti, C. (Ed.). (2001). *L'ascolto dell'abuso e l'abuso dell'ascolto* [The listening of abuse and the abuse of listening]. Milano: FrancoAngeli.

Foti, C. (2007). *Psicoterapia dei bambini e degli adulti vittime di violenza* [Psychotherapy of children and adult victims of violence]. Torino: S.I.E. Edizioni.

Kepner, J. (1993). *Body process: A Gestalt approach to working with the body in psychotherapy*. San Francisco, CA: Jossey-Bass.

Luberti, R., & Pedrocco Biancardi, M. T. (2005). *La violenza assistita intrafamiliare* [Intrafamilial witnessing violence]. Milano: FrancoAngeli.

Malacrea, M., & Lorenzini, S. (2002). *Bambini Abusati. Linee Guida nel Dibattito Internazionale* [Abused children. Guidelines in the international debate]. Milano: Raffaello Cortina Editore.

Militello, R. (2011). Il trauma dell'abuso e il delicato processo della riparazione: come ridare voce e corpo al bambino violato. Intervista a Marinella Malacrea [The trauma of abuse and the delicate process of reparation: How to give voice and body back to the violated child. Interview with Marinella Malacrea]. *Quaderni di Gestalt*, *XXIV*(1), 11–21. DOI: 10.3280/GEST2011-001002.

Onofri, A., & La Rosa, C. (2017). *Trauma, abuso e violenza. Andare oltre il dolore* [Trauma, abuse, and violence. Moving beyond pain]. Milano: Edizioni San Paolo.

Roccia, C. (2001). *Riconoscere ed ascoltare il Trauma* [Recognising and listening to Trauma]. Milano: FrancoAngeli.

Siegel, D. J. (1999). *The developing mind: Toward a neurobiology of interpersonal experience*. New York: Guilford Press.

Spagnuolo Lobb, M. (2013). *The now-for-next in psychotherapy: Gestalt therapy recounted in post-modern society*. Siracusa: Istituto di Gestalt HCC Italy Publ. Co., www.gestalt italy.com.

Spagnuolo Lobb, M. (2015). The body as a "vehicle" of our being in the world. Somatic experience in Gestalt therapy. *British Gestalt Journal*, *24*(2), 21–31.

Spagnuolo Lobb, M. (2016a). Self as contact, contact as self. A contribution to ground experience in Gestalt Therapy theory of self. In J.-M. Robine (Ed.). *Self. A poliphony of contemporary Gestalt therapists* (pp. 261–289). St. Romain la Virvée, France: L'Exprimerie.

Spagnuolo Lobb, M. (2016b). Gestalt therapy with children. Supporting the polyphonic development of domains in a field of contacts. In M. Spagnuolo Lobb, N. Levi, & A. Williams (Eds.). *Gestalt therapy with children. From epistemology to clinical practice* (pp. 25–62). Siracusa: Istituto di Gestalt HCC Italy, www.gestaltitaly.com.

Spagnuolo Lobb, M. (2017). From losses of ego functions to the dance steps between psychotherapist and client. Phenomenology and aesthetics of contact in the psychotherapeutic field. *British Gestalt Journal*, *26*(1), 28–37.

Spagnuolo Lobb, M. (2018). Aesthetic relational knowledge of the field: A revised concept of awareness in Gestalt therapy and contemporary psychiatry. *Gestalt Review*, *22*(1), 50–68. DOI: 10.5325/gestalt review.22.1.0050.

Stern, D. N. (1985). *The interpersonal world of the infant: A view from psychoanalysis and developmental psychology*. New York: Basic Books.

Stern, D. N. (2004). *The present moment in psychotherapy and everyday life*. New York: W.W. Norton & Company Inc.

Taylor, M. (2014). *Trauma therapy and clinical practice. neuroscience, Gestalt and the body*. Maidenhead, UK: Open University Press and McGraw-Hill Education.

Taylor, M. (2015). Uno sfondo sicuro: utilizzo dell'approccio senso motorio nel trauma [A safe background: Using the sense-motor approach in trauma]. *Quaderni di Gestalt, XXVIII*(1), DOI: 10.3280/GEST2015-001002.

Chapter 9

To Be or Not to Be Autistic

From the *Camouflage* Effect to *Élan Vital* – A Gestalt Perspective

Antonio Narzisi

1. What Is Autism Spectrum Disorder?

The identification of autism as a clinical disorder can be traced back to two nearly contemporaneous studies. The first by Kanner (1943) described children characterised by the absence of social interests, the tendency to be alone, intolerance to change, restricted and stereotyped interests, language impairments, and reduced cognitive abilities; the second, in 1944, by Asperger (1944), described equally lonely subjects with restricted interests but without cognitive and language impairment. Kanner's autism and Asperger's syndrome became the two clinical extremes of what are currently referred to as Autism Spectrum Disorders (ASD) and are characterised by two elements: 1) persistent deficits in social communication and social interaction in multiple contexts; and 2) restricted and repetitive patterns of behaviour, interests, or activities (APA, 2013).

According to the Center for Disease Control and Prevention (CDC), the incidence of ASD, which has progressively increased over the years, is 1 child per 54 years (Maenner *et al.*, 2020; Narzisi *et al.*, 2018). This epidemiological report posits ASD as a non-random disorder with important social and health effects. For many years, the etiological hypotheses of ASD were based on the idea that the child was neurologically healthy and that the cause of ASD was to be found solely in the inappropriate relationship with a "refrigerator" mother (Betthelheim, 1967). For almost forty years this etiological hypothesis, now considered inappropriate, has dominated the international clinical scene.

Currently, the Autism Spectrum Disorders are considered the expression of a specific pathological process that, from polygenetic factors (definitely present but only in small part identified), involves an atypical development of the brain architecture responsible for the clinical behavioural disorder. The fact that ASD can be better understood as a genetic and neurobiological dysfunction has progressively led to the development of therapeutic models more consistent and congruent with the specificity of the associated neuro-cognitive and psychopathological deficits. In particular, research on the role that experience plays in gene expression and the construction of brain anatomy is laying the groundwork for treatments that can modify brain function and structure. These are not just simple and/or

DOI: 10.4324/9781003313335-12

forced behavioural modifications. Interventions for ASD can be placed along a continuum with interventions based on behaviourist theory on one end (behavioural approaches) and developmental approaches on the other (developmental approaches). According to this perspective, which is evolving today, all interventions can be placed within a continuum from highly structured, therapist-driven behavioural approaches to less structured approaches that follow the child's interests and intentionality, based on a program that aims to facilitate the child's progress by following a typical developmental trajectory (within the latter type of interventions we can include the Gestalt psychotherapy approach) (Narzisi, 2020; Narzisi and Muccio, 2015; Ospina *et al.*, 2008).

The main purpose of this chapter is to describe the experience of a young girl with ASD through the story of her developmental growth. The passage from the so-called *camouflage effect* to the development of an intra and interpersonal identity identified by the progressive separation of organism and environment will be examined.

2. The *camouflage* Effect in Autism Spectrum Disorder

In contrast to people who receive diagnoses during childhood, some individuals are identified late in life and may fly under the diagnostic radar for many years, in part because of learned strategies to hide social-relational difficulties. Late-diagnosed individuals tend to experience psychological distress attributable to the long-term stress generated by forced adaptation to daily life (Lai and Baron-Cohen, 2015; Lai *et al.*, 2017).

Due to reduced environmental support and pressure to adapt to neurotypical social communication, individuals with ASD may develop dysfunctional coping strategies in the face of developmentally appropriate coping. One such coping strategy is to be able to "disguise" difficulties during social situations (Lai *et al.*, 2017), hiding behaviours that might be considered socially unacceptable in order to "behave artificially" i.e., assume social attitudes that are considered neurotypical. In other words, they pretend not to be autistic (Lai *et al.*, 2019).

Examples of camouflage may include making eye contact during conversation, using learned phrases or pre-prepared jokes in conversation, imitating the social behaviour of others, imitating facial expressions or gestures, and learning and executing strict social scripts (Lai *et al.*, 2017; Lai and Baron-Cohen, 2015). Therefore, it is possible for these individuals to consciously learn to speak more discreetly and/or not stand too close to another person and/or not make personal remarks, perhaps modelling behaviour on a neurotypical peer in order to gain greater social acceptance. However, autobiographical descriptions and clinical observations suggest that camouflage often unfortunately comes at a very high cost in terms of psychological health. It often requires considerable cognitive effort, can be exhausting, and can lead to increased stress, even a developmental breakdown caused by social overload and experienced in terms of social anxiety (Spagnuolo Lobb, 2001, 2016), depression, and even negative impact on one's identity development (Lai *et al.*, 2011, 2017).

Population-based data show that girls are often diagnosed later in life (Lai *et al.*, 2017; Rynkiewicz *et al.*, 2016; Green *et al.*, 2019; Dean *et al.*, 2017; Young *et al.*, 2018) and less easily than boys with autism (Parish-Morris *et al.*, 2017; Schuck *et al.*, 2019), unless there are competing behavioural or cognitive challenges (Lai *et al.*, 2020). One potential reason for this could be the increased tendency to camouflage difficulties in many girls with autism spectrum disorder. When difficulties with social interaction and communication are camouflaged, signs of ASD are less likely to be detected by families, teachers, or primary care physicians who are more unlikely to ask for a specific assessment.

For this reason, clinicians and researchers have described a greater tendency of the camouflage phenomenon in girls as opposed to boys with autism (Lai *et al.*, 2017; Ratto *et al.*, 2018; Cage and Burton, 2019; Hull *et al.*, 2017; Lai *et al.*, 2015; Head *et al.*, 2014). Improving our understanding of camouflage, along with other possible "female autism phenotypes," could further facilitate the identification of diagnostic symptomatology by improving ASD detection and appropriate early support.

Although camouflage has often been described as a major characteristic of girls with autism, it has received surprisingly little systematic scientific investigation (Lai *et al.*, 2017). As reported in the research paper by Lai *et al.* (2017), in a recent qualitative study, Tierney *et al.* (2016) interviewed 10 adolescent girls with autism about the social challenges associated with adolescence and analysed the data using interpretive phenomenological analysis. These girls reported developing explicit strategies for managing social relationships over the years, specifically imitation and *camouflage*.

Hiller *et al.* (2014) compared school-aged boys and girls clinically diagnosed with autism and showed that both groups met clinical criteria in different ways. In particular, some differences could have underpinned or reflected a greater camouflage effect in girls. For example, girls were more likely to be able to integrate nonverbal and verbal behaviours, have better imagery, maintain reciprocal conversation, and initiate (but not maintain) friendships. These characteristics appeared to have an ecological impact, as school teachers reported significantly less concern with girls (compared to boys) with autism regarding their social skills, friendships, and externalising behavioural problems (Hiller *et al.*, 2014).

These pioneering studies indicate that camouflage can be conceptualised as the use of learned social communicative behaviours to mask the underlying difficulties associated with autism.

3. The Meeting With A.

A. is a 19-year-old girl who lives in Rome. She was referred to my office by a psychotherapist colleague who had been working with her for some time. A.'s diagnosis is anxiety disorder. Because of the severity of the disorder, A. is being treated with psychotropic drugs that only partially succeed in alleviating her suffering. The good psychotherapist colleague senses that A.'s diagnosis only partially responds to the girl's need for identity definition.

She feels that in A.'s phenotypic profile there is probably something more correctly ascribable to autistic disorder. For this reason, the colleague talked to A. and asked her if she would like to go to Pisa to investigate her clinical condition. A. accepted and together with her parents spent two days in the city of the leaning tower. During those two days, I saw A. several times, and together we began a clinical-diagnostic process that would involve both the girl and her parents in a setting that integrates the transgenerational component. A. was well-groomed and demonstrated herself to be compliant towards the psychodiagnostic investigation. Her language has a peculiar prosodic tone; it is characterised by a low and tendentially mechanical tone. Her nonverbal communication presents a narrow range of conventional and descriptive acts. In terms of reciprocal social interaction, A.'s gaze is present but does not appear adequately fluid, modulated, and integrated with other communication channels. The quality of the social initiative is reduced; the response to the initiatives of the interlocutor is instead adequate. From a motor point of view, A. is rather static, moves little, and appears extremely constricted. Breathing is intermittent and the girl presents a manifest disorder of state and trait anxiety. She immediately appeared to be very motivated in the dialogue exchange and during the two days of interviews, something unpredictable happened both for me and for her. In the next two paragraphs, I will report: (a) A.'s experience through her personal testimony; and (b) a critical description of the therapeutic process.

3.1 A.'s Testimony: From camouflage Effect to élan vital

Thinking back to my childhood and adolescence, I sometimes wonder what difference it would have made to have been diagnosed with autism when I was younger instead of at 19.

Honestly, I don't know if it would have been a good thing or a bad thing, but certainly my life would have been very different. Even as a child, I taught myself to develop different methods to help me with various difficulties in everyday life, difficulties that my peers didn't seem to have.

This always left me pretty perplexed, because I never even had the option of being able to think that there was an explanation for my differences, and so instead I started to think that my experiences as an autistic child were common to everyone, and that others were just doing a better job of putting up with everything than I was.

I maintained this mindset from elementary school until I was 17 years old. It was far from an easy time, because the social, emotional, and even sensory demands with age only get more complicated. An image that I can use to explain a bit how I felt was that everyone had a manual in which were written all the rules for effective communication with others, and I was the only one who did not have a copy. The only solution was to try it time after time, to see what worked and what didn't, often imitating the behaviours of others to try to blend in better. The other solution was to isolate myself as much as possible by being shy, since that at least was a form of social ineptitude that was relatively more accepted by my peers.

Obviously, this situation leads to a state of extreme loneliness. The only way I could make friends, once I stopped trying in the more traditional method – it was tiring and ended up hurting more than anything else – was to wait for them to somehow drop from the sky into my lap by serendipity, which means I can count all the friends I've ever had on the fingers of two hands. I don't regret it though, and I am absolutely convinced that I made the best choice for me by giving up my clumsy attempts at socialisation. This alone only emphasised my situation, which day by day seemed more alien than what my peers seemed to be experiencing.

I still had no idea why I couldn't socialise, why I couldn't stand the long school days spent in contact with my classmates, and all the difficulties I was experiencing. I was in a state of extreme isolation. I didn't know how to come to terms with it, and here comes to my rescue technology, especially the computer, and even more specifically, the internet. What a lifeline that has been. We've all heard people complain that we young people are always attached to the computer (and later, attached to our cell phones), that we should look around and talk to the people next to us, etc. Certainly this position has some merit in some cases, but for people like me who can't or prefer for whatever reason not to socialise with people close to them, and who need a place to retreat to recharge and better deal with the day's commitments, what better tool can there be than the internet? Do you have a particular interest that people close to you don't share because it's unusual for your age, or maybe because it involves something unfamiliar? If you search for it on the internet, you'll come up with at least four or five forums full of people who are just as excited about it as you are. And that helps. If you can't find someone among your acquaintances who understands you, online someone who shares your experiences in some way, your interests, you find them. So it was for me, too – I have two friends, one from England and one from Canada, whom I would never have met otherwise. Without them, people with whom I could talk normally and from whom I could find support for my everyday life, who knows if I would ever have been able to recognise that, in fact, my experience was not common to the people I knew.

At that point I was 16, 17, and had honestly reached a breaking point. I was burdened with keeping up a facade of normalcy (or rather, a facade of not being autistic, hiding the characteristics that made me stand out as 'different'), I was constantly in a state of anxiety, and I had no idea how I could move forward. No one I knew here understood what I was facing, but the friends I previously mentioned did. And for the first time, I had finally realised that in fact my experience was qualitatively different from others'. A first sigh of relief, after 17 years of living – my problems and social ineptitude were probably not my fault. It was a small sigh of relief though, because as I had mentioned before I was extremely anxious, and who knows, maybe I was faking it all. Obviously, that wasn't true, but it's not like anxiety is the most rational thing ever. I had a beginning, but that was all it was – it explained certain symptoms, but not why I was anxious and depressed in the first place.

And a year later, I am offered what seemed like just a word, autism. Oh. I don't think anyone who hasn't been in that situation can really understand the sense of relief I felt in that moment. Guilt and inadequacy? No More. Doubt that I was faking it? At an all-time low. I was reborn. That's why I'm curious about what would have happened if I'd had that designation earlier. Then again, so many of the problems I had weren't caused by the autism itself, but by the lack of understanding I had of myself.

And now that I know I'm autistic? So much has changed. I have learned to retrieve methods that I developed as a child, and then removed because no one else needed them. I am remembering my body language, which is different from other people. I know what I need, and honestly, in the difficulty that is living in a society that absolutely was not created with autistic people in mind, I now find that doing many things (like taking a train, commuting to Milan to go to university, etc) is much easier, even doable. Also, and this is a point I hold dear, being autistic has brought me many positive experiences. One example is my sensoriality. Sure, I have to carry around really dark sunglasses, because the sunlight is even painful for me, but on the other hand, I have an app on my tablet that is a game of interactive coloured lights, and I can spend hours on it, so much so that it makes my eyes happy. I'm extremely defensive about hearing, but I can listen to one song for weeks if I find the perfect one. And touch, oh, touch.

No one else who isn't autistic can appreciate as much as I do how nice certain textures are, or soft, just perfect. Another example is my heavy blanket – it's a quilt with weights sewn into the squares. Very simple, but it's also one of my favourite things. The feeling of heaviness helps tremendously with stress and fatigue, and it's also one of the most satisfying feelings I can experience. There are many other aspects, such as special interests, or my particular way of thinking in pictures. There are many positive aspects to being autistic that should be encouraged and valued, but of course to do that there would need to be a way to recognise these very special experiences first.

My experience of being autistic is certainly different and more difficult to recognise on the outside than the more commonly shared experience of the young child with a passion for trains, but that is precisely why I find it necessary, indeed, essential that there be variety in the representation of autistic people. We can have completely different interests, voices, aspects of each other, and it is important to recognise this so that it is easier for us to find this word that is so essential to understanding each other. Having the knowledge that I am autistic has not changed my life. It has helped me to live true to myself, and I hope that this opportunity will gradually be open to everyone. Personally, I hope this writing can help someone understand themselves better, or help someone get to know themselves (Original writing by A., faithfully reproduced).

3.2 The Story of A.: From the Experience of the Background to the Definition of the Self

A.'s story, narrated by herself in the first person, is to be considered a manifesto of high functioning autism.

From the point of view of Gestalt therapy, it is possible to describe this testimony through: the experience of the background, the suffering of the *between*, and the evolutionary dynamics from a phenomenological perspective (Spagnuolo Lobb, 2001, 2016).

First of all, the encounter with A., at a therapeutic level, was immediately represented in the form of a significant communicative intentionality towards the therapist of the malaise she herself experienced (synchronic level). During her childhood and pre-adolescence, A. had not found a preferential way of dialogical access to her malaise because of her autistic condition that had affected her developmental experiences (diachronic level).

From the examination of A.'s account, it is possible to identify the suffering of an *ego-function* that, as Spagnuolo Lobb (2001, 2016) asserts, was incapable of deliberation as it was bound by a maladaptive regulatory effort between *id-function* and *personality-function*.

During the pre-adolescent years and those just following, A. presented a significant difficulty in contact between organism and environment. Due to the presence of autism, further aggravated by the camouflage effect, A. had accumulated a confused sensory-motor background in terms of assimilated contacts; she had developed the risk of not recognising her own physiological needs and had not acquired an adequate bodily experience. In terms of personality-function, A. had developed over the years an inability to answer the question "who am I?" When I met A., what was described was the background that distinguished her.

Secondly, A.'s testimony describes the suffering of the "between". This suffering appears to be determined by an intentionality to contact that is nonetheless not sustained at the physiological level and presents an obvious cascading effect on the fluidity of intra- and inter-dialogical reciprocity and thus on the quality of contact (Spagnuolo Lobb, 2001, 2016).

The accumulation of experiences of lack of physiological support of the instances of communicative intentionality constituted for A. the physiological ground of the anxiety disorder comorbid to the autistic disorder. This situation of psychopathological risk had defined the experience of A.'s background in terms of high danger of psychotic organisation. The girl told in narrative terms of a childhood and adolescent life in which a functional separation between organism and environment was not possible for her, thus making it impossible for the self to define itself. This situation had created a background of anxiety that in terms of adaptation did not play an effective long-term function but was represented as an evolutionary breakdown sic et simpliciter (Masi *et al.*, 2020).

A., at a certain point in her young existence, was faced with a suffering defined in terms of interpersonal "betweenness" that rested on a peculiar *neurophysiological ground* characterised by an atypia of brain connectivity described in people with autism (Belmonte *et al.*, 2004) and then by a different use of cognitive priors (Amoruso *et al.*, 2019; Pellicano and Burr, 2012).

Such a characterised neurophysiological ground could have compromised the development of a fluid interpersonal trait significantly affecting A.'s inability to answer the existential question, "who am I?"

Finally, as far as the evolutionary dynamics from a phenomenological point of view is concerned, A.'s testimony confirms that the girl's suffering, although deep, showed a vital impulse that found a privileged ground of expression in the context of the only encounter she had in the setting of diagnostic restitution. The girl's sense of self, significantly at risk of development, could be defined in the experience of the here-and-now of the diagnostic setting. In that setting, A.'s élan vital had the opportunity to begin a process of individuation by experiencing the sense of having felt recognised. As she said, feeling recognised created the basis for the experience of the world that she had been denied over the years. The experience of the diagnosis had a paradoxical effect: the force of the élan vital activated a process of interpersonal "betweenness" that acted in reverse on the ground, reassuring A. and allowing her a gradual organism-environment separation within the personal evolutionary dynamic. The way in which A. made contact in the setting began to restore a sense of herself in contact with the world, triggering an evolution of "betweenness" that allowed her to redefine her experience and organise it as described in her testimony. In addition to this, A. redefined the path of her own existence in terms of life choices and began "to live true to herself."

4. Conclusions

Gestalt psychotherapy (Narzisi and Muccio, 2015) considers experience as something that happens at the boundary of the contact between the 'I' and the 'you' in the act of co-completion.[1] According to this perspective, the "between" becomes the primary unit of analysis and assumes the character of "fundamental existential". This theoretical-clinical position, innovative both in the panorama of psychological developmental theories and in therapeutic practice, moves away from subjectivist reductionism toward a phenomenological perspective defined in terms of the organism/environment field (Wheeler, 1991).

This perspective makes use of a hermeneutics that, within the aesthetic expression of its realisation (rather than within the rigidity of the symmetrical position determined by an a priori), contains the unit of measurement of mental health.

For Gestalt psychotherapy, meeting the other at the contact boundary means being in tension with one's own senses and corporality, and moving towards the novelty and unpredictability of the encounter.

The therapeutic function, based on a phenomenological/gestalt approach, focusses on the between, so as to make the other aware of the differences the person with autism has in their approach to contact.

This is important not only for teaching others how to be with the person with autism, but also for ensuring that the person with autism does not lose his or her particular way of making contact with the environment. The peculiarity of autistic contact can be attributable to a discrepancy caused by the non-intelligibility of his/her behaviour or the risk of the camouflage effect.

Therapeutic work from this perspective means offering to the relationship between organism and environment the possibility of new experiences at the contact boundary. If, in therapy, attention to the "between" were to be neglected in favour of therapeutic programs based on the modification of "pathological" behaviour, in the direction of a typical development that is not always well defined, the risk would be that of continuing to support a "desensitised" and asynchronous organism/environment mode of contact, with inevitable cascading effects on the quality of the encounter.

In keeping with the theoretical assumption of Gestalt psychotherapy, autistic symptoms could be attributed to the lack of sensory modulation and the resulting difficulty in contact. For this reason, it is important to know the individuality of each person with autism in order to understand their way of processing information from the outside world. A person with autism has difficulty in sensory processing and therefore difficulty in creating operating patterns, relevant to meeting the other at the contact boundary.

Autism is a complex and difficult condition that requires meticulous and continuous specialisation (Narzisi, 2014). In the scenario of psychotherapeutic approaches, the Gestalt approach has the epistemological characteristics to make Gestalt psychotherapists, specially trained in autism, important resources in the care of families and individuals with high-functioning autism.

The flexibility of the Gestalt psychotherapy approach, in terms of creative adaptation, the phenomenological perspective of the organism-environment field, the attention to the body (in sensory and motor aspects), and the idea of care as attention to the global constitution of being, offer to those who deal with autistic subjects an advantageous point of view (Narzisi and Muccio, 2021; Bondioli *et al.*, 2021; Fulceri *et al.*, 2018, 2019).

Note

1   Editors' note: in Italian, "con-finire", similar to "confine" (boundary).

References

American Psychiatric Association (APA). (2013). *Diagnostic and Statistical Manual of Mental Disorders* (5th ed.). Washington, DC: Psychiatric Association.

Amoruso, L., Narzisi, A., Pinzino, M., Finisguerra, A., Billeci, L., Calderoni, S., Fabbro, F., Muratori, F., Volzone, A., & Urgesi, C. (2019). Contextual priors do not modulate action prediction in children with autism. *Proc Biol Sci.*, *286*(1908), 20191319. DOI: 10.1098/rspb.2019.1319.

Asperger, H. (1944). Die Autistisehen Psychopathen im Kindesalter. *Archives of Psychiatry Nervenkrankh, 117*, 76–136.

Belmonte, M. K., Allen, G., Beckel-Mitchener, A., Boulanger, L. M., Carper, R. A., & Webb, S. J. (2004). Autism and abnormal development of brain connectivity. *Journal of Neuroscience, 24*(42), 9228–9231. DOI: 10.1523/JNEUROSCI.3340-04.2004.

Bettheleheim, B. (1967). *The empty fortress. Infantile Autism and the Birth of the Self.* New York: Free Press.

Bondioli, M., Chessa, S., Narzisi, A., Pelagatti, S., & Zoncheddu, M. (2021). Towards motor-based early detection of autism red flags: Enabling technology and exploratory study protocol. *Sensors (Basel), 21*(6), 1971.

Cage, E., & Burton, H. (2019). Gender differences in the first impressions of autistic adults. *Autism Research, 12*(10), 1495–1504.

Dean, M., Harwood, R., & Kasari, C. (2017). The art of camouflage: Gender differences in the social behaviors of girls and boys with autism spectrum disorder. *Autism, 21*(6), 678–689.

Fulceri, F., Grossi, E., Contaldo, A., Narzisi, A., Apicella, F., Parrini, I., Tancredi, R., Calderoni, S., & Muratori, F. (2019). Motor skills as moderators of core symptoms in autism spectrum disorders: Preliminary data from an exploratory analysis with artificial neural networks. *Front Psychol, 9*, 2683.

Fulceri, F., Tonacci, A., Lucaferro, A., Apicella, F., Narzisi, A., Vincenti, G., Muratori, F., & Contaldo, A. (2018). Interpersonal motor coordination during joint actions in children with and without autism spectrum disorder: The role of motor information. *Research In Developmental Disabilities, 80*, 13–23.

Green, R. M., Travers, A. M., Howe, Y., & McDougle, C. J. (2019). Women and autism spectrum disorder: Diagnosis and implications for treatment of adolescents and adults. *Current Psychiatry Reports, 21*(4), 22.

Head, A. M., McGillivray, J. A., & Stokes, M. A. (2014). Gender differences in emotionality and sociability in children with autism spectrum disorders. *Molecular Autism, 5*(1), 19.

Hiller, R. M., Young, R. L., & Weber, N. (2014). Sex differences in autism spectrum disorder based on DSM-5 criteria: Evidence from clinician and teacher reporting. *Journal of Abnormal Child Psychology, 42*(8), 1381–1393.

Hull, L., Petrides, K. V., Allison, C., Smith, P., Baron-Cohen, S., Lai, M. C., & Mandy, W. J. (2017). Putting on my best normal: Social camouflaging in adults with autism spectrum conditions. Autism and Developmental Disorders, *47*(8), 2519–2534.

Kanner, L. (1943). Autistic disturbances of affective contact. *Journal Nervous Child, 2*, 21750.

Lai, M. C., & Baron-Cohen, S. (2015). Identifying the lost generation of adults with autism spectrum conditions. *Lancet Psychiatry, 2*(11), 1013–1027. DOI: 10.1016/S2215-0366(15)00277-1.

Lai, M. C., Lombardo, M. V., Auyeung, B., Chakrabarti, B., & Baron-Cohen, S. (2015). Sex/gender differences and autism: Setting the scene for future research. *Journal of the American Academy of Child and Adolescent Psychiatry, 54*(1), 11–24.

Lai, M. C., Lombardo, M. V., Chakrabarti, B., *et al.* (2019). Neural self-representation in autistic women and association with 'compensatory camouflaging'. *Autism, 23*(5), 1210–1223.

Lai, M. C., Lombardo, M. V., Pasco, G., Ruigrok, A. N., Wheelwright, S. J., Sadek, S. A., Chakrabart, I. B., MRC AIMS Consortium, & Baron-Cohen, S. (2011). A behavioral comparison of male and female adults with high functioning autism spectrum conditions. *PLoS One, 6*(6), e20835.

Lai, M. C., Lombardo, M. V., Ruigrok, A. N., *et al.* (2017). Quantifying and exploring camouflaging in men and women with autism. *Autism, 21*(6), 690–702.

Lai, M. C., & Szatmari, P. (2020). Sex and gender impacts on the behavioural presentation and recognition of autism. *Current Opinion in Psychiatry, 33*(2), 117–123.

Maenner, M. J., Shaw, K. A., Baio, J., Washington, A., Patrick, M., DiRienzo, M., Christensen, D. L., Wiggins, L. D., Pettygrove, S., Andrews, J. G., *et al.* (2020). Prevalence of autism spectrum disorder among children aged 8 years – autism and developmental disabilities monitoring network, 11 sites, United States, 2016. *MMWR Surveillance Summaries, 69*, 1–12.

Masi, G., Scullin, S., Narzisi, A., Muratori, P., Paciello, M., Fabiani, D., Lenzi, F., Mucci, M., & D'Acunto, G. (2020). Suicidal ideation and suicidal attempts in referred adolescents with high functioning autism spectrum disorder and comorbid bipolar disorder: A pilot study. *Brain Sciences, 10*(10), 750.

Narzisi, A. (2014). Psicoterapia della Gestalt nella prospettiva evolutiva: linee teoriche e proposta applicativa di un paradigma sperimentale per la valutazione dell'esperienza di contatto Organismo-Ambiente [Gestalt therapy in the developmental perspective: Theoretical lines and application proposal of an experimental paradigm for the evaluation of the experience of contact Organism-Environment]. *Idee in Psicoterapia, 6*(13), 93–101.

Narzisi, A. (2020). The challenging heterogeneity of autism: Editorial for brain sciences special issue "advances in autism research". *Brain Sciences, 10*(12), 948.

Narzisi, A., & Muccio, R. (2015). Autismo e psicoterapia della Gestalt: un ponte dialogico possibile [Autism and Gestalt therapy: A possible dialogic bridge]. *Quaderni di Gestalt, XXVIII*(1), 49–61. DOI: 10.3280/GEST2015-001004.

Narzisi, A., & Muccio, R. (2021). A neuro-phenomenological perspective on the autism phenotype. *Brain Sciences, 11*(7), 914.

Narzisi, A., Posada, M., Barbieri, F., Chericoni, N., Ciuffolini, D., Pinzino, M., Romano, R., Scattoni, M. L., Tancredi, R., Calderoni, S., & Muratori, F. (2018). Prevalence of autism spectrum disorder in a large Italian catchment area: A school-based population study within the ASDEU project. *Epidemiology and Psychiatric Sciences, 29*, e5.

Ospina, M. B., Krebs Seida, J., Clark, B., Karkhaneh, M., Hartling, L., Tjosvold, L., Vandermeer, B., & Smith, V. (2008). Behavioural and developmental interventions for autism spectrum disorder: A clinical systematic review. *PLoS One, 3*(11), e3755.

Parish-Morris, J., Liberman, M. Y., Cieri, C., Herrington, J. D., Yerys, B. E., Bateman, L., Donaher, J., Ferguson, E., Pandey, J., & Schultz, R. T. (2017). Linguistic camouflage in girls with autism spectrum disorder. *Molecular Autism, 8*, 48.

Pellicano, E., & Burr, D. (2012). When the world becomes 'too real': A Bayesian explanation of autistic perception. *Trends in Cognitive Sciences, 16*(10), 504–510. DOI: 10.1016/j.tics.2012.08.009.

Ratto, A. B., Kenworthy, L., Yerys, B. E., Bascom, J., Wieckowski, A. T., White, S. W., Wallace, G. L., Pugliese, C., Schultz, R. T., Ollendick, T. H., Scarpa, A., Seese, S., Register-Brown, K., Martin, A., & Anthony, L. G. (2018). What about the girls? Sex-based differences in autistic traits and adaptive skills. *Journal of Autism and Developmental Disorders, 48*(5), 1698–1711.

Rynkiewicz, A., Schuller, B., Marchi, E., Piana, S., Camurri, A., Lassalle, A., & Baron-Cohen, S. (2016). An investigation of the 'female camouflage effect' in autism using a computerized ADOS-2 and a test of sex/gender differences. *Molecular Autism, 7*, 10.

Schuck, R. K., Flores, R. E., & Fung, L. K. (2019). J brief report: Sex/gender differences in symptomology and camouflaging in adults with autism spectrum disorder. *Autism and Developmental Disorders, 49*(6), 2597–2604.

Spagnuolo Lobb, M. (2001). The theory of self in Gestalt therapy. A restatement of some aspects. *Gestalt Review*, *5*, 276–288. DOI: 10.5325/gestaltreview.5.4.0276.

Spagnuolo Lobb, M. (2016). Self as contact, contact as self. A contribution to ground experience in Gestalt therapy theory of self. In J.-M. Robine (Ed.). *Self. A poliphony of contemporary Gestalt therapists* (pp. 261–289). St. Romain la Virvée, France: L'Exprimerie.

Tierney, S., Burns, J., & Kilbey, E. (2016). Looking behind the mask: Social coping strategies of girls on the autistic spectrum. *Research in Autism Spectrum Disorders*, *23*, 73–83.

Young, H., Oreve, M. J., & Speranza, M. (2018). Clinical characteristics and problems diagnosing autism spectrum disorder in girls. *Archives de Pédiatrie*, *25*(6), 399–403.

Wheeler, G. (1991). *Gestalt reconsidered.* New York: Gardner Press, Inc.

Chapter 10

Adolescents in Eclipse
Journey Notes From the Labyrinth of Social Withdrawal

Michele Lipani

1. The Eclipse of Social Life

Matteo is thirteen years old. His parents say he was always an introverted child but with a relational life sufficiently adequate for his age.

Now that he is older, you would expect him to build ever closer relationships with his peers and enjoy the carefreeness of his teenage years, but instead he prefers to stay at home, with no interests or hobbies to keep him motivated. He spends entire afternoons in his room, especially when people come to visit his parents or his elder sister. He does not go over to anybody's house and invites nobody home.

A couple of months before the summer holidays, he started saying that he did not want to go to school. Initially he would give some timid excuse not to go, but faced with his father's firm opposition, and after some scolding, he clearly stated he was not well and hated it at school.

He was not having any particular problems with his marks at school, and he did not appear to be troubled by anything specific, such as teasing by his school mates, for instance, or some form of bullying.

Despite a high number of absences, he managed to finish the school year. Throughout the school holidays, though, Matteo continued to spend his days confined to the home. Concerned, his parents tried to encourage him to go out with a friend of his or a cousin who would often call, but Matteo flatly refused, saying constantly, "I'm happy at home."

The months went by and Matteo's depressive decline was matched by a rising sense of helplessness and anxiety in his parents, with moments of misunderstanding alternated with vain attempts to find solutions. The two parents began moving in random, often contradictory directions.

After a few months, tensions in the family were running high and the father was becoming determined to force his son to go out. But at a certain point, Matteo started going out on his own. He would leave home around six o'clock and come back just after eight, telling his parents he had stayed outdoors and hung out with his friends.

One day, however, his mother discovered by chance that, in reality, when Matteo went out, he would go upstairs to the top floor of the building and stay there,

DOI: 10.4324/9781003313335-13

on the landing before the terrace, where nobody ever went. He would sit there on the stairs, on his own, before coming back home a couple of hours later.

At that point, it became clear to the two parents that Matteo's troubles were much greater than they had thought, and they decided to seek professional help.

Faced with the difficulty of dealing with the developmental challenges presented by his age, Matteo, like many of his peers, seeks a solution by withdrawing from social life and confining himself to the home.[1] Although such developmental pressures normally encourage adolescents to open up to the world, some take a different direction, shunning the social horizon.

Hikikomori is a phenomenon that is fairly well known these days. After emerging in Japan in the 1980s, it has since taken root in Italy, as in many Western countries, and appears to be on the rise. Although it is perhaps more widely associated with young adults, in clinical practice I often observe situations of social withdrawal among adolescents and pre-adolescents. I meet parents whose children seem to live in solitary labyrinths, as though having given up all hope.

Here I would like to contribute a few journey notes, a thread of sorts to help us guide any modern young Theseus out of their struggle with the Minotaur of solitude.

2. Retreat: Phenomenology and Diagnosis

A first aspect of the journey into reclusion by an adolescent raises the question of the sense and meaning of such a dystonic relational attitude when compared to the developmental changes we would expect. Just like Matteo, other teenagers I have met displayed no clinically significant difficulties in their childhood. It is only when they become adolescents that they start retreating into a labyrinth, initially built on the rejection of the occasions offered by social life; for instance, they prefer not to go to friends' parties or they do not go out on a Saturday night. The first steps of retreat may be accompanied by headaches or tummy aches whose frequency is correlated with school attendance or activities they formerly took part in willingly. The urge for isolation is often attributed to vague motivations connected with relations with peers or with teachers. Then they progressively, or suddenly, abandon school. One refusal after another finally makes it clear that their life is confined only to the home, if not only to their own bedroom.

The onset of withdrawal therefore does not come suddenly, such as in response to a traumatic event, but unfolds slowly and is often underestimated by adults. Although every family's story is different, parents are usually left disoriented, beginning what may turn into a long string of all too often fruitless efforts to reopen an adolescence that has folded in on itself. As highlighted by some authors, the onset of withdrawal may be triggered by some "precipitating factor" present in the school setting or more generally, in the setting with peers. It may be a string of bad experiences, which often leave the adolescent feeling frustrated, but they do not always have the characteristics of bullying (Adorno and Lancini, 2019).

I remember the case of Gabriele and his slide into isolation at twelve years of age, when he started saying he did not want to go to school on Mondays and Thursdays, to avoid gym class. The PE teacher had started organising "matches" rather than exercises, but Gabriele, in his awkward lankiness, could not bear the idea of being the loser in those "contests" with his classmates. He then went on to progressively avoid all situations in which he perceived any chance of potential "humiliation".

We know that the impoverishment of social life is an element of various psychiatric conditions, and so an in-depth diagnostic assessment and differential reading of capabilities and fragilities is fundamental to identify, for example, neurodevelopmental, psychotic spectra, depression, anxiety, or avoidant personality disorders. Many adolescents, however, do not appear to fall into specific psychopathological profiles, nor do they display the fluidity of the transitory withdrawals that are fairly frequent in adolescence. Some authors are in favour of recognising a new disorder, albeit with indicators common to other pathologies (Adorno and Lancini, 2019). There is still no diagnostic recognition defining the disorder of social withdrawal, in its descriptive aspects at least. Even the *Diagnostic and Statistical Manual of Mental Disorders* (DSM-5) (APA, 2013), the most recent edition of the manual, does not propose any specific diagnosis.

Independently of its nosological collocation, as a therapist I am interested in grasping the new developmental paths and forms of expression taken by suffering in young people that are emerging from changes in the cultural setting, which seem to me today, more than in the past, to seek some form of protection in the avoidance of social life. The adolescents I am speaking of strike me as prisoners of a developmental impasse.

I do not possess sufficient elements to assess the complexity of the phenomenon and the multiplicity of variables that come to bear on each family's story; thus, I will only touch on some aspects which have no causal value but which strike me as a constant in many of the cases I have heard. Reclusive behaviours, as they are usually described, do not take on the form of a decisive rejection of the other. Rather, they suggest the need to protect oneself from some perceived threat. Thus, although dysfunctional in terms of the developmental process, withdrawal from social interaction with others assumes an adaptive value. The protective value of the strategy appears to be found first of all in the possibility it offers for lowering anxiety. At the beginning of the slide into the labyrinth, there is a prevalence of experiences that appear to be seeped in anxiety. It is as though each teenager approaches the relational experience with a solitary burden of anxious inadequacy.

It is well known how many adolescents are plagued by insecurities and a sense of emptiness and helplessness. The long, hard process of becoming oneself is often tough and wearisome, with the risk of one humiliation after another. The psychological reorganisation involved in adolescent experience has always entailed the concept of a *work in progress* as well as vulnerable situations – all this does not seem to have changed. What does seem to have changed, however, is the map of the territory of growth, which has become more complex, and the quality of the journey companions, today more uncertain of themselves and less confident. Perhaps teenagers who withdraw into themselves cannot bear the adolescent struggle of reorganising their existence and feel they cannot share that struggle with anyone.

Sixteen-year-old Federica is merciless in her judgement of herself, anticipating the risk that others may see through her fragilities, tearing open a wound she believes unbearable. She does not dare expose herself by seeking advice about her difficulties, even from her peers, because she is too afraid of being teased; rather, she looks for information from web sites.

As Pietropolli Charmet (2013) argues, exposing oneself becomes a powerful detonator that threatens to blow up the narcissistic myth of childhood. These are kids who do not feel ready to take the plunge into growing up, and rather than run the risk that it entails, they would rather mortify their vitality and sacrifice their growth. Often, it is only the parents who ask for help, because the adolescent may not want to see a therapist – the request for help may be seen as confirmation of failure.

The early stages of clinical work require a strong alliance to be built with the mother and father. Given that social withdrawal can be a way of dealing with one's anxiety and an extreme attempt to save one's psychic health (Lancini, 2019), a first, fundamental objective of therapy is to support the parents in remodulating the meanings they attach to their child's behaviour, helping them see it from an adaptive and developmental perspective.

3. The Dark Side of Narcissism and the Dissolution of the Childhood Myth

Changes in adolescence are often destabilising, but the vast majority of teenagers find a counterweight to them in creativity, opportunity, and confidence; above all, though, they are transitory. So we might ask: how come they are instead so potentially devastating for some? Without denying the complexity of the various situations, I believe it can help to reflect on the parenting models that have underpinned the growth and upbringing of recent generations. Given the space available here, I will address only one element that can be correlated with the solitude that is often found paired with vulnerabilities.

In parenting styles today, less emphasis is placed on ethics and norms (and hence on sacrifice and the sense of guilt), to the advantage of narcissistic values that, by comparison, have amplified the sphere of subjectivity and the relativity of limits (La Barbera *et al.*, 2007). Narcissistic parenting models have fuelled expectations in parents that at times border on the grandiose, cultivating an image of the child that is legitimate in its confidence but often lacking in the capacity to support him.

On the other hand, kids often do not withstand the impact with the reality of adolescence. Adolescents who withdraw are grappling with the reorganisation of a self-perception that, especially in relation to their peers, sends back an image to them that is often very diverse from their childhood expectations. Every day we see adolescents in the grips of a permanent anxiety, hungry for visibility, in the spasmodic search for "likes" and "followers"; teenagers who appear to struggle to keep up in the continuous race of "exceptional performances" that prove their value; kids busy in measuring the quality of their existence through the constant connection with others, as the fear of failure becomes a daily constant. Thus, they remain trapped in an exasperated search for recognition, in an age when, like never before, the nod of social approval seems so decisive for them to feel they have value.

The relationship with the peer group is often a strong alliance, but for many, it seems instead to have become a contest that is increasingly harder and harder to compete in. A contest permeated, for example, by themes such as beauty and personal success, which have become fundamental as meaning organisers but are unattainable for most. Some, despite feeling a powerful need for recognition, cannot bear the shame of possible failure and find themselves slowly but surely stepping back in retreat. These absences and fragilities need to be reckoned with, but for many kids, that road becomes unsustainable, as the gap becomes too great between the shadow of themselves and reality, between what the adolescent expected himself to become and what he actually risks becoming (Lipani, 2016). That sense of inadequacy that that has almost "physiologically" and perpetually accompanied the life of many adolescents now merges with a new climate, one that does not admit any weakness or vulnerability (Ammaniti, 2018).

Adolescent transformations, in cases of social withdrawal, are a mix of ingredients, therefore, that do not blend – an identity too thin-skinned and slight in its structure; a relational context that is too complex and charged perhaps with expectations; the bitter taste of inadequacy and humiliation; the risk of unbearable narcissistic wounds; boundaries and bonds that easily evaporate; and a shame that sounds the alarm and the withdrawal into a hidden corner in which to take shelter and recover one's breath (Lipani, 2014).

The risk of disappointment and the feeling of shame are two themes that help me make sense of the difficulty of growing up in modern society:

> shame in the adolescent world today seems to refer no longer predominantly to transgression and guilt, but to the issue of not being successful. Thus there is no shame in showing off, but there is shame if showing off at any cost should fail and we are not admired, or even just noticed.
>
> (Battacchi, 2002, p. 12)

From a Gestalt therapy point of view, shame seems to me a relational message. It is like drawing a veil over fragilities and perceived limitations, to hide away from the eyes of others, considered too demanding and not at all sympathetic.

For Roberta, the desire to be "seen" and accepted has veered, after countless attempts, she says, towards a pervasive anguish that she mitigates through self-exclusion.

In Gestalt terms, we might say that in contacting the environment, it is as though the energy of the developmental process has been cramped into a depressive space, a position it accepts for a greater good, that of maintaining some sort of psychological stability. The price she risks paying, however, is too high, with the progressive contraction of her psychic ground and the mortification of her growth.

Frequently, the flood of anxiety that invades the family is handled by the parents through attempts, at times quite clumsy, to eliminate the reclusive behaviour, thereby underestimating the adaptive message it gives. The request for help is most likely to come when the unexpressed vitality of the teenager and his unsupported anxiety slowly give way to a depressive dimension. Therapy work and the support of the parents should help rebuild the adolescent's confidence in accepting a gap between how he would like to be and how he manages to appear, opening up space for him to affirm his own fragilities (Spagnuolo Lobb, 2016c).

4. Fragile Grounds Affect Developmental Processes

The parenting models we have mentioned in turn merge into the complex web of the cultural ground of society (Lipani, 2016). And we can, in fact, look for a framework of meaning for the developmental process and the troubles faced by isolated kids even in the characteristics of the cultural fabric. The weakening of social links, as is often commented, bears an impact on bonds, on parental roles, and on the possibility of finding containment in moments of difficulty. On the other hand, the social life of many families is often circumscribed to the private sphere, while the school system fumbles to find new ways to fulfil its role in supporting growth and in orienting the choice of values. I believe we can echo those who see social withdrawal as a kind of cultural syndrome by saying that it is a loss of contact with the society to which we belong.

I often consider social isolation as an indicator of the fragility of two grounds – the social/cultural ground and the family/personal ground. Social retreat would appear to point in part to the fragility of the cultural ground, reflecting the difficulties of a society that is demanding in its expectations but lacking in its sense of belonging and capacity to give support, and in part to the fragility of the teenager in remodulating the ground of his adolescent Self. There is undoubtedly a fragility in many kids and in their families, but there is also the difficulty our society shows in admitting and containing vulnerability. When the challenges of adolescent development become a hurdle, social withdrawal will strike some as the only means of protection left to them.[2]

Therapeutic intervention needs to find ways to offer support on both the social/cultural plane and the family/individual plane.

> If decades ago, in the narcissistic society, it was obvious for humanistic psychotherapists to focus on the figure, today it is obvious to focus on the ground. . . . What our clients need today is to be supported in their experience of the ground.
>
> (Spagnuolo Lobb, 2016a, p. 272)

The Gestalt vision of suffering, as a process that is relational, implies the need to care for the entire experiential ground of the family. My clinical experience suggests that social withdrawal cannot be addressed through intervention based solely on a traditional clinical model, limited to therapy activity on an individual basis with the adolescent. The positive therapy work conducted with Matteo's family, for instance, mobilised resources on a number of fronts, including the intensive involvement of both parents, the help of a home education worker, and the cooperation of teachers.[3] Various projects confirm that intervention is more effective when it builds on the work of a coordinated team, based on an interdisciplinary model involving various professionals, such as a psychologist, social workers, youth workers, and teachers (Adorno andLancini, 2019).

5. The Suffering of the Family Field

The difficulties of an adolescent who cannot bring himself to leave the home clearly concern a suffering in him, but such suffering cannot be reduced solely to the intrapsychic or behavioural dimension, as it profoundly touches the quality of the relational process within the family field. As a process of the field, understood in phenomenological and relational terms, it concerns the complementary experiences of the parents and the adolescent (Fogarty, 2016; Francesetti, 2015).

Parents often feel a jumbled mix of emotions, thoughts, and sentiments, swinging between a sense of confidence that it will all turn out okay, because they trust in the capacities the child once showed, and the anguish of no longer recognising a child now so stubbornly shut up in himself. At the same time, they may underestimate or even overestimate their concerns; indeed they often say they feel lost in their child's same labyrinth.

Nicola is a seventeen-year-old whose father says he sometimes feels like giving up on the idea of seeing his son go to university, but at other times he feels it is still too soon to relinquish his future. However, he also says he cannot understand or find ways to stop his son's progressive slide into the shadows of the world, where he is becoming little more than a shade.

Sofia's parents find themselves envying the parents of other seventeen-year-olds, who have to battle with their children to make them come home at a reasonable hour; instead they anxiously stress over seeing their daughter hanging around home all day, every day.

In the complementary game of the psychological movement between the *inside* and *outside*, in the division of roles it is usually the adolescent who pushes to break free and set sail towards new horizons, while the parent is the custodian of the safe harbour of the home, of the family that gives support and repair, if necessary. Instead, with the reclusion of the adolescent in the home, those roles and developmental paths are thrown out of whack.

Sometimes, the parents seek a solution in making suggestions and proposals, for instance by organising to contrive more or less spontaneous encounters with their child's companions, or they may find it plausible to blame the Internet, as the child may spend a considerable amount of time online.

During an argument at Oscar's house, the PlayStation was hurled to the floor, giving rise to a certain relief in his mother, who hoped it would help break what she considered a bad habit. Instead all it marked was a two and half month break in all communication between father and son, and even then, Oscar did not appear to show any interest in talking to his father again. For him it was just another wall raised.

The therapy process usually begins when the parents come to realise that their child's refusal to go out may be a problem that will not sort itself out on its own with time. The expectations of therapy held by parents are generally that of a priority intervention targeting the reclusive behaviour, in the hope of "unblocking" the situation and thereby resolving the problem. We can sympathise with the parents and feel the easy temptation of imagining the symptom of *not going out* as a "block to be removed," a behaviour to be eliminated. However, the symptom of *reclusion* is just one aspect of a more complex psychological-relational arrangement in which the priority for us concerns the modes of being in relation with the other and the quality of contact with the environment.

Involving the parents is the "essential background in order to understand any unexpressed and blocked intentionalities in the field – and to support them by helping them develop their own resources and relational competences" (Conte and Tosi, 2016, p. 102). An important – if at times by no means easy – step in the therapy process is, therefore, to agree on the idea that the therapy plan should embrace all of the family. A correct nosological diagnosis is of course indispensable to avoid the wrong intervention; however, it is just as important to accommodate the understanding the parents have of the problem and to discuss the functionality, or lack thereof, of the relational approaches adopted up to that time.

While considering the family as the initial target of the therapy plan, the therapist may modulate the setting in various ways, according to the situation, the resources, and the possibilities available. Meetings may be held with different family members or solely with the parents, while it is unlikely that individual meetings with the adolescent will initially be possible. In some cases, a brief period of work with the parents will not be sufficient, and specific individual or couple therapy with the parents may be necessary.

Family therapy can unfold on two planes that intersect and progress together, where on the one hand, there is the fundamental work on the relationship between the parents and child (as well as any siblings), and on the other there is the exploration of specific issues that emerge in the daily life of a family with a reclusive adolescent. The fundamental aspect of therapy concerns analysis and activity on the modes of contact between parents and children. Interest in how the child and parents interact should be guided by phenomenological observation, which helps us understand not only the experience of the adolescent but also the complementary experience of the parents, who together will have devised styles of contact, or ways of expressing anxiety, but also flexibility and the possibility of experiencing novelty (Spagnuolo Lobb, 2016a).

Recent studies by the Istituto di Gestalt HCC Italy have focussed on a proposal for observing parenting skills, known as *dance steps*, with the objective of describing the movements performed in contact between parents and children, in the unfolding of the co-created contact process (Spagnuolo Lobb, 2016a).[4] The use of such criteria leads us to understand the quality of the relationship and in the case of social withdrawal, for example, the fragile sense of security towards the world outside the family, the anxiety felt in venturing towards new experiences, and the possibility of letting go of control over interaction.

Gestalt therapy activity is guided by the capabilities of the family; it supports the parents in understanding the suffering of their child, his anxieties, and his attempts to relieve them. A reorganisation of the existing relationship around the issues of adolescent development and the context of growth is helpful in strengthening the ground of experience and supporting the recovery of the developmental process. Work to support the parenting role can vary in duration, depending on a variety of factors. This is not the time or place to look further into those factors, but such work is fundamental in opening up the possibility of involving the adolescent directly.

6. A Thread for Theseus: Therapy With the Adolescent

6.1 The Courage to Take on the Labyrinth of Isolation

The request for help is often hidden in the folds of a fragile awareness. The adolescent may not perceive his reclusion as a difficulty in his relationships and as a way to protect his fragilities.

Sixteen-year-old Federico prefers to speak of choosing and wanting isolation, which he says comes from not endorsing the lifestyle of his peers; or he says he feels no motivation for encountering others. He feels happy on his own, and if he wants to, he knows where to find his friends. For the moment, though, he hovers in permanent stand-by mode. He has inverted his sleep/wake cycle, and when his parents are at work, he sleeps. He gets up around lunch time, then spends most of his time holed up in his room, avoiding going out even for the small occasions of daily life (his grandmother's birthday, to buy himself a top or shoes). At night he has been going to bed later and later, absorbed by a video game or something online.

Progressively, even interaction with parents and siblings may become impoverished in its content or frequency, exposing the adolescent to the risk of developing other psychopathological ways of being, especially of an anxious or depressive nature.

When Federico first agreed to meet me, he showed the discouraged attitude of someone who is convinced nobody can help him, and so it is not worth even trying.

The priority for me was to find a way of meeting him that was flexible enough to adapt to his comfort zone and respectful of his current limits. Initially, there was no therapy contract, and we set each appointment as we went along, and sometimes the session lasted less than the time available. I never asked him for more than he was prepared to share, nor to do anything he could not do. The basis of our arrangement was to contact and reach him only to the point with which he felt comfortable.

In these cases, the direction therapy takes is that of consolidating the sense of contact, where the objective is to enrich the quality of awareness, which is often compromised by a desensitisation to feelings and emotions, and to restore the quality of the intentionality for contact. In general, the ground of the therapeutic relationship is shaped by the principles of Gestalt therapy with clients in developing age groups, and its central fulcrum turns on the theory of the self.[5] In the Gestalt paradigm, the therapist and the client are involved in an intersubjective dimension, where each and every experience can create new, dynamic equilibria between the stable aspects of the self and new elements introduced in the encounter with the other.

We should be mindful that social withdrawal, the symptom and problem to be resolved, is instead a solution to a difficulty for the adolescent, contributing to the organisation of interaction and the regulation of emotivity. While at the start of the therapeutic process, it is the resonance of the therapist that offers itself in contact, as the relational ground lays the bases for trust, the adolescent's capacity for attunement will grow, and he will be a bit more willing to question his habitual repertoire of meanings and modes of interaction. In the therapeutic context and from a field perspective, the fragilities of the adolescent become part of the co-created relationship with the therapist, which allows him to calibrate the pace and distance, while respecting the emotional state of the client.

6.2 Fears and Courage Become Allies in the Therapeutic Relationship

The attention focused on the sensations that the two bodies express – what Spagnuolo Lobb calls "aesthetic relational knowing" – can progressively help establish an attunement that aims to restore the spontaneous reaching for full contact.[6] In therapy work, developmental changes intersect with three fundamental functions of contact, which in turn reorganise the adolescent's experience of himself and the world.[7] A first fundamental dimension of Gestalt therapy work is the attention paid to the ground of bodily experience, grasped in its phenomenological making (Frank, 2001; Lipani and Conte, 2014). Thus, the therapist takes care of the way each adolescent enters into the relationship – his sensations (watching, listening, touching), the way he moves and breathes, shows curiosity, and interacts. Work on the ground of the id-function implies grasping the awareness of bodily feeling.

The first sessions can be rather tough going, as the constant state of anxiety is paired with a tendency to desensitise bodily experience in an effort to regulate oneself, which can crystallise and transform into rigid modalities.

*In my meeting with the sixteen-year-old Diego, for instance, a muffled atmos-
phere formed between us, as though space and time had stopped. Everything
appeared to be "suspended." While on the one hand he said he was putting off all
the challenges typical of his age to the definitive, magical threshold of adulthood,
on the other, right now he mobilises no energy and no motivation. It was hard for
both of us to find elements to share. I had the impression that he was living in the
shadows even of himself.*

The depressive atmosphere often pervades other capacities as well, as thought
is impoverished and the range of emotions and interests narrows. Another element
of the ground in the contact process is given by the personality-function, which
is guided in the contact by the fund of experiences assimilated in the past, ones
which shape the perception of one's social self and the quality of one's roles.[8] If
the id-function takes the form of a chronically depressive experience, the
personality-function will shape experiences of helplessness, eliciting shame in
relation to what one could do but is not able to do, at least in the expectations of
the teenager and those of his significant others.

Sofia says she has always known how shy she is, but now she also feels inept,
like when she convinces herself to go out with other girls her age (fifteen) but
then is always awkward and clumsy, a complete misfit. According to her, her
friends do what they can to include her, but it is her own fault if she does not
know what to say and how to act. Every time she sees them, she cannot wait to
get back home.

The construction of the sense of self is a slow process of assimilation of
the contact experiences that enrich the ground and form the basis for new figures. Exposure to repeated "failures" of contact can weaken the sense of self-
effectiveness in managing one's relationship with the environment, while the
personality-function assimilates the anxiety of projecting oneself towards full
contact and the retroflection of the action, with its need to pull back. In the
activation of the ego-function, the adolescent experiences a progressive loss
of vitality, interest, motivation, and sense of purpose, and so identifies with
the inevitable urge to retreat and withdraw. The anxiety of projecting oneself
towards the environment turns into a retroflection to protect oneself and one's
integrity, which feels threatened.

6.3 Trust in the Encounter Opens Up Glimmers of Hope and Possibilities

The therapeutic encounter offers support in modulating sensations and their intensity, keeping them within a "window of tolerance" that Gestalt therapy describes
as "safe emergency," to limit the risk of retreat from experiences of novelty and
growth (Taylor, 2014). By following aesthetic criteria,[9] the therapist manages to
keep arousal within a window of tolerance so that the adolescent remains present
and open to contact, while at the same time seeking to explore and expand that
comfort zone (Taylor, 2014).

The therapeutic value of the encounter lies more in the process than in a method or technique (Fogarty, 2016). To help manage anxiety, alongside the numerous techniques of Gestalt therapy (relaxation exercises, breathing exercises), we can take inspiration from a variety of techniques and activities developed in other theoretical contexts (art therapy and psychodrama, for instance), providing that they are then used consistently with the epistemological framework of Gestalt therapy.

Individual therapy work, as part of a broader project of care, intersects with the work done in parallel with the parents and with the social context of the family (the school, for instance). In short, the fundamental objective is to enrich the contexts of experience for the adolescent by balancing his tendency for defensiveness and avoidance with possible new ways for him to satisfy the drive for openness and experimentation, to allow his curiosity and fear to find new equilibria and new creative adjustments.

7. Conclusions: There Cannot Be a Theseus Without a *Polis* to Support Him

Social withdrawal can be understood as an expression of a suffering born of a new narcissism. It seems to signal the difficulties faced by adults and the social ground in supporting the physiology of contact with the adolescent and with his vulnerabilities, while enhancing his creativity and vitality at the same time. Family therapy can help resolve issues and obstacles and create occasions for positive experiences that encourage an opening towards the world. The therapeutic relationship with the adolescent helps build a significant barrier to the risk of an insidious regression in skills and capabilities, something which is often feared in these cases. Therapy can help the adolescent find new hope and direction and build a map of the world to be explored and discovered.

I would like to conclude this chapter by stressing how giving a voice to the absence of these kids from social life implies not only complex and structured therapy work but also the assumption of "political" responsibility by psychologists towards the community. The complexity of our cultural and social scenarios and the rapid pace of change in relational styles often render parenting and teaching roles quite fragile and disorienting. Perhaps we could promote more projects and activities to foster discussion and debate on parenting models and teaching styles, so as to encourage their remodulation and greater attunement with the developmental processes of today. In that way, relationships between adults and adolescents could find new meanings, new means of support, and new alliances.

Ultimately, I believe that the social withdrawal of many youngsters signals a need to rethink the relations between the generations.

Notes

1   In this chapter, my use of the masculine pronoun to refer to the adolescent is only a form of shorthand, an expedient in writing, for while the phenomenon of social withdrawal

in adolescence is in fact more widespread among males, it is rapidly on the rise among females, too.

2　Developmental issues for this age group include, for example, the reorganisation of bodily experience, the individuation process, and social rebirth (Lipani, 2016).

3　Since social withdrawal is considered a Special Educational Need (Italian Ministerial Decree of December 2012), flexible educational arrangements can be put in place to help the adolescent not feel completely excluded from school.

4　In the observational approach proposed, contact between the adolescent and parent is marked out, following aesthetic and phenomenological criteria, in "dance steps," where "the two create the feeling of a secure ground, in which they mutually perceive and recognize the intentionality of the other, they adapt to one another, and can take courageous steps, having fun, reaching each other, and opening up to the world" (Spagnuolo Lobb, 2016a)

5　On Gestalt therapy with children, see Spagnuolo Lobb et al. (2016) and essays published in Quaderni di Gestalt, XXIX (2016).

6　As a relational process, contact takes place through dynamic functions known as functions of the Self. These functions are expressed in the emerging of an excitement from the ground of bodily and socio-relational schemas already assimilated (id-function and personality-function), in the development of an intentionality that, by identifying with an appropriate action, leads to full contact (ego-function), and, finally, through subsequent withdrawal and the assimilation of the new quality of the experience accomplished.

7　The analysis of the modes and quality of contact represents a basic therapy "tool," as psychopathology can be viewed as both a dysfunction in contact processes and an alteration in the vitality and spontaneity of the organism. Over the years, Gestalt therapy has theorised different acceptations of the concept of contact and the suffering of contact. For the position taken by the founders see Perls et al. (1951/1994).

8　More recent interpretations of contact propose redefining losses of the ego-function (introjection, projection, retroflection, and confluence) as "experiential dominoes," or the different modes of contact of which a child is capable, and which he brings to the relationship (Spagnuolo Lobb, 2012). We can understand the id-function and the personality-function as two grounds of the experience of contact, and the ego-function as the experience of figure.

9　For a discussion of aesthetic criteria see Spagnuolo Lobb, 2018.

References

Adorno, F., & Lancini, M. (2019). Autoreclusione volontaria. Proteggersi dalla vergogna [Voluntary self-enclosure. Protecting oneself from shame]. In M. Lancini (Ed.). Il ritiro sociale negli adolescenti. La solitudine di una generazione iperconnessa. Milano: Raffaello Cortina Editore.

American Psychiatric Association (APA). (2013). Diagnostic and statistical manual of mental disorders (5th ed.). Washington, DC: Psychiatric Association.

Ammaniti, M. (2018). Adolescenti senza tempo [Timeless Teenagers]. Milano: Raffaello Cortina Editore.

Battacchi, M. W. (2002). Vergogna e senso di colpa. In psicologia e nella letteratura [Shame and guilt. In psychology and literature]. Milano: Raffaello Cortina Editore.

Conte, E., & Tosi, S. (2016). Between spontaneity and intentionality of growth: Gestalt therapy and children. In M. Spagnuolo Lobb, N. Levi, & A. Williams (Eds.). Gestalt therapy with children. From epistemology to clinical practice (pp. 101–122). Siracusa: Istituto di Gestalt HCC Italy.

Fogarty, M., Bhar, S., Theiler, S., & O'Shea, L. (2016). What do Gestalt therapists do in the clinic? The expert consensus. *British Gestalt Journal, 25*(1), 32–41.

Francesetti, G. (2015). From individual symptoms to psychopathological fields. Towards a field perspective on clinical human suffering. *British Gestalt Journal, 24*(1), 5–19.

Frank, R. (2001). *Body of awareness. A somatic and developmental approach to psychotherapy.* Highland, NY: Gestalt Press.

La Barbera, D., La Cascia, C., & Guarneri, M. (Eds.). (2007). *Patologie del limite e narcisismo* [Pathologies of the limit and narcissism]. Palermo: Flaccovio.

Lancini, M. (Ed.). (2019). *Il ritiro sociale negli adolescenti. La solitudine di una generazione iperconnessa* [Social withdrawal in adolescents. The loneliness of a hyperconnected generation]. Milano: Raffaello Cortina Editore.

Lipani, M. (2014). "Mi sento taroccato". Identikit per un preadolescente in affanno ["I feel mugged". Sketch for a struggling pre-teen]. In G. Francesetti, M. Ammirata, S. Riccamboni, N. Sgadari, & Spagnuolo Lobb (Eds.). *Il dolore e la bellezza. Atti del III Convegno della Società Italiana Psicoterapia Gestalt* (pp. 165–168). Milano: FrancoAngeli.

Lipani, M. (2016). Disagio sottovoce. Fragilità e risorse in una famiglia alle soglie dell'adolescenza [Discomfort in a whisper. Fragility and resources in a family on the threshold of adolescence]. *Quaderni di Gestalt, XXIX*(2), 31–48. DOI: 10.3280/GEST2016-002004.

Lipani, M., & Conte, E. (2014). Giovani funamboli: esperienze depressive in adolescenza [Young tightrope walkers: Depressive experiences in adolescence]. *Quaderni di Gestalt, XXVII*(2), 95–108. DOI: 10.3280/GEST2014-002006.

Perls, F., Hefferline, R. F., & Goodman, P. (1994). *Gestalt therapy: Excitement and growth in the human personality.* New York, NY: The Gestalt Journal Press, or.ed., 1951.

Pietropolli Charmet, G. (2013). *La paura di essere brutti. Gli adolescenti e il corpo* [The fear of being ugly. Adolescents and the body]. Milano: Raffaello Cortina Editore.

Spagnuolo Lobb, M. (2012). Toward a developmental perspective in Gestalt therapy, theory and practice: The polyphonic development of domains. *Gestalt Review, 16*(3), 222–244.

Spagnuolo Lobb, M. (2016a). Self as contact, contact as self. A contribution to ground experience in Gestalt therapy theory of self. In J.-M. Robine (Ed.). *Self. A poliphony of contemporary Gestalt therapists* (pp. 261–289). St. Romain la Virvée, France: L'Exprimerie.

Spagnuolo Lobb, M. (2016c). L'esperienza adolescenziale nella società post-moderna. Intervista a Michela Marzano [The adolescent experience in post-modern society. Interview with Michela Marzano]. *Quaderni di Gestalt, XXIX*(2), 11–18. DOI: 10.3280/GEST2016-002002.

Spagnuolo Lobb, M. (2018). Aesthetic relational knowledge of the field: A revised concept of awareness in Gestalt therapy and contemporary psychiatry. *Gestalt Review, 22*(1), 50–68. DOI: 10.5325/gestalt review.22.1.0050.

Spagnuolo Lobb, M., Levi, N., & Williams, A. (Eds.). (2016). *Gestalt therapy with children. From epistemology to clinical practice.* Siracusa: Istituto di Gestalt HCC Italy Publ. Co., www.gestaltitaly.com.

Taylor, M. (2014). *Trauma therapy and clinical practice. Neuroscience, Gestalt and the body.* Maidenhead: Open University Press.

Chapter 11

Addiction as Persistent Trauma of the Ground Experience

Neuroscience and Gestalt Psychotherapy

Giancarlo Pintus and Marialuisa Grech

1. Addiction and Gestalt Psychotherapy: Possible Clinical Procedure

As Proust wrote "Perhaps the immobility of the things that surround us is forced upon them by our conviction that they are themselves, and not anything else, and by the immobility of our conceptions of them" (1922, p. 8). In a historical period like the one in which we are living, it could seem hyperbolical to define the spread of addictions as a pandemic. And yet the epidemiological and clinical data tell us that this is not a long shot. It is a common experience, in both the public and private sphere, to encounter an exponential increase in reports of addiction, with regard to both substance abuse or that of psychotropic pharmaceuticals, and that of addictions to do with objects (shopping, gambling, internet . . .), experiences (sex, work, sports, . . .) or persons ("love addiction" in all its various forms). We are dealing with a growth phenomenon, which concerns not only adolescents or youth, but adults and the elderly more and more. These are often unbreakable bonds, of which often people are not clearly aware or do not acknowledge. This often makes difficult the work of the psychotherapist, who can sense resistance on the part of the patient but also the quality of seduction, or the fear of undermining these relationships that have become absolute and inviolable ("Because an addict is someone who suffers from nostalgia" – Renato Zero, *Più Su*, 1974).

During training in psychotherapy, it therefore becomes essential to develop a specific sensitivity for going beyond the surface, for understanding such attachments and providing the necessary support so that the person may develop more diverse relational modalities in a world in which the Other is always experienced more as a danger or a burden. We are dealing with a type of suffering with multiple and complex neuro-bio-psycho-social implications, where the will of the patient might be reduced to the minimum, and the hoped-for change is simultaneously feared as a real bereavement.

Consequently, in this chapter, we wish to provide some knowledge relative to the neuro-biological and clinical-psychological dimensions of pathological dependencies; we will delve into the hypothesis of addiction as a persistent traumatic experience right from the onset; finally, we will accompany the reader in

DOI: 10.4324/9781003313335-14

this dramatic process of grasping the evolutionary aspects, which often amount to a failure of recognition in a primary relationship.

Along the way, we will offer a reading of the clinical case of Carla, in order to see in what way it is possible to restore a sense of relational security necessary for change.

2. Gestalt Psychotherapy, Neurosciences, and Addiction

The suffering related to the addictive experience is at the moment a largely unexplored clinical sphere and for which there exists a rather meagre reference bibliography in Gestalt psychotherapy.[1] Yet, we think that an integration of our clinical approach and neuroscientific knowledge is extremely justified and functional, all the while respecting specific epistemologies.

In his early work, Perls (1942) speaks about addiction in terms of the "dummy complex", namely the difficulty of completing the passage from sucking to that of biting, which represents the surrender to one's own physiological and healthy aggressiveness. The addicted person revives his need to belong to a relationship (which is his intentionality of contact left open), but he/she does it through the convergence with an object, surrendering to the aggressive force needed to manipulate the environment, and finding in the object of the bond a crutch and a relational surrogate. In fact,

> the lack of containment in the primary relationships and the uncertainty which characterizes daily life, have created a crucial change in people's way of life. Our clients . . . are unsure of what and who they are, what they want, if it is worthwhile to live since they do not know whether they will be alive tomorrow.
>
> (Spagnuolo Lobb, 2016a, p. 272)

Faced with such existential angst, the addicted person's attitude

> is to prevent the achieved behaviour [*Authors' note*, the use of the addictive object] from being snatched away (by weaning). The jaw is set in the hanging-on bite of the suckling with teeth, who could go on to other food, but won't. . . . This muscular paralysis prevents any sensation.
>
> (Perls *et al.*, 1951/1994, pp. 231–232)

In actual fact, the addicted subject moves from sensation towards action skipping the normal process of the growth of excitement, incapable of orienting himself appropriately within the environment. In short, the drug addict would seek, through substance use, to desensitise him/herself from the anxiety generated from the physiological increase of excitement in the contact process with the environment (Clemmens, 1997) and thus "The use of the toxic substance does not make them feel capable of independence, but is sought in order to feel their own bodies, to feel that they are living persons" (Spagnuolo Lobb, 2013, pp. 208–209).

In our view, addiction could be the adaptive result, the specific complementary psychobiological and social vulnerabilities, of a primary relational process in which the person taking care of the child is living a ground experience[2] that is full of anxiety or one that is perhaps desensitised, so as not to be able to be adequately attuned to the contact boundary (Pintus and Pappalardo, 2019). We therefore believe that the early relational deficiencies in the pre-personal phase of the building of the self may be an important factor of vulnerability at the onset of an addiction; the anxiety perceived in the field and created precisely by the significant adult can alter the spontaneous and vital presence of the Other at the contact boundary, causing a lack of that sensorial base upon which the self is built; in this way, primary relationships, in which the ability to contain angst fails, and in an ever more unpredictable world (cf. Spagnuolo Lobb, 2014), represent markers of vulnerability at the onset of addictive experiences and of a desperate need for belonging and recognition, which represents an unfinished intentionality of contact (cf. Pintus, 2011, 2015).

3. Carla and Her Shopping Cart Filled with Emptiness

When I meet[3] Carla, she is 39 years of age. She lives alone, has a bloated body, and carries herself awkwardly. She speaks with a strident tone of voice. She is disinclined to smile, and yet she still exudes a kind of yearning with a vestige of vitality. She often goes around with a shopping cart that she wearily drags along as if she were carrying within it the entire weight of a tortured life.

Carla is one of the 4 millions of Italians who, in 2019, it is estimated have occasionally or continuously made use of substances (cf. DPA, 2020). But Carla is also a heroin addict. She belongs to that clinical population in treatment, representing in Italy around 4% of consumers (around 130,000 people). As in a large segment of cases, Carla began her relationship with abused substances at a young age – at 11 years old: she drank alcohol, smoked cigarettes, and soon after tried cannabis. At 13, she got her first introduction to heroin: an explosive experience!

Carla is the youngest of three sisters, in a family in which the atmosphere is cold, aggressive, demeaning, characterised by the quarrels between the parents and an uncommitted attitude towards the daughters. No sense of connection, no warmth has ever been created among the sisters, and the memories of playing together are vague. The parents separate when Carla is 16 years old. From that moment begins the pilgrimage of moves from one house to another, from one city to another in an attempt to win the heart of her father. Carla has never had significant friendships. She struggles to remember the name of a few friends; as an adolescent she often runs away from home to find refuge in the only context in which she is able to find a place and an identity: the street.

For a girl not yet of age, the street is an extremely difficult setting in which to survive. Carla is a vagabond/beggar continuously in search of a man/father to protect her, support her, and provide warmth and safety. She is not searching for excitement when she trips. She doesn't need the "hit" of psycho-stimulants. Hallucinogens would alter a perception of reality already compromised; she is sad, angry, alone, and she seeks a hypnotic balm which might make living in this world more bearable. Heroin quickly offers this possibility, and Carla likes it because it can finally assuage her anguish, at least as long as the heroin flows hot and reassuring in her veins. At 19, she falls in love with another addict met at the corner of some street, and with whom she has a daughter, but just as in a poorly-written script, this man too will leave her due to an overdose.

At this memory, Carla stops, sinks into her seat, sighs, and for a moment seems far away from me, from this room, from everything. I feel cold. I have to swallow. I move my neck to feel my presence. I attune myself to her respiratory rhythm, and slowly her narrative continues. She remembers again being alone and even angrier. She "commits" to a love story with the drug, with the zeal, and the dedication that one has for a trusted lover. She often hangs around the street because it is there that she finds her "stuff" and is surrounded by other companions in solitude; *"with them I found warmth and closeness"* she says, *"the fix is a way to share something important. I wasn't alone. I was part of a tribe of desperate people that loved each other."* Carla is seeking a role, a family, a home, and heroin gives her a sense of belonging and the identity of a *"drug addict"*, which is how she still defines herself. With her cold and hard words, she describes this as an important period: *"Drugs were a constant discovery, the only certainty and stability that I could have. Heroin was a buffer for me. It extinguished every worry, every pain, even that of having left my daughter to my mother; heroin and I – we're all one.*

4. Brains, Minds, Relationship

Let us leave Carla for a bit with her reflections on the meaning of life and consider a few things. Numerous studies demonstrate that the relational detuning of the adult would result in a minor development of the mesolimbic area and a deficit in the decoding of the emotions and of the push towards experimentation, contributing to the turning of these children into fragile and insecure adults (Pintus and Pappalardo, 2019). In contrast, early involvement in a system of secure attachment, characterised by a sense of protection and security, stimulates, in the central nervous system, the production of neuropeptides (among which oxytocin) and monoamine (Pulvirenti, 2007), fundamental to the regulation of a sense of security (Porges, 2017), to the perception of danger and joy, and to the formation of cognitive maps. In some ways, their neuro-availability helps the building of affective certainties and trust in relationships, while their lack activates processes of insecurity and of the search for experiences, potentially at risk for dependency (Cozolino, 2006; Porges, 2017), as factors of compensatory affective modulation;

the use of substances, however, perpetuates the dysregulation in the release of oxytocin, crystallizing an already dysfunctional situation.

The modernity of the Gestalt model emerges precisely in this dialogic and fluid inter-exchange with the neurosciences[4] outlining effective hermeneutic and treatment keys in the field of addictive experiences as well.[5] Addiction, in fact, appears as one of the possible creative adaptations when the relationship with the significant Other fails, a relationship for which there was an absence of support, in a complicated experiential ground, for a vigorous awareness (Siegel, 2007) of one's own presence at the contact boundary. In addiction, we are dealing with a brain that could not tune in to other brains (Rizzolatti and Sinigaglia, 2006; Cozolino, 2006; Iacoboni, 2008; Rizzolatti and Vozza, 2008), because they were not spontaneously and totally present in the phenomenological field.

Brains not able to be shaped via the vital impetus of nurturing relationships remain deprived of a network of support and in a void of significant contacts. Interdependence is the natural condition of a human, and his/her brain is modified thanks to stimuli and relationships to which he/she is exposed from the very first phases of development. One who is raised within relationships that provide adequate recognition (in other words, those that support the intentionalities of the field), without distorting them with the anxieties of the figure of reference, is the fundamental premise of a nurturing and therapeutic relationship wishing to promote the growth of the person (Cavaleri, 2007): from birth to death, all of us need others who discover us, who are interested in learning who we are, and who help us to feel safe and secure (Cozolino, 2006).

By contrast:

> In the absence of the other, to be recognised will be the object that I consume, the object that I buy, the object upon which I become dependent. New dependencies are born out of the "nostalgia for the other", out of the dependency on another that isn't there. The other is not there and I become dependent on an object, on something, which instead is there, and which I can find anytime I want. New dependencies are the pathologically "transfigured" desire of the legitimate desire to be recognised by the other.
>
> (Cavaleri and Pintus, 2010, p. 45)

Recognition, in a culture that wishes to promote mental and social well-being, must become a basic function of educational and therapeutic programmes, because it is before a You that recognises me that is born an I, and upon which the mind is built – a possible phenomenon only within a co-constructed relational field. The mind then becomes a boundary event, because only at the contact boundary can a nurturing encounter be realised between an I and a You likely to stimulate growth and achieve the ultimate human pursuit: relational reciprocity (Cavaleri, 2007; Iacoboni, 2008).

The experience of addiction, on the other hand, inhibits growth and becomes a vicarious surrogate experience: moreover, addiction is a betrayal of love. The addicted person, in the first phases of his substance journey, is in all respects similar to a person in love, where the object of dependence is the surrogate of the relationship with the environment that has been neither warm nor nurturing, and has inhibited experiences of genuine recognition.

5. Addiction Therapy: Revitalise the Self, Perceive the Security and Safety of the Ground, and Provide Genuine Recognition

The intake and abuse of substances is usually associated with the adolescent period of evolution, but this fact is only partly true and takes on specific contours, although today, the styles of consumption, the types of substances and addictive experiences, and the significance of this relational style may be profoundly changed and involve transversally all ages and all socio-environmental conditions (cf. UNODC, 2016; EMCDDA, 2019; DPA, 2020; ESPAD, 2020).

Adolescence certainly remains the preferred period for transgression and the use of substances, a life phase in which the developmental themes of autonomy and dependence are reintroduced into the person's experiential field. Present-day adolescents, over-sheltered and deprived of the risk of engaging in experience, undoubtedly appear much more dependent on the adult than in the past; today, an adolescent has to deal with the imperative of proficiency, a constant demand on his/her own body/mind to perform, a demand that does not envisage normality or waiting (Spagnuolo Lobb, 2014). For the contemporary adolescent, finding his/her own space in the adult world, his/her evolutionary purpose, does not only have a social value, it is a genetic task; the adolescent lives a paradigmatic passage of time from the educational to the relational, and this latter time of creating a relationship with an adult is often bound up with performance. Failures are experienced as inabilities, limitation experienced as abnormal, and talent has become a central theme; in adolescence, the person contends with the fallibility and personal humanity of the significant adult.

Youngsters who have not been allowed to experience their own fallibility are more subject to enormous amounts of anxiety and angst. In this no-man's-land, the occasional encounter with the effects of a drug, the ability to experience nonfeeling, the pleasurable sensation of mood change, are almost always the reasons why a teenager will continue to use drugs. It can happen that at a certain point the addictive behaviour may no longer be pleasurable and becomes egodystonic, and it is usually in this moment when the adolescent asks for help. Adolescence represents a complex period for the difficult developmental task of self-definition, a moment of confusion between an identity no longer relevant and a new one in the process of being defined: if upon the teenager's request, the intentionality that he/she is requesting is not supported, and on the contrary, a raft is provided for the identity based on the symptom, one risks facilitating the process of dependence, equipping the youngster with a pathological label for the pain he/she is feeling.

Carla is an example of this: she was certainly a difficult little girl, born and raised in a metropolis, which does not offer much when faced with loneliness and pain. Shy, angry, and solitary, she wanders along the streets like an urban animal, in search of new experience, of new excitement, perhaps of love. There is no warmth in her house, or at any rate, it cannot be felt. After their separation, Carla's parents seem to be competing for who ignores her the most on the emotional plane, while their expectations for her academic performance, continually on the rise, must remain disappointed and frustrated: Carla pays back the absence of love and care with the worst grades in school and with disorderly behaviour. Of this period, she will afterwards say: "the greater their cold pretence that I was who knows who, the more I became aware of their non-involvement with me, and I reacted by denying their expectations. They were two strangers. I denied that they were part of my life if they could not give me affection, warmth, and a smile. As usual, in the end, I was the one who paid the price. I would have liked to continue my studies, and perhaps get a degree, but obviously destiny had other plans for me. I will never forgive my parents for never having truly loved me."

Heroin at 13 did the rest: it gives her warmth. It placates her past anger and solitude. It pampers her. At that time, there is no difference between the person and the substance. The borders are confused. The ground is invaded by the explosive pleasure of heroin (Pintus, 2011, 2014), and the rest of the world is excluded from it, and subsequently there will be no space even for her daughter, thus perpetuating the spiral of exclusion which had made her suffer so much as a child. Her interests steadily fade away. Human relationships evaporate into the background that is more and more pervaded by the obsessive pursuit of pleasure (or mostly the search for peace and tranquillity by then); the daily rhythm is marked by the constant ritual of "the search for money, the search for drugs/consumption/pleasure". She abandons every job she embarks on. She cannot handle the weight and the boredom of work. She however also begins to sense that her beloved drug is two-faced (pleasure and pain), but when she reduces her use of it, she cannot help but turn to alcohol.

Heroin, with which she begins to have some problems of tolerance and abstinence, will overwhelmingly return to her life at 24 years of age, almost like an old flame that is reserving a bitter surprise for her, because Carla, via the practice of taking the drug intravenously and due to the poor hygienic conditions in which she often lives, soon contracts Hepatitis B and C, which will force her to reassess her own life and her own autonomy. Even more devastating will be her encounter with the HIV virus: Carla's face becomes dark and serious when she hints at this page in her life, a moment that seems to her etched into her cognitive and emotional memory. The discovery of her seropositivity becomes for Carla the circumstance of a desperate cry of rage and pain, of fear and suffering for herself (and for her daughter), a trauma of consciousness from which she will only recover after many years.

In all of these years, Carla's parents never called into question their own role in the addiction suffering of their daughter, not even the mother who up until her death pointed her finger at that rebellious, stubborn, and angry child. From this clinical example, in this historic phase, it also seems urgent to reflect socially and clinically upon the support to parents in their intentionality of raising their child, in their competence at being in a conscious and syntonic way at the contact boundary, and then perhaps we will be able to see the number of young drug users diminish. In fact, a young person's treatment process is unthinkable if it does not see that the contextual, if not primary, obligation is to take charge of the parents. Only when the adolescent will feel safe and secure that someone is taking care of his/her parents, that he/she no longer has to do it, then will he/she be able to breathe, ask for help, and be in turn supported.

Supporting a parental couple whose child lives in a situation of pathological dependence means working, in therapeutic terms, by taking into account the fragile ground from which the two prevalent figures emerge: a sense of guilt and a sense of inadequacy with respect to role. Of the two figures, the sense of guilt is the most obvious, and the angst unleashed because of it, is what drives the couple, individually or together, to participate in an active way in their child's treatment process. When the parents reach out to social services or to the professional assigned to their son or daughter, the first thing they say is: "Because I don't understand. Where did I go wrong?" Thus, in order to get the anxiety over failure to retreat and leave space for a lucid vision of the lived experiences, the first intervention to undertake is to rid the field of the feeling, which is, on the one hand, omnipotent, in order to be able to decide in full about the child's life and destiny, and on the other hand, one of handing power over, for which the thought and the strategy that the couple offers is: "I have failed. You take care of it now." The dance with the parents entails these steps: a necessary closeness in the beginning so that they may be able to breathe and relax in a setting that does not judge the error that took place during the upbringing process, one that does not seek out a response no matter what, but one which stimulates a new question in the here-and-now of the relationship with the child. In this sense, in the parenting support process, there is also a need for the right distance, so as to allow the emergence of the new and competent parental figure. This important aspect is correlated to the second figure, which is inadequacy in terms of role. Being a parent today, as it has been over the last ten years, means fulfilling a role for which not only has one not been prepared but for which one has not been supported. Being a parent today means knowing what "you do not want to be", which essentially means not wanting to be like your own parents. However, it is not yet ingrained as a collective social experience how one can be a mother or a father today. Therefore, the parents of millennials are trying to be parents through "not being" rather than "being". From this, we see the importance of giving space to the experience of being a parent in one's own style, and of reinforcing, during the parenting support process, the originality of the individual person as a resource in the relationship with their son or daughter.

5.1 What Is the Aim in Addiction Therapy?

Let's go back to Carla: disappointed in heroin, a lover that she denies herself but one she cannot do without, Carla turns to the Servizio Tossicodipendenze (Drug Addiction Service) to be placed within a care community, but after a few months she discontinues the therapeutic programme in order to live with one of the other residents that she has met in the facility. In this period, Carla begins to take high maintenance dosages of Methadone. It feels like a dream of a real family, of a relationship of mutual support without the crutch of heroin but under the pharmacological cover of Methadone; however, the still fragile dreams drift away when her partner begins to use again, also dragging her once more into the abyss of heroin. As always, every attempt to discipline her relationship with the drug seems extremely difficult due precisely to the memory of pleasure.

The relationship becomes strained also because of the presence of her daughter, whom Carla wanted with her again after leaving the care community; she reached an awareness that the role of mother, no matter how awkward and inexpert she feels, is perhaps the only element of stability upon which she can count, and with this confidence she tries to survive despite the conflicts, and the betrayals of her partner, the financial difficulties, and her liver problems, related to her use of intravenous heroin. The couple crisis gets deeper and deeper, so she turns once again to the Drug Addiction Service for an integrative pharmacological treatment with Methadone and gradually carries out various therapeutic and socio-rehabilitative interventions, but she is always aloof, aggressive, and full of anger towards everyone, repeating her usual way of conducting herself: the quest for protection, relational diffidence, and the desire for autonomy. It is impossible for her to manage the attempt to stop using heroin in the presence of her partner, who uses their house as a place to deal and consume drugs, retriggering in Carla a most powerful and never-dormant craving. She tells in words issuing out of this primitive force: "Seeing him in that state, I would want to put his blood into my veins, so strong was the call of the stuff (heroin) and the anger for what he was feeling in his body with the heroin, while I was trying to give meaning to my life and that of my child." It is at this point that, with her tired shopping cart always with her, I become acquainted with Carla.

Let us immediately clarify a point: Gestalt psychotherapy in the treatment of addictions does not primarily aim at the subject's sobriety and abstinence, as much as, at the restoration of relational competencies based on the spontaneity of the self at the contact boundary. Having considered the neurobiological isomorphism between the cerebral areas involved in the genesis of a dependency, and the areas involved in the acquisition of relational competencies, we believe that a therapy to do with dependencies must be rooted in deep relational work that aims to provide containment (Spagnuolo Lobb, 2012) and to increase the person's crucial competence in making contact in a salutary and spontaneous way. However, Gestalt work with addiction experiences does not aim towards the management of the addictive object (the figure) as much as towards the promotion of a healthy and real experience of recognition and towards the mobilisation of the ground and the perception of time.

In pathological dependencies, the obsession with the object of love is so intense, so capable of nullifying the certainties acquired in the ground, that in the treatment it is necessary to work creatively in order to revitalise the ground; the treatment is therefore accomplished thanks to a strong relational rootedness, a place of settling down in which to be able to surrender one's own pain and shame, to support new and small excitements, to restore spontaneity at the contact boundary (Spagnuolo Lobb, 2013), and to co-create an experience of genuine recognition (cf. Pintus, 2011, 2014). Every attempt to make of therapy a management of the relationship with the substance risks disastrously foundering, because the object, or better the memory of the relationship with the object, is a much too strong antagonist with respect to the therapist-patient relationship, especially in the first phases of the therapy. Consequently, the goal of the treatment cannot be that of taming the relationship with the substance, as much as providing occasions for experimenting with the excitement of contact with the therapist-environment, so that the person may acquire the confidence and the competence to live the new experience in a salutary way.

Pleasure is, in fact, a hunger for nurturing experiences. Only in the novelty of full contact is there enjoyment and growth (Perls *et al.*, 1951/1994). Appeasing this hunger for pleasure, which is hunger for pleasurable relationships, is equivalent then to a return to the most intrinsically human condition, the condition of being a person-in-a-relationship, because there, where there is no environment capable of supporting this primary intentionality, the person with an impoverished ground will turn to relational surrogates. This constitutes what is implicit in terms of addictions in Gestalt psychotherapy: work based on relational containment (the ground) and not on the symptom (the figure). True healing is experiencing that one can fill the void left by the object, which is a void of nurturing relationships, through a relationship that trains one to achieve experiences of recognition and belonging.

The relational field that is created with an addicted patient seems, in fact, very demanding; characterised by anesthesia of the border, contradictions, rigidity, and emotional short circuits. Seduction, cynicism, contempt, disqualification, and ambivalence are all part of the acquired behavioural repertoire that the patient also brings to the therapeutic setting. A very interesting role is played, for example, by deception, at which it is necessary to look, not as an attempt to obtain a secondary advantage but as a symptom itself of the pathology of dependence. The chronic use of substances creates a cognitive distortion over time, almost a delusional misperception, because of which the person that is lying is absolutely convinced that what he/she is stating is the truth. Knowing this allows one to protect the relationship, giving up judgemental and misleading interpretations. The therapist must run the risk of being in what Stern (1985) defined as the intersubjective space ("I know that you know that I know") and use the wait as an integral part of therapy and the competencies of the clinician.

5.2 Clinical Treatment of Addiction as the Work
With the Ground

We have seen how the chronic use of addictive substances irreversibly alters the cells of the ventral tegmental area of the mesencephalon, of the nucleus accumbens, and of the entire dopamine system, which, when hit by waves of dopamine of exogenous origin, inhibits, through homeostasis, endogenous production, rendering the designated areas hypoactive. This would explain, on a neurobiological level, the hypophoric destiny of the post-drug-addicted personality in which the restoration of a physiological level of arousal of the dopaminergic system is slow and agitated, having as a consequence a tendency towards mood deflection and the risk of relapse.

The saturating power of the substance has occupied every space for reflection, every affective dimension, polarising and crystallising the immobile and the immutable perception of a time that is marked along the substance's search-consumption-effect rhythmic pattern. Carla's speech is pervaded by exclamation points, unshakeable categories, rationalisations in search of confirmation; everything is rigid, but there is no action, no movement. Excitement and vitality are lacking. Listening to her, one has the impression of an experience of an immobile and immutable world (Polster, 1987). Every attempt to make her therapy a management of her relationship with the drug will inevitably fail.

So much rigid compulsion and so little spontaneity could discourage any therapist, but "the Gestalt therapist not only observes these patterns but also tries to intuit the now-for-next, the intentionality concealed in the client's habitual, desensitised pattern of contact, via an aesthetic relational knowledge" (Spagnuolo Lobb, 2016b, p. 276).

In addiction, the ternary dimension of time seems abolished; all the tension seems to be turned towards the external (towards the search for the love object) or towards the internal (towards the enjoyment of pleasure or the relief from pain): the mobility of the border is traumatised (Pintus, 2016, 2017). Time becomes a blocked process in an eternal present, which is nostalgia for the past. The fixity of the figure does not allow for the mobilisation of the ground. There is nothing new. There is no other excitement. There is no assimilation. There is no growth.

This means that the patient is reliving a fixed script in which every day is the same as the last in the constant repetition of a rhythm no longer marked by chronological time, but by the urgent need to resort to the object of attachment: for an addicted person, there is no difference between work days and holidays. Each day, the anxiety must be quelled, and the memory of pleasure, lived in the first phases of the encounter with the drug, must be tenaciously pursued. The involvement is such that the mental and emotional space for every other desire, excitement, and motivation is progressively reduced, ultimately rendering the relationship with the object an absolute relationship (Pintus and Crolle Santi, 2014).

For these reasons, addicted people, and particularly drug addicts, seem to have lost the capacity to embrace change, to assimilate new knowledge, to update their own definition of themselves. Most of the time, even after an effective period of therapy, perhaps in a community setting, they are able at best to define themselves as "ex"-addicts. It is precisely in this moment that relapse into addiction is most easily discernible. Leach and Kranzler (2013) specifically demonstrate how the relapse is often triggered by experiences of rejection, abandonment, and relationships with hypercritical partners, for which, even if therapy enables one to have a reparative experience, the scar from the wound can reopen whenever unfavourable conditions arise. Carla is an expert in this: she has avoided prison but she has undertaken, as we have seen, various community programmes, therapies, and treatments. In the so-called "cage" where the users of The Drug Addiction Service station themselves in between conversations, coffees, fights, and laughs (especially those that want to escape the very sweet and lethal call of the street and those that have nothing to do and no one who expects them), Carla is considered an important and authoritative person – certainly not for her appearance. The beauty, which perhaps once graced her face and her body, is by now a faint memory. Carla is bloated, heavy, slow, ragged, and yet she has the attitude of a Roman matron that lends her dignity, respect, and authority in that circus of solitude and pain that is the "cage".

5.3 Therapy as the Experience of Recognition

Carla accepts, after much struggle and reflection, to pursue methadone treatment combined with admission to the Day Centre of the Drug Addiction Service initially with her usual diffidence and an air of challenge that one, who has learned to distrust the world, often adopts. Little by little, by means of the reading and commentary of the morning journal, the daily programming spent with the other inmates and care professionals, the care and maintenance of the facility's rooms, and through the participation in cultural or sporting initiatives outside of the Centre, Carla discovers new excitement, a new enthusiasm for the daily activities finally flowing through her, even if she feels the need to discredit them in order to protect herself from all the novelty.

One day she knocks on the door of the Centre, late as usual, and she displays a bag full of balls of wool and knitting needles; she enters dragging her feet but with an unusual light in her eyes. After the management business of the Centre, Carla asks if she can finish the scarf that she is making for her daughter and she shows me the knitting needles. I remember well the sensations I experienced, an accumulation of excitement and doubt, because Carla displays 4 knitting needles, looking me in the eyes in a challenging and ironic manner: I feel all the excitement and the risk involved with this new activity, while her eyes seem to penetrate mine for a time that seems infinite, but it comforts me to feel the vibrations at the contact boundary finally alive and throbbing.[6] I feel my breathing and hers little by little finding synchronicity – a harmonic rhythm. My muscles relax. I swallow and I see new mobility in Carla's face: I welcome the invitation to co-create something *together*, her intentionality never before fully realised; she will be the one to show me the right way to tie the wool to a knitting needle and to lift the other in the air, like swords. I give support to this skill of hers. She thanks me. Her body relaxes. She feels at home, and she opens herself up to this new creative experience. This is once more a *sword*, as drug addicts call the needle of the syringe, but a sword that gives life to something, knot after knot, centimetre after centimetre, knitting memories, hopes, pains, and fears.

With this novel project that Carla is offering at our contact boundary, I feel her confidence in taking a risk with me, in her new way of being in the here-and-now of the relationship. Accepting for me means supporting "the excitement for contact which has lost its spontaneity in development" of the patient (Spagnuolo Lobb, 2016a, p. 273).

This knitting, day after day, becomes our creative way of being together, while she narrates at the same time her troublesome past history and the renewed consciousness of her present, of her creative resources, of her fragile work plans, of her ambiguous relationship with heroin, made up of love and hate.

It is true that for the healthy organism "the present is always novel" (Perls *et al.*, 1951/1994, p. 22) but we have seen that this does not apply where the ternary process of time and the figure-ground dynamic have been crystallised around a single figure, the ever-present and de-contextualised result of the craving. Faced with this new gestalt, which timidly emerges from the ground, I grasp the sense of Perls' phrase for which in psychotherapy "the patient does not remember himself, merely reshuffling the cards, but 'finds and makes' himself" (Perls *et al.*, 1951/1994, p. 10).

5.4 The "Dance of the Words": Spontaneity and Reciprocity at the Contact Boundary

Caught in the continuous resolution of a proprioceptive emergency, which does not permit space for other intentionalities, or in the anxiety over the possibility that this emergency might suddenly come up, addicts live in the constant imperative of finding a solution to this distress that involves the entire psychic/physical apparatus with the immediacy and the inevitability of an instinct.

To the agonising question: "Who am I? Whom have I become?" the substance, already part of the neurobiological and emotional processes of the patient, allows for only one response, even if it is loaded with complex resonances: "*I am a drug addict, what else?*" At the same time, after therapy, self-definition risks being clarified not for what it has become but for what it is no longer, and Carla says it with her usual toughness: "*I am an ex-drug-addict, in some way I will always be one, for good or bad, my life is with heroin, and it will never leave me even if I won't seek it out anymore*".

Self-definition represents the clinical and social challenge for every addiction therapy, where the object of dependence has become one with the person, integrating itself into the identity. Consequently, every therapy, aimed at coming between the person and what he depends on, turns out miserably destined to fail by feeding the impotence of the therapist and the anger and frustration of the patient (cf. Pintus and Crolle Santi, 2014). The struggle and the fear of being able to assimilate something new renders the therapeutic action extremely taxing due to the difficulty in having an effect on the life and on the definition that the patient can provide for him/herself: the action risks not being able to assume that temporary form of the self, which we call assimilation, and so the self-regulative process, which is basically one's mental life, cannot achieve its full expression.

The real live presence of a significant other at the contact boundary, equipped with a non-judgemental attitude, and one that is open to the new and the beautiful, hidden by the symptom, can become for the addicted subject an opportunity to positively retrace dysfunctional pathways of attachment, which have created the conditions for a specific vulnerability at the encounter with highly restraining (initially), saturating (at the cognitive, emotional, and relational level), and dysfunctional experiences like addictions. But unlike an immobile and unchangeable object, the invigorating and real presence of the therapist can be a reparative occasion for achieving the interrupted intentionality. Thus, concepts like contact boundary, situational field, and aesthetic relational knowing represent an extraordinary and actual bridge to what the neurosciences have always outlined in the field of understanding the functioning of the cerebral processes and of the physiological pathogenesis of an addiction.

Meanwhile, from the muscular paralysis, which for years has characterised Carla's attitude, a timid but significant gesture of creative vitality is surfacing; in that contact boundary, prepared at length and skilfully avoided, emerges a creative action, which reconfigures the awareness of her needs, the growth of excitement, the ability to orient herself and manipulate that experience with a sense of fullness (Cavaleri and Lombardo, 1993). That action, which belongs to the final contact, is the result of a free and directed growth of movement towards the environment: a full intentionality that is consciously searching for its own active realisation in the contact with the environment, which Carla now deliberately savours with pleasure.

The hour of the "dance of the swords", as we decide to call that moment of unusual therapy based on the reciprocal, creative, and alive presence, becomes an appointment awaited with the pleasure of belonging together and of a full recognition – a moment in which Carla's existential themes are reactivated, lukewarm requests for guidance, plans to also share with the other care professionals in a flowing stream of awareness. Carla, perhaps for the first time, discovers herself capable of hesitant desires, capable of making requests that are at least a little confident, and capable of mobilising her own intentional energy towards action. During our meetings, what re-emerges in Carla, and between us, is that long-dormant spontaneity, which is "the art of integrating the ability to choose deliberately (ego-function) with two types of experiential ground: the acquired bodily certainties (id-function) and the social – or relational – definitions of the self (personality-function)" (Spagnuolo Lobb, 2013, pp. 71–72).

Thus is born the proposal to transform that manual skill of hers into an occupational opportunity in which Carla wants to play an active part, and it is incredible to watch her slowly thrive in her body as well (better looked after), in her appearance (more feminine), in her language (more articulate and less stiff): in this new spring, gratitude is being renewed for that "therapeutic art" (Spagnuolo Lobb, 2013, p. 131), which makes the taking care of others' wounds continually new, risky, and fascinating.

The desire for personal and financial autonomy extends towards the rediscovered capacity for wanting a better future for herself and her daughter, one made up of little things, exactly those elements that addiction caused her to lose. In the assimilation of this new *gestalt*, Carla has the possibility, in a protected environment, such as the therapeutic relationship, to become self-aware, detect desires, explore new and creative possibilities, by expanding the boundaries of self-definition, of her own responsibility, and transforming the lived experience into enriching knowledge for the relational ground.

Carla will always be marked by her relationship with heroin. The nostalgic craving will never abandon her, but for her this is clear, after years of therapy, and months and months of "dances" with the swords, that the old and dazzling love that annihilated every pain and delivered her to an inexpressible pleasure is long gone. It remains a bright and fearful memory of that abyss of synaptic pleasure, but her road today is driving her to push her cart onto quieter streets, ones that are less exciting, and in which she will be able to experience not being alone on a journey, and not being only an addict.

In this, and in a thousand other ways of living, the reciprocity between therapist and patient (Spagnuolo Lobb, 2019), in the aesthetic and phenomenological gaze of the therapist (Spagnuolo Lobb, 2012, 2016b, 2018), turned towards capturing and supporting the awkward harmony and withheld vitality, which emerges in the relational process, Gestalt psychotherapy becomes a fertile approach, and one still to be developed, in part, in the treatment of addictions.

Notes

1 On this subject see Pintus and Crolle Santi, 2014, p. 11.
2 For an in-depth study of the concept of "ground experience" see Spagnuolo Lobb, 2016b.
3 The clinical case reported here was followed by Giancarlo Pintus in a public service facility for addiction.
4 See Spagnuolo Lobb and Cavaleri (2011); Cavaleri (2013).
5 Gestalt psychotherapy founded upon a solid relational model (individual, group, residential) and upon reciprocity, in fact, allows people to repeat the primary experience of feeling accepted and cared for, facilitating the release of oxytocin and stimulating the processes of learning and the assimilation of the new (Panksepp, 2012).
6 When we say "the importance of being seen" we are referring to the experience of the other's gaze, which, without the use of words, allows us to have the experience of recognition, that experience that Carla has always lacked. That gaze, which, without words, tells us: "I am here, and I am here for you, because you are important to me now."

References

Cavaleri, P. A. (2007). *Vivere con l'altro. Per una cultura della relazione* [Living with the other. For a culture of relationship]. Roma: Città Nuova.

Cavaleri, P. A. (Ed.). (2013). *Psicoterapia della Gestalt e Neuroscienze. Dall'isomorfismo alla simulazione incarnata* [Gestalt therapy and Neuroscience. From isomorphism to embodied simulation]. Milano: FrancoAngeli.

Cavaleri, P. A., & Lombardo, G. (1993). In principio era l'azione. Riflessione sull'azione in Gestalt therapy [In the beginning was action. Reflection on action in Gestalt therapy]. *Quaderni di Gestalt, 15*, 25–39.

Cavaleri, P. A., & Pintus, G. (2010). "Essere-con" nel mondo di oggi. Dialogo sulla cultura della relazione ["Being-with" in today's world. Dialogue on the culture of relationship]. *Quaderni di Gestalt, XXIII*(1), 35–49. DOI: 10.3280/GEST2013-001006.

Clemmens, M. C. (1997). *Getting beyond sobriety. Clinical approaches to long-term recovery*. San Francisco: Jossey-Bass Inc. Publishers.

Cozolino, L. (2006). *The neuroscience of human relationships. Attachment and the developing social brain*. New York: W.W. Norton & Co Inc.

Dipartimento per le Politiche Antidroga – DPA. (2020). *Relazione annuale al Parlamento sul fenomeno delle tossicodipendenze in Italia anno 2019* [Annual report to Parliament on the phenomenon of drug addiction in Italy year 2019]. Roma: Presidenza del Consiglio dei Ministri.

EMCDDA – European Monitoring Centre for Drugs and Drug Addiction. (2019). *European drug report 2019: Trends and developments*. Luxembourg: EMCDDA Joint Publication.

ESPAD Group – European School Survey Project on Alcohol and Other Drugs. (2020). *Results from the European school survey project on alcohol and other drugs*. Luxembourg: EMCDDA Joint Publication.

Iacoboni, M. (2008). *I neuroni specchio. Come capiamo ciò che fanno gli altri* [Mirror neurons. How we understand what others do]. Torino: Bollati Boringhieri.

Leach, D., & Kranzler, H. R. (2013). An interpersonal model of addiction relapse. *Addictive Disorders and Their Treatment, 12*(4), 183.

Panksepp, J., & Biven, L. (2012). *The archaeology of mind: Neuroevolutionary origins of human emotion*. New York: W.W. Norton & Company Inc.

Perls, F. (1942). *Ego, hunger and agression: A revision of Freud's theory and method*. New York: Random House.

Perls, F., Hefferline, R. F., & Goodman, P. (1994). *Gestalt therapy: Excitement and growth in the human personality*. New York: The Gestalt Journal Press, or.ed., 1951.

Pintus, G. (2011). Tempo e relazione nel vissuto dipendente. Percorsi ermeneutici e clinici [Time and relationship in dependent living. Hermeneutical and clinical paths]. In M. Menditto (Ed.). *Psicoterapia della Gestalt contemporanea. Esperienze e strumenti a confronto* (pp. 203–210). Milano: FrancoAngeli.

Pintus, G. (2015). Processi neurobiologici e riconoscimento terapeutico nell'esperienza addictive [Neurobiological processes and therapeutic recognition in addictive experience]. *Quaderni di Gestalt, XXVIII*(1), 63–71. DOI: 10.3280/GEST2015-001005.

Pintus, G. (2016). Neurobiological processes and contact competence in addictive experience. *International Journal of Psychotherapy, XX*(3), 23–29.

Pintus, G. (2017). Addiction as persistent traumatic experience: Neurobiological processes and good contact. *Gestalt Review, 21*(3), 221–232.

Pintus, G., & Crolle Santi, M. V. (Eds.). (2014). *La relazione assoluta. Psicoterapia della Gestalt e dipendenze patologiche* [The absolute relationship. Gestalt psychotherapy and pathological addictions]. Roma: Aracne Editore.

Pintus, G., & Pappalardo, N. G. (2019). Sintonizzazione genitoriale, riconoscimento degli stati affettivi e vulnerabilità alle addiction: alcuni dati di ricerca [Parental attunement, recognition of affective states, and vulnerability to addiction: Some research data]. *Quaderni di Gestalt, XXXII*(2), 79–97. DOI: 10.3280/GEST2019-002005.

Polster, E. (1987). *Every person's life is worth a novel*. New York: W.W. Norton Co Inc.

Porges, S. W. (2017). *The pocket guide to the polyvagal theory. The transformative power of feeling safe*. New York: W.W. Norton & Company, Inc.

Proust, M. (1922). *In search of lost time*. London: Chatto and Windus.

Pulvirenti, L. (2007). *Il cervello dipendente* [The addicted brain]. Milano: Salani.

Rizzolatti, G., & Sinigaglia, C. (2006). *So quel che fai* [I know what you do]. Milano: Raffaello Cortina.

Rizzolatti, G., & Vozza, L. (2008). *Nella mente degli altri. Neuroni specchio e comportamento sociale* [In the minds of others. Mirror neurons and social behavior]. Bologna: Zanichelli.

Siegel, D. J. (2007). *The mindful brain: Reflection and attunement in the cultivation of well-being*. New York: W.W. Norton & Co Inc.

Spagnuolo Lobb, M. (2012). Toward a developmental perspective in Gestalt therapy theory and practice: The polyphonic development of domains. *Gestalt Review, 16*(3), 222–244.

Spagnuolo Lobb, M. (2013). *The now-for-next in psychotherapy: Gestalt therapy recounted in post-modern society*. Siracusa: Istituto di Gestalt HCC Italy Publ. Co., www.gestalt italy.com.

Spagnuolo Lobb, M. (2014). Web: il richiamo dell'altrove, tra riconoscimento e definizione di sé [Web: The call of elsewhere, between recognition and self-definition]. *Etica per le professioni, 2*, 21–28.

Spagnuolo Lobb, M. (2016a). Self as contact, contact as self. A contribution to ground experience in Gestalt therapy theory of self. In J.-M. Robine (Ed.). *Self. A polyphony of contemporary Gestalt therapists* (pp. 261–289). St. Romain la Virvée, France: L'Exprimerie.

Spagnuolo Lobb, M. (2016b). Gestalt therapy with children. Supporting the polyphonic development of domains in a field of contacts. In M. Spagnuolo Lobb, N. Levi, & A. Williams (Eds.). *Gestalt therapy with children. From epistemology to clinical practice* (pp. 25–62). Siracusa: Istituto di Gestalt HCC Italy, www.gestaltitaly.com.

Spagnuolo Lobb, M. (2018). Aesthetic relational knowledge of the field: A revised concept of awareness in Gestalt therapy and contemporary psychiatry. *Gestalt Review, 22*(1), 50–68. DOI: 10.5325/gestalt review.22.1.0050.

Spagnuolo Lobb, M. (2019). The paradigm of reciprocity: How to radically respect spontaneity in clinical practice. *Gestalt Review, 23*(3), 234–254. DOI: 10.5325/gestaltreview.23.3.0232.

Spagnuolo Lobb, M., & Cavaleri, P. A. (2011). Psicoterapia della Gestalt e neuroscienze: il perché di un dialogo [Gestalt therapy and neuroscience: The reason for dialogue]. *Quaderni di Gestalt, XXIV*(2), 5–9. DOI: 10.3280/GEST2011-002001.

Stern, D. N. (1985). *The interpersonal world of the infant: A view from psychoanalysis and developmental psychology*. New York: Basic Books.

UNODC – United Nations Office on Drugs and Crime. (2016). *World drug report*. New York: United Nations.

Chapter 12

Conflict in Couple Relationships as Space for Recognition

An Opportunity that is Still Possible in the Post-Pandemic World

Pietro Andrea Cavaleri

1. The Global Economy and a Smartphone as a Friend

Like a hurricane that devastates everything in front of it, the pandemic has also hit the lives of many couples hard.[1] Compared to the previous period, divorces and separations have increased, there has been more conflict and more diverse forms of violence in family relationships (cf. Longo, 2021). The loss of work, forced cohabitation for long days, and sudden social instability have seriously altered precarious relational balances and brought to light already existing vulnerabilities (cf. Cavaleri, 2020). This is what emerges from the story of Giuseppe and Francesca, from which this reflection on couple conflict as a possible space of recognition begins (cf. Cavaleri, 2018).

Giuseppe has been speaking non-stop for over ten minutes now, his tone of voice loud and aggressive. It is as though he is reciting the same old speech for the umpteenth time, a script he knows off by heart. Francesca sits still and silent without even trying to interrupt. Her eyes blink in and out of focus, first on her husband, then on me, almost as though checking how much credence I am giving his accusations. The atmosphere becomes increasingly stifling, but what their bodies are telling me implicitly attracts my attention much more than the monologue that is becoming increasingly annoying. Giuseppe is a banker, whereas, after years of working in accounts for a company, Francesca is now unemployed. They have been married for ten years and have two daughters. Their married life was smooth and peaceful, but for the last two years their relationship has been in crisis. He is obsessed with the idea that his wife, through Facebook, has become mixed up with a dubious group of people and suspects that she is already cheating on him. His jealousy has reached such a point that he has wiretapped the house, without, however, obtaining "sufficient proof." Nevertheless, he cannot rid himself of the idea that she has "a friend," and is growing more and more convinced of it by the day.

Stoking Giuseppe's jealousy is the fact that, ever since she has lost her job, Francesca spends extensive amounts of time on her smartphone, and with a recently divorced neighbour. The two women would appear to spend so much

DOI: 10.4324/9781003313335-15

time together, that Giuseppe has even begun to suspect they have a lesbian relationship. Their life together is deteriorating day by day. He is growing increasingly obsessive and overbearing. She shuts herself up in a deathly silence for days on end after every argument, which only makes her husband's suspicions worse. Their sexual intimacy has become non-existent, and that, for him, is further proof that she must be having a relationship with another person, whether a man or a woman. Francesca is worn out by what she calls her husband's "unfounded" and "obsessive" jealousy. Their immediate families and a handful of friends know of their troubles, but after their initial, unsuccessful attempts to help, they have all abandoned them. They are alone and confused. The state of confusion and turmoil between them is now out of control. But then, that is hardly surprising! The context of their relationship is typical of our times.

We have here a highly "liquid" context, unstable and insecure, marked by isolation, solitude, and the absence of tight-knit social networks able to support the couple in their moments of crisis. But in the place of relatives and friends, there is something else – there is the invasive presence of social media networks, a relational world that is entirely virtual and frustrating in its illusory inconsistency. And then there is extensive financial and job instability. Changes in the working world and the economic recession of recent times have left their toll on many families, upsetting many private situations and straining the balance of many relationships.

The evident "fragility" of the couple relationship is perhaps tied to how our very conception of the marital bond has changed. From the "social" event it once was, marriage has been transformed into a "private" affair, where the ties between a couple are no longer underpinned by a legal bond or a strong sense of responsibility, but rather by a sentiment, by a simple affective relationship (see Bauman, 2003; Cavaleri *et al.*, 2013). If that "sentiment" vanishes, there is no longer any reason for the formal "bond" to exist, or for informal cohabitation to continue (Miller, 1997). The "bond" can simply be dissolved, but not without suffering and rifts.[2]

2. Gestalt Intervention and the Complexity of the Organism/Environment Field

Giuseppe and Francesca are opposite me. One raves on obsessively; the other is locked away in silence. Their emotions have an impact on me – I am part of their same *field*! I share it fully, co-creating it together with them through my presence. What can I do to help them? Where do I start? What Gestalt therapy tools can I draw on? Working with couples, I have learnt how important it is to orient myself by four cardinal "Gestalt" points. They have become a sort of "compass" for me, helping me find my way in the *field* that is co-created with the couple at every instant. Those "four cardinal points" are: focus on the *ground*; pay attention to *aesthetic relational knowing*; support *mutual recognition*; and revitalise the *integrating and regulatory function of the self*.

2.1 A Ground to be Revealed and Lots of Unfinished Business Waiting for an Answer

From the very first session, couples that come for counselling or therapy are entirely focussed on their own "figure," or what they judge to be the cause of the crisis. In general, they present contrasting versions of that "figure," where each party provides a different description of it. Nevertheless, both partners will agree that what is brought to the session is the "figure" they need to work on and be helped with. For the couple in our example, the "figure" is without a doubt constituted by the obsessive jealousy of the husband, which is legitimate and entirely justified for Giuseppe, whereas it is unjustified and delusional for Francesca. What is certain, in reality, is that if the therapist concentrates on the "figure" brought by the couple, without shifting the focus onto the "ground," he or she will not get very far. For it is in the "ground" that the polarities lying in the shadows of the conflict are regularly found – forgotten traumas, denied emotions, hidden needs, emerging intentionalities. Buried deep in the "ground" lie personal fragilities and vulnerabilities that are not accepted and then projected onto the other, requests that each partner would like to make but which they are too ashamed to even express.[3] To better understand how important it is to focus on the "ground" and all that is buried in it, let's return now to our couple and see what they can reveal to us in this regard.

In the first session, Francesca's agitation is palpable, and it is clear she has something important to say. She has discovered that her husband "drinks." Giuseppe is highly embarrassed, but then justifies himself by saying, "everyone does it," and that there is nothing wrong with having a drink. It is a way of "picking [himself] up" when he gets home after a stressful day. At work, he has been under pressure for months. He absolutely has to make a good impression on the boss, because there is talk of staff cutbacks. But it is "all under control," and he can stop whenever he wants. I ask him how he can be so sure. He stares at me, almost piercing me with his gaze. His eyes are lost in the void, as though captured by a remote, yet intense memory. He replies that it has happened before, at various times when he was younger, and he has always had the willpower to stop. This sudden reference to the past comes with something of a grimace, a hint of a bitter smile, almost as though he wants to open up to me, as though he wants to tell me something unpleasant that Francesca knows but I do not. There is a "secret" there, one which he might do well to bring out in the open. As he speaks, his eyes begin to moisten. I understand he is about to tell me something very important. In the *field* between the three of us, there suddenly emerges a sort of "positive" tension, made up of an intense urge to listen, silent expectation, and focussed attention.

He was just over eighteen years of age and he was going to the beach with a female friend one Sunday towards the end of summer. All of a sudden a car cut across the road and he was unable to brake in time. The collision was inevitable, and his friend was killed on impact. Although investigations by the police found that he was not at fault in any way, the event devastated him and for a long time he was wracked by a deep sense of guilt, haunted by nightmares, and subjected to panic attacks. His first experience with alcohol abuse goes back to that time. Then came his routine, orderly job at the bank, and his meeting meek and reliable Francesca, marking the start of a new life of stability and certainty. Suddenly, Giuseppe interrupts his story and stops, as though snapping out of a dream. A tense, lost look returns to his face. He looks at his wife, as though wanting to return to the crude reality of today. For him, the real problem is not that he has started drinking again, but that his wife is no longer the person she was before. The *field* changes abruptly. The climate of fear and anger that seemed to have vanished just before returns. Giuseppe's voice resumes its resentful tone and he accuses his wife of having drastically changed. Before she was kind and considerate, a woman "with a head on her shoulders." Now she has changed beyond all recognition, she is "out of her mind!"

Francesca, who up to this point has seemed absorbed by her husband's words, becomes jumpy again and starts wriggling nervously in her seat. I ask her to take a deep breath and only after that invite her to speak, addressing her husband directly and looking him in the eyes. A few seconds go by. Then, with an assertive attitude that for me is completely unexpected, she begins to speak. It is not true, she says, that she is "out of her mind" and that she has changed. She was just fourteen years old when her father died from a terminal illness. Widowed, her mother sought affective support and concrete help from her. To help the family, she was forced to drop out of university and start working straight away. When she met Giuseppe, for her it meant a return to a normal life. In him she found that emotional stability and sense of security and containment that she had lost with the death of her father. But now it is as though she needs something else, something opposite perhaps. She feels the need to go beyond her family responsibilities, beyond the safety of patterns that have long shielded her from her fears. Hence the friends on Facebook and the time spent with the divorced neighbour, representing a sort of desire to get to know the lives of others, whose approach to life has been very different from hers, free from the stifling duties imposed on her first by her widowed mother, then by her husband, initially a safe haven, now an oppressive prison.

The couple's "ground" is revealing all its hidden wounds, all its "unfinished business," all the skeletons that seemed to belong to the past, but which still have the power to materialise anew, with the same destructive force as before. Giuseppe carries within him a trauma that continues to gnaw at him after all these years. The tragic death of his friend brought him prematurely face to face with how unpredictable life is and how that can make us feel so infinitely vulnerable. To deal with that traumatic discovery, he seems to have learned to take obsessive control of everything and everyone, including Francesca. In describing how he feels when his wife is intent on her smartphone, Giuseppe says, "It's as though she's left reality behind and stepped into a movie. A movie where what happens is no longer under my control. It makes me feel powerless and inadequate."

Even Francesca appears to have forgotten something in the "ground." She is unable to see and reconcile herself with a part of her that was stolen prematurely from her adolescence. Too early in her life she was denied the chance to transgress, to experience life without the emotional blackmail and duties of all sorts imposed on her from the outside. It is highly likely that, just like Giuseppe, she lives in a dream world. In response to her husband's jealousy, she often will not say a word, shutting herself away in silence. She relates: "I feel oppressed, like I'm in a prison I can't escape from!" Perhaps she is reliving the oppression of an old prison, in which she was locked away for years, before getting married. Giuseppe initially was a "tower" in which to recover her lost sense of security, but now that "tower" has become a grim prison.

The "co-created ground" shared by the couple and the therapist is decisively too insecure and unreliable, weighed down and shaken by an unsustainable anxiety. What assessment can we give of it? While we observe our couple from a Gestalt therapy perspective, it could be of great help to draw on the analysis proposed by Margherita Spagnuolo Lobb (2016) to describe the experience of the "co-created ground" under different types of perception at the contact boundary. If in normal conditions the environment is perceived to be reliable and the ground is clear and transparent to the self, experienced as a safe and secure existential base, in a framework where the ground is experienced with anxiety, that clarity, security, and reliability are dangerously missing.

In the light of this, we can hypothesise that the traumatic experience of a sudden loss, such as that suffered by Giuseppe, produced the perception in him of a ground that is insecure, unstable, and unreliable, a ground that the self is no longer able to control and predict in a sufficiently adequate way. The sudden trauma modified the entire figure-ground relationship, leaving the self unable to assimilate the novel state of affairs and incapable of processing and integrating the change. On the diagnostic plane, such an understanding of the "ground" induces us to consider Giuseppe's tendency for control as an adaptive strategy to deal with the trauma, as an attempt to survive it and stem the sense of insecurity that has pervaded his life ever since; whereas on the therapeutic plane, it directs us to intervene in order to support the self in its creative ability to process the loss and accept the novel state of affairs.

The loss of her father, the premature imposition of duties and responsibilities, and the impossibility of fully exploring adolescence produced in Francesca the experience of a ground perturbed by anxiety, which in this case, however, assumes neurotic connotations. The ground, in fact, continues to be sufficiently clear and secure for her. The anxiety with which it is perceived is not always experienced at such an elevated level. Nevertheless, a certain degree of spontaneity has been lost; the equilibrium between active and passive presence is upset, and no clear vision can be had of the other. All these elements will steer our therapeutic intervention towards greater support for the ego-function of the self, the legitimisation of spontaneity, and the capacity to be fully present to the senses.

2.2 How to Draw on "Aesthetic Relational Knowing"

Slowly, the couple's co-created ground is revealing itself to us and becoming a little clearer and less confusing. A careful reading of it will now help us orient our work better. But that is not enough. How can we continue to "see" the ground through the initial figure imposed by the couple? What can we draw on to move in the right direction? To answer those questions, we need to focus on the second "cardinal point" of our "compass," which is *aesthetic relational knowing*. To understand the constantly shifting situation of the couple and focus constantly on the "shared phenomenological field" constituted by the couple itself and the therapist, it is essential to draw on a special form of knowing, which Margherita Spagnuolo Lobb (2018), borrowing in part from Stern (2010), calls *aesthetic relational knowing* of the field. Aesthetic relational knowing is a knowledge that revolves around two fundamental experiences of the couple and the therapist in the first person – embodied empathy and resonance. As we all know, there are many ways of knowing the world in which we are immersed. In general, the cognitive type of perspective, which refers, as Schore (1994) would say, to the left hemisphere, is given precedence. What we are talking about here, instead, is a knowledge that refers to the right hemisphere, one which gravitates towards the aesthetic dimension, towards spontaneity at the contact boundary, i.e. the way in which reality reaches our senses, the empathetic vibrations of the body, and emotional resonance as sensitivity to the *phenomenological field co-created* in the therapeutic encounter.

Drawing on this type of knowing is a strategic choice for the Gestalt therapist, especially when working with couples, where the atmosphere that fills the field and the implicit, non-verbal elements of the relationship prove particularly decisive (cf. Cavaleri and Spagnuolo Lobb, 2017). It is a type of knowledge that is integral to the Gestalt therapy framework and its phenomenological approach to the *field*, but which also rests on solid neurophysiological bases. In fact, it is rooted, on the one hand, in the discovery of mirror neurons and in research concerning *embodied empathy* and *embodied simulation* (Gallese, 2006), and on the other, on discoveries by Porges (2017) concerning *neuroception* and *social engagement*. In contrast to individual settings, in a couple setting, the two partners tend quickly to forget they are in a context of professional care and often engage with each other in a spontaneous way, thereby manifesting the habitual interactions acted out in private, and giving way to a verbal aggression that can be quite violent at times, as well as to explicit or poorly concealed attempts at manipulation. All this heightens the conflict, feeds the dynamics of the rupture, triggers archaic "attack and escape" or "freezing" mechanisms, and renders the atmosphere stifling and the co-created field treacherous and unsafe. Thus there is a need to work on the *field*, to create the necessary conditions to foster more secure and reliable "social engagement" (Gottman and Schwartz Gottman, 2018). To achieve this objective, the fundamental key lies in focussing on *aesthetic relational knowing*.

A good part of the relational involvement experienced constantly by a couple is managed automatically through neuroception – the acute sensitivity to detecting the intonation of the voice and facial expression of the partner, and to signs of danger or safety coming from the physical environment, sounds, and noises. Both the system of social involvement and attack-and-escape or freezing behaviours are connected with neuroceptive automatisms. In order to make the setting for the couple more reliable, it is necessary to introduce into the co-created field key elements of safety. Elements such as attentive listening, the use of a low vocal tone, a direct, relaxed gaze, a regular breathing pattern, and game-playing have a non-negligible effect on the therapeutic plane, calming the physiological state of tension and supporting social interaction, thereby fostering processes of awareness (Dana, 2018).

It should also be stressed how promoting mutual engagement and bidirectional communication, fostering an understanding of bodily reactions, and drawing attention to affective processes in the co-created field are all key to enabling all three people in the session to connect and co-regulate themselves better, building more positive and secure relationships. At the same time, all this helps open up access within each person to a level of knowledge, which is aesthetic relational, and which draws its most important clues from the qualitative elements of the relationship itself (safe or unsafe, reliable or unreliable), at the preverbal (facial expressions, tone of voice, breathing patterns) and intercorporeal levels. All these clues can only be grasped if we learn to be "open to the senses" and be fully present at the organism/environment "contact boundary" in the co-created field. They are all "aesthetic elements" that allow each of the three players to "know" what is happening inside their own organisms through interoception and what is happening outside, in the co-created field, through exteroception.[4]

In the decisive session related earlier, the "aesthetic clues" in the field that suggested I should put aside the "figure" – the problem of obsessive jealousy – and turn towards the husband's ground came to me with great intensity from Giuseppe's eyes. Even before he started speaking of his "tragedy," his eyes were lost in the void and glazed over, almost as though expressing a deep suffering and the surging of an intense emotion. What I saw elicited a strong "resonance" in me. I felt a sudden sense of compassion towards him and was overcome with emotion! Giuseppe noticed me for an instant. He had yet to say a word, but our eyes met and spoke volumes. That mutual "preliminary knowledge" allowed him subsequently to start to relate his secret, his tragedy, in a climate he sensed to be safer and more reliable, as he would later tell me.

2.3 A Sisyphean Task, or the Continuous Struggle for Recognition

In the life of the couple as well as in the therapeutic setting, knowledge of oneself and the other is an acquired knowledge that soon reveals itself to be precarious and provisional. No sooner have we acquired it than it appears to apply no more, lacking any truth and ability to explain a relational reality that in the meantime has already changed and which calls for new cognisance, to be "re-cognised." When conflictual tensions emerge in a co-created field, the state of conflict often signals a flaw of cognisance, the lack of a re-cognition that is necessary but late in coming. From that point of view, the conflictual rift constitutes a positive relational event, which calls for each partner to adapt to the novel situation and overhaul their knowledge of the other. In short, it calls for "mutual re-cognition".[5] And thus we have arrived at our "third cardinal point," or *mutual recognition*.

Maria and Giovanni have always been the classic "perfect couple," envied by all. They recently celebrated their twenty-fifth wedding anniversary. They have been together ever since they were teenagers, when she was still the shy, insecure daughter of divorced parents, and he a cocky engineering student, the son of a successful property developer. A long time has passed since then, and their roles seem to have been inverted. Today, she has a successful career managing a chain of stores selling oriental carpets. He, after taking over the family business, was forced to close it down due to the economic crisis that hit the building sector. To avoid remaining unemployed, he started managing one of his wife's stores. While secretly playing with her father's smartphone one day, the youngest of their three daughters discovered he was having an extramarital affair and she immediately told her mother, who now wants a divorce. Giovanni claims he ended the affair ages ago, that it was just a "moment of weakness!" – he loves his wife and would never leave her. In recent months he has felt neglected by his wife, and he only cheated on her to feel "more like a man!" Maria is furious and wants to kick him out, but a part of her is also afraid for her daughters, as she does not want them to suffer the way she did when her parents broke up.

At the start of their relationship, they felt sure they knew each other well. Now, they have suddenly discovered they have changed and are struggling to re-cognise. Giovanni is frustrated with his professional identity and finds it difficult to recognise and accept his wife's "assertive" side, to the point he fears being "crushed" by it. Maria refuses to make contact with her more insecure side and so does not recognise her husband's hidden fragilities and his shame at having failed in his career. Each of them misrecognises the other in the part of the ground that has re-emerged, but at the same time, they each refuse to identify as their own the polarities in the shadows, hidden within themselves.[6] A sort of blindness prevails in each of them, inhibiting them from recognising their own wounds and recognising the wounds of the other. In this shared darkness, the suffering that spills from each of their wounds is attributed to the other, such that Giovanni dramatically feels "neglected," to the point of having to do something to "feel more of a man," while she has been patently "cheated on" by an ungrateful husband, who therefore has to go.

As Zinker (1977) would say, Giovanni and Maria have divided up their polarities and each fills the "dark" polarity of the other. Each attacks the other from the position of the polarity that is dark to them, thus transferring into the couple relationship their own unresolved polarity conflicts.[7] Giovanni attacks Maria from the position of the "failed businessman," who feels humiliated and neglected by a "career woman." Maria attacks Giovanni from the position of the "insecure adolescent," destabilised by the unsuspected fragility of the "rock-solid man" she married years ago. The intentionality of a "failed husband" in need of help cannot be reconciled with the intentionality of an "adolescent wife" in need of secure certainties. If each of the partners can be helped to identify with their own "dark polarity," to embrace it and nurture it, it will be easier for them to recognise and accept the intolerable side of the other. In that way, their separate intentionalities can be integrated together, opening up space for a clearer and more vital "intentionality of the couple".[8]

The gift of recognition can be given to the other, if we ourselves have already received it from someone, and if, with time, we have learnt in some way to give it to ourselves.[9] Recognising the other, being recognised by him/her, and recognising ourselves are closely interconnected experiences. They are all different aspects of the same relational alchemy that sparks our humanity. If that precious alchemy is lost, we risk losing not only our humanity, but also our mental equilibrium, our psychic well-being, the harmony of our couple relationships, and even the peace of the communities and the world in which we live. Siegel (2007) claims that the areas of the brain activated by an experience of "interpersonal empathy" are the same as those activated in the experience of "intrapersonal empathy." This confirms how the capacity to recognise the other is closely connected with the experience of being recognised, but also with the capacity of recognising ourselves – of identifying with our own personal history, with the fragilities and the wounds it has left in us, and of learning how to process them, embrace them, and integrate them so as to build a "consistent vision," a Gestalt of ourselves, a complete and meaningful figure.

Thus there is a "triadic perspective" to constantly bear in mind – recognising the other, being recognised by him/her, and recognising ourselves.[10] All three constitute "foundational" human experiences, on which depend the humanisation of every relationship, the regulatory quality of the co-created field, and the mental health of every single organism that interacts within it. The central importance of recognition in a broad sense, and especially mutual recognition, has come to constitute a basic fact not only for Gestalt therapy, but for the greater part of contemporary psychological and neuroscientific research.[11] And although we are cognisant of all this, a question, however, still remains. What approaches can be taken to promote and foster recognition?

From a phenomenological point of view, while I am with Maria and Giovanni, I might sense what they must be experiencing in that moment by "analogy" with what I would be feeling if I were in their shoes. Or I might entirely neglect my previous personal experience and let myself be totally overtaken by their presence, and be overrun by their questioning faces (Lévinas, 1969). Or, again, I might concentrate on what is happening "between" us, which means focussing my attention on a "third dimension," which is not only mine or only theirs but is made up of "midway" realities – the continuous exchange of moods, implicit meanings, emotions, and aesthetic elements that emerge and impact "between" us (Ricoeur, 2005). This "third dimension" (Benjamin, 2017) which constitutes a good part of the co-created field is the elective sphere of recognition. It is the clearing from which it is possible to regenerate co-regulation and support ways to promote mutual recognition within the couple relationship, the place from which a Gestalt emerges, a unitary yet unmerged form, capable of integrating mutual differences and imbuing them with new meaning. Spagnuolo Lobb (2013, p. 195) identifies this step in the couple's ability to differentiate in the other's behavior the intentionality that determines it, separating it from the wound it causes in her/him.[12] But even here, as with aesthetic relational knowing, if I hope to grasp all that, I need to be "open to my senses" and fully present at the "contact boundary." I need to be so as the therapist, and I have to teach the two partners in the couple relationship to be so, session after session.

Even mutual recognition is never an accomplished and definitive experience, but regularly reveals itself to be an ongoing "Sisyphean task," marked constantly by the frustrating realisation of having to start all over again. Mutual recognition is what nourishes the life of a couple and much more, yet its fragile and precarious dynamics seem destined in fact to lead us constantly to a "rift," to an inexorable and extenuating failure.

Benjamin (1988, 2017) offers a highly original take on the defeating experience of rifts in the dynamics of mutual recognition. Building on the work of Stern (1985) and Beebe (1985), she argues that, just like in the mother-infant relationship, the bond in every affective relationship, especially in couples, is always precarious and destined to fail, but the "reaching for recognition" and the capacity for resilience in each of the partners are such that "making up" is always possible, underpinning the step from "breaking-up" to being newly "reunited again." Human beings and couples of any kind, just like all the mothers and infants in the world, are made to experience relational conflict and rift, but also to survive those experiences, knowing each time how to repair and restore a reunited bond.

Conflict in couple relationships and rifts are not, therefore, the antechamber to definitive break-up or irrefutable evidence that the bond between the couple has fallen apart, the proven proof that two people are just not made to be together and all is irretrievably lost. Conflict in couples and the experience of rift are instead "natural," all part and parcel of every significant affective bond and of the dynamics of mutual recognition, which generate and re-generate that bond. Conflict is the indispensable space in which we experience our own and the other's true "subjectivity." It is the clearing from which something "new" always emerges in one or both the partners – something that is still waiting to be recognised, welcomed, and integrated. The rift that emerges from conflict compels us to acknowledge the diversity of the other, forcing us out of our "cocoon" and to "refresh" our perception and representation of the other and our shared bond.[13]

Every rift, therefore, can be handled by us in one of two different ways.

One is to open ourselves to the other with a positive affective reaching, driven by acceptance, compassion, and the willingness to forgive.[14] The other is to "resist" the diversity of the other in an attempt to continue treating the other as an object, a "thing" over which to exercise power and manipulation. The first way makes it possible to generate mutual recognition and co-regulation in the couple; the second opens the way for the failure of recognition, for a persistent rift that becomes chronic, for the desensitisation and dysregulation of the couple, and for major forms of dissociation in one or both the partners. The "triadic perspective" and the "circular dynamics" activated by the experience of mutual recognition heal the rift and reactivate the self-regulation of each of the partners and the co-regulation of the couple. But for that to happen, it is first necessary to grasp and process the "perturbing events"[15] that originated the rift, and to support – especially through the activation of the "right hemisphere" – recognition of the polarities in conflict, the processes of affective self-regulation and co-regulation, and an openness to compassion and forgiveness towards oneself and the other (cf. Molinari, Cavaleri, 2015).

As happens in the mother-infant relationship, the more immediate our capacity to acknowledge and welcome the novel situation and the diversity of the other, the more incisive "healing" will be (cf. Gottman and Schwartz Gottman, 2018). Instead, the longer we wait, the more our resistance will grow and the more difficult it will be to "heal" the relationship and thus "re-generate" the affective bond of the couple. In Gestalt therapy terms, we can say that the painfulness of the limit constituted by the rift goads the couple to new "creative adjustments" each time, revitalising in each of the partners the integrating and regulatory function of the self. And so, we come to the fourth point of our "compass," *the integrating and regulatory function of the self.*

2.4 Reanimating the Self to Mutually Recognise Each Other and Return to Co-regulation

Even Maria and Giovanni can deal with their conflict and their rift in a constructive way. To do so, however, they need to be helped in regaining possession of the integrating and regulatory function of the self (Perls *et al.*, 1951/1994) and guided along a gradual path towards the recognition of each other and themselves,[16] learning how to be "open to the senses" and present at the "contact boundary" in their couple relationship (Spagnuolo Lobb, 2013, pp. 189–193). Over time, they have both forgotten how to talk to each other, looking each other straight in the eye, and giving a name to the emotions that each elicits in the other, with the courage to ask, spontaneously and confidently, what each wishes for themselves from the other. Without realising it, they have slowly withdrawn from the real intimacy they shared, to each retreat into their own world of shadows and spectres, which the other cannot see, and which have the power to ensnare them further and further into a distressing sense of exclusion, loneliness, and helplessness. Every day that passes, they each learn to slip further away from the other, to "desensitise" themselves that little bit more from a life as a couple that is becoming increasingly tenuous, hazy, and distant. If that is the case, then my therapeutic objective now lies in restoring their capacity to be "sensitive" to each other once again, to re-cognise and re-generate their affective bond. To achieve such an objective, it will be necessary, session after session, to focus on reanimating the integrating and regulatory function of the self on both the personal and couple planes (self-regulation and co-regulation).[17]

Building on the Kantian concept of synthetic unity, while remaining faithful to the insights of Goldstein, Perls and Goodman identify in the self the "integrator" of the experience of contact that takes place in the co-created field, at the contact boundary "between" organism and environment (Cavaleri, 2013). The self "is the contact boundary at work," which "organises" life from one moment to the next, "It is the artist of life" (1951, p. 235). The self fully expresses itself in its capacity to integrate and synthesise every single element that contributes to shaping the experience of the co-created field and organism-environment interaction, giving it all shape and unity in a single, meaningful Gestalt.[18] The self "always integrates perceptive-proprioceptive functions, motor-muscular functions, and organic needs. It is aware and orients, aggresses and manipulates, and feels emotionally the appropriateness of the environment and organism" (Perls *et al.*, 1951/1994, p. 373). Thanks to the typical capacity of the self to integrate, "organic excitation expresses itself, becomes meaningful, precisely by imparting meaning and motion to percepts, as is obvious in music" (Perls *et al.*, 1951/1994, p. 374). Such integration effected continuously by the self is never "otiose" but is the outcome of ceaseless creative adjustment, where "the self is the power that forms the gestalt in the field; or better, the self *is* the figure/background process in contact-situations" (*ibid.*).

The validity and profound insight of these theoretical definitions formulated by Perls and Goodman remain intact after all these years, continuing to constitute a fundamental touchstone for all Gestalt therapists, and others (see Stern, 2010). But how can all these conceptualisations be translated in practice in the therapeutic setting to support the self, especially when it itself is fragmented and has lost its ability to function fully, when it is no longer able to outline complete figures and integrate the myriad parts of the contact experience into a unitary and meaningful whole? To help me orient my practical work, especially in couple settings, over the years I have put together a sort of grid of reference that I like to call the "Gestalt therapy pentad of the self" (perception, feeling, intentionality, action, learning-narrative). In the classical tradition of the Gestalt therapy approach, a more well-known "pentad" is that used for the phenomenological analysis of each contact episode (confluence, introjection, projection, retroflection, egotism).

Alongside the original pentad, I refer to the "Gestalt therapy pentad of the self" to monitor and constantly revitalise the various forms through which the self "integrates," "organises," and regulates the experience of organism-environment contact in the co-created field. In fact, it is thanks to the self and its functions (the id-, ego- and personality-functions) that, in every contact experience, the reality of the body and the reality of the environment are integrated and take the form of *perception*; that the excitation of the body and the resulting emotional experience take the form of a *feeling* of emotion; that the will, orientation, and direction are unified to give form to *intentionality*; that the movement towards the environment and its manipulation take the form of deliberate *action*; and that the assimilation of what is novel, its integration with past experience, and the imparting of meaning give rise to the form of *learning-narrative*. This "pentad" should never be grasped and utilised in "monadic" terms, referring to the single individual. Rather, it should always be interpreted in a relational key and with reference to the field.[19]

If the intention is to achieve the objective of reanimating the self and restoring its self-regulatory and co-regulatory functions, then I need to focus on certain of its *vital capacities*, namely its capacity to perceive, to feel emotions, to want, to act, and to narrate.[20] From a "triadic perspective," therefore, during the session, it will be useful to ask myself: Are I and the couple present at the contact boundary and open to our senses? Are we able to perceive and perceive ourselves? That is, can we give a clear, sharp form of *perception* to what is happening "between" us in the shared field? Are we able to recognise the emotions we experience as mine, yours, and ours, to give them a name and fully identify ourselves with the *feeling* of the emotions that are emerging "between" us? Are we being aware of the *intentionality* that is taking shape from the experience of perception and from the feeling of emotions? Do we know what we want and whom to ask for it? What can we "do together" to transform the emerging shared intentionality into a clearly precise *action*? In sharing the experience of a co-created field, are we receiving new *learning*, which can be related with pregnant words and become the subject of a shared *narrative*?

What are the techniques, the experiments, the metaphors, the games, and the stories that the couple and I can place in the field to develop *perception, feeling, intentionality, action, and narrative*? What can we do together to revitalise the specific forms through which the self organises and integrates our interaction in the field, forming a complete whole, a single, meaningful Gestalt? These are the questions that I asked myself in every session with Maria and Giovanni, throughout the rather testing work we did together for some time, even in the difficult months of the pandemic.

In the end, they decided to stay together but with a new awareness of the parts of themselves hidden "in the shadows," and with a renewed capacity to re-cognise and re-generate themselves and each other.

Despite the pandemic and its wearisome climate of suspension for those who live by trade, Maria and Giovanni were able to transform their fragility into an extraordinary opportunity for growth.

The pandemic, like any other critical and unexpected event, demonstrated that the power of conflict doesn't lie in the destructive and frustrating effect of the "breaking" of human ties but rather in the generativity of their "repair", in other words, in the possibility of creating new relationships, new forms of integration between belonging and difference, and new opportunities for mutual recognition (Tronick and Gold, 2020).

Notes

1 In this chapter, the term "couple" is used regardless of gender. Although the clinical examples reported concern only heterosexual couples, it is believed that the

psychotherapeutic interventions described can be applied to any couple relationship regardless of gender.

2 The disappearance of the formal and institutional aspects of the traditional family has made possible the emergence of new ties. Intimate relationships are now less conditioned by gender diversity and more anchored to emotional ties. If, on the one hand, this social change has placed affectivity as an essential support to the life of a couple, on the other, it has led to the emergence of contradictory and fragile situations.

3 On intimacy and shame in couple life from a Gestalt perspective see Lee (2008); Wheeler and Backman (1994).

4 For Gestalt clinical work on the relationship between enteroception and heteroception, see Spagnuolo Lobb and Gallese (2011).

5 On recognition from a philosophical perspective see Honneth (1992) and Ricoeur (2005).

6 The dynamics we are describing here often have to do with "dissociation"; in this regard see Bromberg (2011), Fisher (2017), and Van der Hart et al. (2006).

7 On conflict and the polarity dialectic in the Gestalt therapy model see Cavaleri (2003, 2007)

8 On intentionality in couple relationships see Spagnuolo Lobb (2013, pp. 177–200).

9 In couple relationships, the gift of recognition is often expressed in the special form of the "gift of forgiveness"; see Molinari and Cavaleri (2015).

10 With reference to the experience of "recognising oneself," the concept of "earned-secure attachment" can be useful; see Fisher (2017) and Siegel (1999).

11 In this regard see, among others, Benjamin (1988, 2017), Beebe and Lachmann (2002), Stern (1985, 2010), and Tronick (2008), Ammaniti and Ferrari (2020).

12 In order to support the couple in this delicate step, Spagnuolo Lobb suggests, on a practical level, the *illogical leap of the game*. That is, leave the problem temporarily unresolved to do something else. Playing, for example, is an excellent tool to help the couple to recover "the spontaneous creativity which characterizes every significant relationship. The Gestalt couple therapist's goal is not that the partners not quarrel, but that they be able to enjoy themselves and feel alive, whole, creative at the contact boundary of their relationship" (2013, p. 191).

13 In outlining their theory of self and the concept of contact itself, the founders of the Gestalt model state: "Contacting is in general the growing of the organism . . ., conflicting . . ." (Perls et al., 1951/1994, p. 151).

14 For a detailed discussion of the concept of compassion in a psychotherapeutic perspective see Siegel (2007); Gilbert (2010); Kabat-Zinn (2013); Wollants (2012).

15 By "perturbing events" that provoke a "rift," here we mean a whole set of components, including parts in the shadows that emerge from the ground and implicit memories and states of insecurity activated through neuroception (cf. Bromberg, 2011; Porges, 2017; Ammaniti and Ferrari, 2020).

16 Spagnuolo Lobb underlines: "Recognising the experience of the other in her/his diversity and at the same time in her/his interweaving with our fears leads to the differentiated perception of the other, and helps the partners to contact each other" (2013, p. 189).

17 On affect regulation see Hill (2015). On co-regulation see Dana (2018).

18 For a further discussion see Cavaleri (2013).

19 The angle the pentad takes, from both an epistemological and clinical point of view, is that of the "triadic perspective" of mutual recognition (recognising the other, being recognised by him/her, and recognising oneself) and the "circular dynamics" that drive it.

20 For a neuroscientific reference see Damasio (2010).

References

Ammaniti, M., & Ferrari, P. F. (2020). *Il corpo non dimentica. L'Io motorio e lo sviluppo della relazionalità* [The body does not forget. The motor ego and the development of relationality]. Milano: Raffaello Cortina.

Bauman, Z. (2003). *Liquid love: On the frailty of human bonds*. Cambridge: Polity Press.

Beebe, B. (1985). Mother-infant mutual influence and precursor of self and object representations. In J. Masling (Ed.). *Empirical studies of psychoanalytic theories*. Hillsdale: Lawrence Erlbaum.

Beebe, B., & Lachmann, F. M. (2002). *Infant research and adult treatment: Co-constructing interactions*. Hillsdale, NJ: The Analytic Press/Taylor & Francis Group.

Benjamin, J. (1988). *The bonds of love: Psychoanalysis, feminism, & the problem of domination*. New York: Pantheon Books.

Benjamin, J. (2017). *Beyond doer and done to: Recognition theory, intersubjectivity, and the third*. New York: Routledge.

Bromberg, P. M. (2011). *The shadow of the tsunami: And the growth of the relational mind*. London: Routledge.

Cavaleri, P. A. (2003). *La profondità della superficie. Percorsi introduttivi alla psicoterapia della Gestalt* [The depth of the surface. Introductory paths to Gestalt psychotherapy]. Milano: FrancoAngeli.

Cavaleri, P. A. (2007). *Vivere con l'altro. Per una cultura della relazione* [Living with the other. For a culture of relationship]. Roma: Città Nuova.

Cavaleri, P. A. (2013). Dalle parti degli infedeli. Per un dialogo fra saperi diversi [On the side of the infidels. For dialogue between different knowledge]. In P. A. Cavaleri (Ed.). *Psicoterapia della Gestalt e neuroscienze. Dall'isomorfismo alla simulazione incarnata* [Gestalt psychotherapy and neuroscience. From isomorphism to embodied simulation] (pp. 22–41). Milano: FrancoAngeli.

Cavaleri, P. A. (2018). La vulnérabilité relationnelle [Relational vulnerability]. *Cahiers de Gestalt Therapie, 40*(1), 87–101.

Cavaleri, P. A. (2020). A Gestalt therapy reading of the pandemic. *The Humanistic Psychologist, 48*(4), 347–352. DOI: 10.1037/hum0000214.

Cavaleri, P. A., Augello, D. M., Buscemi, D., & Spanò, A. (2013). *Quando l'amore è un'arte* [When love is an art]. Roma: Città Nuova.

Cavaleri, P. A., & Spagnuolo Lobb, M. (2017). Estetica dell'alterità: l'esperienza del conflitto e il reciproco riconoscimento nel campo terapeutico [Aesthetics of otherness: The experience of conflict and mutual recognition in the therapeutic field]. *Idee in psicoterapia, 10*(1–2), 69–82.

Damasio, A. (2010). *Self comes to mind: Constructing the conscious brain*. New York: Pantheon.

Dana, D. (2018). *The polyvagal theory in therapy: Engaging the rhythm of regulation*. New York: W.W. Norton & Co Inc.

Fisher, J. (2017). *Healing the fragmented selves of trauma survivors: Overcoming internal self-alienation*. New York: Routledge.

Gallese, V. (2006). Corpo vivo, simulazione incarnata e intersoggettività. Una prospettiva neuro-fenomenologica [Living body, embodied simulation, and intersubjectivity. A neuro-phenomenological perspective]. In M. Cappuccio (Ed.). *Neurofenomenologia. Le scienze della mente e la sfida dell'esperienza cosciente* [Neurophenomenology. The sciences of mind and the challenge of conscious experience] (pp. 293–326). Milano: Bruno Mondadori.

Gilbert, P. (2010). *Compassion focused therapy. Distinctive features*. London: Routledge.

Gottman, J. M., & Schwartz Gottman, J. (2018). *The science of couples and family therapy: Behind the scenes at the "love lab"*. New York: W.W. Norton & Co. Inc.

Hill, D. (2015). *Affect regulation theory: A clinical model*. New York: W.W. Norton & Company.

Honneth, A. (1992). *Kampf um Anerkennung. Grammatik sozialer Konflikte* [Struggle for recognition. Grammar of social conflicts]. Frankfurt am Main: Suhrkamp Verlag.

Kabat-Zinn, J. (2013). *Full catastrophe living: Using the wisdom of your body and mind to face stress, pain, and illness*. New York: Random House.

Lee, R. G. (2008). *The secret language of intimacy. Releasing the hidden power in couple relationships*. New York: Gestalt Press.

Lévinas, E. (1969). *Totality and infinity: An essay on exteriority*. Pittsburgh, PA: Duquesne University Press.

Longo, A. R. (2021). Amori in emergenza [Emergency loves]. *MIND. Mente & Cervello, 197*, 24–31.

Miller, M. V. (1997). *Intimate terrorism: The crisis of love in an age of disillusion*. New York: WW Norton & Co Inc.

Molinari, E., & Cavaleri, P. A. (2015). *Il dono nel tempo della crisi. Per una psicologia del riconoscimento* [The gift in the time of crisis. For a psychology of recognition]. Milano: Raffaello Cortina.

Perls, F., Hefferline, R. F., & Goodman, P. (1994). *Gestalt therapy: Excitement and growth in the human personality*. New York: The Gestalt Journal Press, or.ed., 1951.

Porges, S. W. (2017). *The pocket guide to the polyvagal theory. The transformative power of feeling safe*. New York: W.W. Norton & Company, Inc.

Ricoeur, P. (2005). *The course of recognition*. Cambridge: Harvard University Press.

Schore, A. N. (1994). *Affect regulation and the origin of the self: The neurobiology of emotional development*. Hove, UK: Psychology Press.

Siegel, D. J. (1999). *The developing mind: Toward a neurobiology of interpersonal experience*. New York: Guilford Press.

Siegel, D. J. (2007). *The mindful brain: Reflection and attunement in the cultivation of well-being*. New York: W.W. Norton & Co Inc.

Spagnuolo Lobb, M. (2013). *The now-for-next in psychotherapy: Gestalt Therapy Recounted in Post-Modern Society*. Siracusa: Istituto di Gestalt HCC Italy Publ. Co., www.gestaltitaly.com.

Spagnuolo Lobb, M. (2016). Self as contact, contact as self. A contribution to ground experience in Gestalt therapy theory of self. In J-M. Robine (Ed.). *Self. A polyphony of contemporary Gestalt therapists* (pp. 261–289). St. Romain la Virvée, France: L'Exprimerie.

Spagnuolo Lobb, M. (2018). Aesthetic relational knowledge of the field: A revised concept of awareness in Gestalt therapy and contemporary psychiatry. *Gestalt Review, 22*(1), 50–68. DOI: 10.5325/gestalt review.22.1.0050.

Spagnuolo Lobb, M., & Gallese, V. (2011). Il now-for-next tra neuroscienze e psicoterapia della Gestalt [The now-for-next between neuroscience and Gestalt therapy]. *Quaderni di Gestalt, 24*(2), 11–26. DOI: 10.3280/GEST2011-002002.

Stern, D. N. (1985). *The interpersonal world of the infant: A view from psychoanalysis and developmental psychology*. New York: Basic Books.

Stern, D. N. (2010). *Forms of vitality. Exploring dynamic experience in psychology and the arts*. Oxford: Oxford University Press.

Tronick, E. Z. (2008). *Regolazione emotiva. Nello sviluppo e nel processo terapeutico* [Emotional regulation. In development and in the therapeutic process]. Milano: Raffaello Cortina.

Tronick, E. Z., & Gold, C. M. (2020). *The power of discord: Why the ups and downs of relationships are the secret to building intimacy, resilience, and trust*. London: Scribe UK.

Van der Hart, O., Nijenhuis, E. R. S., & Steele, K. (2006). *The haunted self: Structural dissociation and the treatment of chronic traumatization*. New York: W.W. Norton & Co Inc.

Wheeler, G., & Backman, S. (Eds.). (1994). *On intimate ground: A Gestalt approach to working with couples*. San Francisco: Jossey-Bass.

Wollants, G. (2012). *Gestalt therapy. Therapy of the situation*. London: Sage.

Zinker, J. (1977). *Creative process in Gestalt therapy*. New York: Brunner/Mazel.

Chapter 13

Working with the Family in Gestalt Psychotherapy

Giuseppe Sampognaro

The opening words to *Anna Karenina:* "Happy families are all alike; every unhappy family is unhappy in its own way" (Tolstoj, 1877) bring us back to the sense of malaise that lurks within the family nucleus and which possesses unique and irreplicable characteristics, just like every living organism is unique and irreplicable. And the family is a living organism. It is born, grows, and dies, infusing parts of itself into family nuclei that have their origin in it.

1. The Clinical Treatment of the Family Today

For some time, we have been sharing in the idea that the family is the place in which one learns to *be-with* (Spagnuolo Lobb, 2013, p. 242) and to build a relationship with the world. This is why more and more importance has been correspondingly attributed to the emotional climate within the domestic walls, where the intra and intergenerational dynamics (within the parental couple, between parents and offspring, and between the same siblings) possess the power to have an impact on the mental health of the individual members, besides the abilities of the entire nucleus to carry on a healthy contact with the environment.

At the same time, the family in turn serves as a sounding-board for the social climate and tensions that pervade the environment of which it is the embodiment. In an era like our own, already feeling the effect of liquidity and fragmentation typical of a society defined as "borderline" for its ambivalence (Spagnuolo Lobb, 2013, p. 33; Sampognaro, 2021, p. 35), the explosion of the pandemic has accentuated the growing sense of external danger and the agonising imperative to distance oneself and defend oneself from a threatening and treacherous "other than oneself". The lockdown has ratified the role of the protective shell that the family plays in everyone's life, especially that of minors. The external enemy is the same pandemic that has materialised in the risk of contagion at the hands of others, experienced as enemies to guard against (The Family Studies and Research University, 2020).

This aggravation of the bond within the nucleus has made the use of the family setting itself even more necessary during the therapeutic journey of children and

DOI: 10.4324/9781003313335-16

adolescents "following the principle that the child is an integral part of the family-*gestalt*" (Sampognaro, 2016, p. 181), given that

> this is where the discomfort of children is born, and also where the therapist tries to promote a "reparative" process, acting as a facilitator of the relationships that make up the family-*gestalt*. . . . This idea of child therapy as a search for good form in the relationships within the family rests on the assumption that the symptom expressed by a distressed child is the creative adaptation of *that* specific child within *that* specific context.
>
> (*ibidem*, p. 175)

Recently, the pandemic situation has contributed to the idea of no longer deeming the support to the removal from a family totality, which is experienced as regressive, as the therapeutic objective of the work with families. Rather, the aim has become that of supporting the members and developing/consolidating a sense of belonging, as well as real and nurturing affective bonds with the nucleus, so as to be able to calibrate the distances (times and ways) of the relationships in emergency situations as well, such as the one we are living through. This represents therapeutic work especially directed at youngsters, in order to facilitate their entry into the social context with enough basic confidence and competence to open themselves to the world, as well as to fashion significant and caring relationships in the attempt to overcome diffidence and fear for their own safety – the great obstacles to growth which keep young people chained within their own family grouping.

Therefore beyond its own protective function, the family, in the time of the coronavirus (and of the new habits linked to distancing), has been perceived, especially in cases of relational problems, as a "prison" for its members, forced into contact – the continuous and exclusive contact with the same members of the family nucleus – and into a deprivation of social relations considered dangerous and potentially pathogenic. We must underscore, in this context, the surge in cases of domestic violence, recorded precisely during the periods marked by lockdowns. This has occurred to such an extent as to cause the international research bodies to speak of a "shadow pandemic" (Loi and Pesce, 2021; ISTAT, 2020). It is this ambivalence (a place of care but also of suffering) that makes the clinical work with the family complex and more problematic.

2. The Gestalt Perspective on the Family

Within the family setting, the coordinates developed over the years of theoretical debate relative to our model are still valid:

- The *family life cycle*, marked by the physiological events of existence within every human nucleus, but which can be altered and "personalised" by unforeseeable experiences as well (bereavement, separations, loss of a parent's work, organic or psychiatric illnesses of one of the members, etc.).

This first parameter refers to the phase of development, which the nucleus undergoes when the decision is made to ask for help from a psychotherapist. We have already defined the family as a living organism, which grows over time and which faces a series of physiological changes (Spagnuolo Lobb, 2013, Chapter 8). "Examples of predictable and chosen events are weddings, births, adolescence, children leaving home, retirement. Practically speaking, those represented by the entry, exit, and development of the family members" (Terkelsen, 1980, cited in Bogliolo, 2012, p. 13). We should add to these customary and natural junctures of existence moments of crisis that are part of the unpredictability of the human condition: the sickness of one of the members, the possible loss of work (or instead promotions and professional successes that change the socio-economic balance), an emotional crisis experienced by the parental couple, an accident, a natural event that damages the house. Every emotionally significant episode along the family journey cannot help but have repercussions, from the relational point of view, among the members of the nucleus, and between the family Gestalt and the outside world.

One of the first tasks of therapy is precisely that of making the family members aware of the significance of their being there in relation to what is happening – or what has just happened – in the history of the family as a sensitive organism. The greater the emotional impact of an event, the greater the necessity of adjustment, of a rebalancing, and the choice of doing therapy is read as a necessary reaction in order to tackle these abrupt movements triggered by unforeseeable facts, sometimes obvious and clear, sometimes imperceptible, and of which the family has little to no awareness.

The family life cycle in turn should be framed within a broader cycle, relative to the historical-political context in which the family lives. Margherita Spagnuolo Lobb (2013, pp. 151–154) categorises in a more detailed way the great epistemological changes of the history of psychological thought in relation to the social sentiment of the time, attributing as well the variations in the familial emotional climate to factors connected to the relational experience typical of every era: a narcissistic society (the Fifties-the Seventies) marked by the effort of the individual to break free of any type of subjection, including the familial; a technological society (the Seventies-the Nineties); a fluid society (the Nineties-2010); a fragmented society (from 2010 to today).

- The *observation of the intentionality of contact* between the members and between the family and the environment, and the subsequent observation of the abilities to co-create the contact boundary.

Since it is well-established that the existence of an overdetermined motivation (achieving a satisfying contact with Otherness) which animates every human being and which within the family group should be manifested in a fuller way and without censure, the question is: how does each member of the family nucleus advance his/her own intentionality of contact in relation to the other members?[1] It is the *how* that represents the heart of our hermeneutics, and so in the work with families, the therapist is an attentive observer of the ways and rhythm in which the participants relate to each other within the setting, in order to discover the relational code which differentiates the family life of each one of them, and then of the entire nucleus vis-à-vis the environment. In deference to the principle of the Figure/Ground dynamic, the therapist, at the same time, perceives the other side of the coin and looks for the answer to this question: in what way do the members of this family avoid contact? In other words, in what way do they disrupt their intentionality, thus obtaining a *weak* figure, according to the definition of Perls *et al.* (1994)?

The movements between the members, and between the members and the outside world, build the contact boundary, namely the space for the encounter. To what are we referring with this concept? We are referring to what happens when the people who interact try to connect with each other, at the precise point, in which this connection happens: a meeting of looks, a touching of bodies, a shared smile, the temporal space of a greeting, a nod of the head to another family member. And what is the contact boundary between the family and the outside world in the therapeutic setting? It is surely that space co-created between the family and the therapist, for whom – in the presence of the professional who is taking care of them – they simply do or not do some things: their posture, the intensity of their communications addressed to him/her (and therefore silence as well), the closeness/distance, and the figure that they form by shifting themselves within the shared space, the liveliness or the immobility on the physical and/or verbal level, and the way in which they listen, in which they ask questions, in which they relate with each other with the awareness of the Other, who certainly affects their interacting; their punctuality or lack of it in their arrival, the way in which they leave the setting at the end; the rituality of their greetings. These are all events that create the contact boundary and that represent the material with which the therapist works, with the purpose of making all of it known to the family.

3. The Goal of Gestalt Family Intervention[2]

In the context of clinical work with families, the therapist's intent is to:

Return sensitivity to the intra- and extra-familial contact boundaries (the restoration of spontaneity in the promoting of the intentionality of contact).

Facilitate the visibility of each member and mutual recognition.

Develop a critical sense (and thus supported by awareness) of belonging to the nucleus, but also of a differentiation from it.

Stimulate the energy and vitality of the family gestalt.

4. A Clinical Example

In illustrating the case of Sandro, we are trying to apply the therapeutic actions and the theoretical principles that guide our work with families in this time period, marked by great social upheaval caused by the virus but also by important developments in Gestalt thought applied to clinical treatment.

Sandro is a boy of 12. Bright, intelligent, to a certain extent precociously adult (he speaks in articulate Italian, collects vintage videogames, and has a profound knowledge of twentieth century history, etc.), he is the second of three children belonging to a family, which has recently been broken apart. He has a sister of 15 and a little brother of 8. The parents, both 45 years of age, after various "on again off again" moments, separated for good the year before, during the full lockdown. However, they have remained on good terms, and the father, a business man, maintains daily contact (especially via the phone, given that he is often travelling) with his children. The mother doesn't work, but she is a very dynamic person and is only waiting for her little son to grow up so that she can look for a job that will satisfy her and occupy her days, at the moment absolutely dedicated to the family.

The problem that the parents point to – during the first meeting without the children – is the disproportionate aggressiveness of Sandro with regard to Luca, the little brother. It seems that, annoyed by Luca's boisterous way of playing, and by his sometimes noisy presence, he pounds him to a pulp, especially when they are home alone. This situation is so prevalent that the parents avoid leaving little Luca unsupervised and continuously monitor that the fights between their sons do not get out of hand. The mother most of all is severely tested by this situation: she often witnesses their clashes; she is often forced to intervene in order to tear the younger from the clutches of his older brother, and she cannot explain why Sandro has these outbursts of violent fury. Above all, she notices the enormous difference in Sandro's attitude and behaviour when he is at school or simply outside the house: "He's beyond reproach, a little man, a kind and responsible person, to the extent that his teachers and the parents of his friends compliment me on his good nature and good manners."

It seems that these violent behaviours may have begun precisely during the long quarantine that marked 2020 (just before the couple's separation). However, they did not die out when the situation improved. A year later, they are persisting and upsetting the entire family. Sandro, when asked about his conduct during a preliminary individual meeting, is only able to justify himself by blaming Luca. "He's a pain in the neck," he states, "and sometimes he becomes unbearable." He admits to overdoing it, but he says that this happens because 'my parents can't make him stop, and when he gets worked up, he makes fun of me or makes a mess in my room. Only punching him can stop him." When it has been argued that surely this is not a solution, he says that he has tried to take a kinder approach, but his brother seems to enjoy provoking him and won't stop. "He's the problem, not me."

So it is decided to embark on a path of family therapy aimed at understanding into what overall dynamic the pattern of the conflict between Sandro and Luca has been implanted.

Everyone takes part in the first session, just as in the following ones: father, mother, Enrica (the fifteen-year-old eldest daughter), Sandro, and Luca.

4.1 Step 1

Always fascinating for the therapist, in the work with families, is the discovery of what is *beyond* – beyond the appearances of the first meeting with its formalities and rituals. Beyond the forced smiles, or instead the sulky expression of some of the family participants who are showing their displeasure and unwillingness, since they feel coerced into coming. It is natural to wonder: what will happen in a few sessions? Or even after only a few seconds? And this sensation of exciting curiosity provides the best energy for being with what we see and feel, in deference to the phenomenological principle of taking at face value what is there – a principle that does not exempt us from harbouring the expectation of "what else will happen". The sensation is like that evoked by the paintings of Edward Hopper[3]: you observe the scene depicted by the artist, and you have the feeling that something disturbing and unpredictable is about to happen.

This feeling is always with us, during the work with the family. We know that the other polarity will emerge. We know that the one who is silent will speak, that he/she who expresses him/herself in an affected and mild-mannered way will lose it and shout, that the one who uses sarcasm will cry, and the one who appears cooperative could also get up and walk out, slamming the door. And this knowledge comes from the teachings of Gestalt psychology that has made us aware of the perceptive strength of the ground that supports what appears as the figure: in the very famous "Rubin's vase", the white profiles exist thanks to the black goblet, and vice-versa. What appears is visible because the ground supports it and allows the very contours of the form to stand out. In this way, within the gestalt-family, the attitudes and behaviours of the individual members are supported by the relational context.

The figure/ground dynamic is, however, exactly that – dynamic – and therefore nothing can ever be taken for granted. There are micro-movements, which a watchful eye perceives during the session, and for which the psychological characteristics of a member have variability and vibrations because of what takes place at the contact boundary between the participants of the nucleus. The therapist, as well, with the way in which he welcomes the group (the words he uses, and the non-verbal expressions that characterise the way in which he/she speaks, looks at them, and moves) is an integral part of the relational situation. In this initial phase, however, it is still possible for the therapist to maintain the role of observer, like the spectator able to appreciate the alternation in tonality and pitch, which generate a music that characterises *that* family in *that* moment.

And it happens like this during the meeting with this family. Despite the therapist's warm enough welcome, the atmosphere is characterised by a sense of palpable tension in the parental couple, anxious about the behaviour of their children: Sandro is serious, calm and collected; Enrica seems annoyed, fiddles with her cell phone, sighing deeply as if to say "what am I doing here?"; little Luca is clearly bored, and in an autonomous way explores the room on the lookout for a source of stimuli that might attract his attention. He finds it when he becomes aware of a table on which there are some blank sheets of paper and a pencil case with coloured felt tip pens. He asks if he can use them, and before receiving an answer is already seated at the table and colouring.

They give the impression of a family which is adjusting itself in this first phase of making acquaintance and orientation: each one introduces him/herself, one with a long monologue (the mother), another with barely two words forced out of them (Enrica). One can perceive, in the background, the effort, the conflicts, and the lengthy negotiations that surely preceded the decision to all come and live this experience. As Spagnuolo Lobb states (2013, p. 202), the process through which the family determines to go into therapy is particularly important for selecting the intervention of choice with *that* family.

The therapist plays an active part. He specifies the reasons for the choice of setting, asks each member of the group to declare his/her own state of mind and intentionality in being there, and suggests some moments of free dialogue among the members of the group. In so doing, he has the chance to observe even more "from within" what happens at the contact boundary of the various individuals in the family. He learns *the language* which characterises the nucleus, observes the displacement of the members within the space of the room, and the micro-movements which each one of them carries out, notices who speaks and who doesn't, and tries to grasp the *intentionality of contact* of each person present with regard to the others.

The Gestalt domains, as they have been set down by Margherita Spagnuolo Lobb (cf. 2013), represent the emotional/relational base from which the family moves in its contact with the environment. Faithful to the principle in which the whole is greater than the sum of its parts, and by means of which the family is understood as an entity endowed with life and its own psychological peculiarities, the configurations of the domains (and for this very reason defined as "polyphony") characterises the being-with of the nucleus, its way of interacting, which indicates the relationship between its members and that of the group with the outside. It is not just about pinpointing which modalities emerge during the course of the interaction, but also how, when, how intensely, and with what nuances.

In relation to the case at hand, the family Gestalt presents a range of relational modalities which go from the retroflective attitude of Sandro, who speaks little and listens with involved attention (perhaps he realises that he is the cause of this experience engaging the entire family); to this particular juncture, which Enrica seems to be living with her own thoughts, which keeps her distant from what is happening around her; from the introjecting of the two parents, who seem to be hanging onto the therapist's every word, in the execution of their job as "good patients"; up to the projecting of Luca, who is exploring, touching, and goes to be held, first by his mother, and then his father, interrupts whoever is speaking, bounces into the centre of the room, asks if there are any toys, and then sits down at the table and starts to colour. What emanates from this polyphony of competencies of the ground, however, is a composite way of *being-with*, but it is, all in all, calm and adaptive. The family is there, with its internal differences, but also with its spontaneity.

In order to give support and impetus to this phase, the therapist suggests a "game" to the family: each person will take a turn and say to the others what he sees as the positive qualities in each of them, without an "if" and without a "but". He/she will be able to point out the physical characteristics which he/she perceives as particularly beautiful, as well as qualities relating to the nature, attitude, or behaviour of the others – in short, everything about the family member that he/she likes. This suggestion is met with curiosity and apprehension by the family.

It is the father who begins the game. His breaking the ice kicks off the experience, which is then revealed as being extremely significant, with respect to the perception of the image that each individual in the family has of the other.

The moments of exchange reveal the not-said, which – in the moment itself, in which it is expressed – is highlighted in all of its relational potency and "moves" the intrafamilial boundaries. Significant is the contact between little Luca and Sandro. The child enumerates his brother's qualities: "Sandro, I like your long hair. You have a beautiful face. You're smart and you make me laugh. . . . And I also like that you hit me". Everyone looks at each other in puzzlement, and Sandro asks his little brother: "But what are you saying?! You like being hit by me?" Luca answers: "Well, I think it's one way to get you interested, and when I'm big, I'll remember that at least you spent time with me." Sandro is stunned by this declaration, and when it is his turn, it is as if he is making a concerted effort to find positive elements in Luca's behaviour, perhaps in answer to that statement that has disoriented him. The sister, Enrica, on the other hand, remains taciturn, and marginally participates in this exchange, devoting few adjectives to each family member.

Everything gets livelier when it is the turn of the mom and dad who – according to the rules of the game – have the opportunity to reveal what they consider to be mutual positive aspects. Both of them do it with great pathos. The father's voice is broken while he says to the mother how much he has always appreciated her capacity to manage the family. He praises her energy and her beauty. The mother cries when expressing to her ex-husband her admiration for the caring he has always bestowed on everyone, and reveals her nostalgia for those moments of joy that he knew how to create within the family.

While the parents exchange such "caresses", Sandro silently and lovingly embraces his little brother – who is now giving signs of restlessness – and holds him tightly to him, stroking him, as if to keep him quiet, ensuring that he doesn't interfere with that moment of great emotion; Enrica, who, up until a moment ago, seemed detached from the context, lowers her mask down to the bridge of her nose, and reveals her eyes full of tears. The therapist verbalises all this, and the family's response is a moving silence. At the end of the go-around, each one expresses having been pleasantly surprised by the course of the meeting. Everyone, except for little Luca, who candidly declares: "It went exactly how I thought it would: I was bored".

4.2 Step 2

During the next session, the family takes off again from where they left off – the sense of fullness subsequent to the exchange of "love-strokes" related to the exercise suggested by the therapist the time before. Little Luca immediately moves towards the same table where he finds again papers and coloured pencils for drawing, which he undertakes to do, but always with his ear tuned into what is happening among the members of his family; Sandro seems livelier and more relaxed. He intervenes and highlights with banter and clever observations the fullness of his being present. Even Enrica seems more involved, and sometimes keeps her cell phone in her pocket without becoming distracted and flaunting her indifference. The mother and father are always lively and active in their contact with the therapist and the children, and the feeling that they had revealed earlier seems to persist between them.

The therapist suggests another exercise, inviting each person to express to every other family member a personal demand, which, if satisfied, could better their relationship of two. Therefore, it represents a formulation of a request for change. "In order for us to improve our relationship, I would like you to . . ."

In this phase, too, the emotional climate becomes intense. Luca expresses to the others concrete desires (as is typical for his age); but when it is his turn to talk to Sandro, he asks him to play with him without getting angry, showing that he perfectly grasped the meaning of the exercise. In contrast, Sandro asks his little brother to respect his privacy more, and also expresses his need to have quiet to pursue his hobbies without Luca getting on his nerves by behaving in a provocative and noisy way. The other family members listen in silence. Once again, the exchange between the mother and father – centred on reciprocal requests for help in carrying out their relative tasks related to their role in bringing up the children – becomes the focus of interest for the children, who vibrate with emotion as they listen to their parents talk to each other with respect and affection. Enrica finally takes her place and asks all the family members to accept her mood swings, and sometimes, her desire for solitude, without forcing her to be different and more engaged.

The father has something to add. He asks permission and then says: "Luca, I have thought about what you said last time to Sandro: you like it when he hits you because then he shows interest in you, and one day you will remember that you were together. You know, I thought that maybe what's important for you is to feel the presence of the others, and I'm asking myself whether I make you feel mine, in a way you would like." And then, towards Sandro: "I would like to tell you that I suspect that this anger that you sometimes exhibit towards your brother is maybe something that I have triggered in you. I mean, I wonder if it was my leaving the house that has made you become so short-tempered." Neither of his sons answers him.

The therapist observes, listens, and listens to himself, allowing the emotions to pass through him, the emotions pervading each person in the family with respect to the intentionality of contact disclosed by each one of them. He is aware of a feeling that seems to relate to an all-encompassing and an older experience with respect to what is happening in the here-and-now.

We call this special feeling – with respect to the individual members and with respect to the social life of the entire family – the *aesthetic relational knowing* of the therapist (cf. Spagnuolo Lobb, 2016, 2018).

The family in therapy co-creates with the professional a phenomenological field which ritualises in the here-and-now situations lived in the there-and-then. It is the therapist, with his/her sensitivity and adaptability, who readily absorbs the two aspects relating to the emotional attunement (empathy with one or more members) and to the resonance of the field (perception of the existential drama already experienced by the nucleus in other moments of the past).

Therefore, a phenomenological field exists, one which is articulated and reflected in the dynamic of contact that the family nucleus is experiencing with the environment (in this case, the therapist is the family's environment).

Always starting from the experiential field created by the family, it is as if the therapist perceives and experiences the emotional resonances that the family members are creating with each other, between themselves and the environment with which the family enters into contact. The aesthetic relational knowing of the therapist allows, as Spagnuolo Lobb states, a view of "the other side of the moon" (Spagnuolo Lobb, 2018), namely an aspect of the family's psychological life, which usually stays hidden to someone who does not possess this clinical sensitivity.

The use of such a refined therapeutic tool presupposes a basic trust and there-fore a consolidation of a therapeutic relationship that already has behind it several hours of sessions between the professional and the family.

It is precisely this particular way of perceiving the family situation which allows the therapist – now – to verbalise what he has discovered. "You have made known your desires for what would improve your reciprocal contact. I should feel relieved because of these important and sincere exchanges between you. How-ever, I feel that, in this family, there is something else. I sense that there is some-thing painful that is not being expressed, and which concerns all of you as a group. It is a sensation that has been reinforced after your dad said those things to Luca and Sandro. Can you tell me if what I am feeling actually exists, or is it only an impression of mine? Is it true that there is a sense of suffering in you which has not yet come out, which has not yet been clearly expressed?"

Once again, a profound silence highlights this important moment. The mom and dad lower their heads. Enrica lifts up her mask until it covers her eyes. Sandro becomes serious and crosses his arms. Luca stops drawing and looks at each indi-vidual in his family one after the other. He seems curious and concerned.

It is Sandro who shatters the silence. "We feel bad since mom and dad sepa-rated. We've never said it, but I think that's what is hurting us."

On hearing Sandro's words, Luca begins to nod and it seems as if he won't stop, even though he goes back to drawing. The father puts his head in his hands. The mother gets up and goes over to Enrica to comfort her because she is sobbing. But the mother, too, is very distraught.

The therapist gives everyone a chance to express what they are feeling, underscoring how this event – the breakdown of the family – has perhaps not been well assimilated yet, and that perhaps they have not talked about it in a satisfactory or long enough way, as it deserves.

The session ends with a go-around during which each, in turn, confirms the therapist's perceptions, and demonstrates their suffering and their readiness – in this phase – to face this issue, which has always been taboo for them.

4.3 Step 3

From what has emerged in the two previous sessions, it appears evident that the family has undergone a double trauma: the pandemic erupted exactly in their moment of crisis, which – although it had begun earlier – materialised in the separation of the mother and father. This unexpected and destabilising change has had as an effect the necessity – on the part of the group – to adapt itself creatively and quickly: face the fears and restrictions imposed by the Covid emergency, in a phase of great tension within the couple, culminating in the determination to separate. Precisely in the moment when the generational line of the children would need much support and solidity, the break-up came, and therefore the collapse of security, which the parents, with their loving presence, have always guaranteed.

The therapist is well-aware of this reading but mentions it without imposing it upon the family. His "interpretation" is not important. What is important is how the family sees itself, and above all, their own *next*.

In order to make this fundamental aspect emerge, he suggests a technique, which Gestalt therapy borrows from the systemic model, readapting it according to its own theoretical arrangement: the *"sculpture of the family"*.

Each member will be a sculptor, positioning the others in the central space dedicated to the representation of the intrafamilial relationships. He/she will mould the bodies of the others like raw material to which to give shape. He/she will also model the facial expressions, and in the end will place him/herself within the "sculptural group", thus expressing his/her own idea of how the family currently makes contact internally. Subsequently, the sculptor will reproduce his/her work, this time representing how he/she would like the family to be (and so he/she will change the posture and expressions of the various members depending on his/her own intentions).

The group becomes animated. The emotion is palpable as is the desire "to make something", and everyone gladly participates in this game. The mother begins, and then little Luca (who really enjoys himself, and with his laughter and liveliness passes on his good humour to the others). Then comes the father, then Sandro, and the last one is Enrica. As a variant of the traditional exercise, the therapist suggests (and the family accepts with enthusiasm) photographing with a cell phone each sculpture, in order to preserve the memory of it, and make subsequent comparisons.

In the end, the atmosphere is serene, even if – thanks to the comparison between the sculptures – everything seems to be converging towards the same goal: achieving a sort of family unity that might give continuity to the sense of an "us", and taking into account as well the separation of the parental couple. The variants expressed by the sculptures of each person are significant: the father who positions himself slightly far from the group but with a loving look towards the other family members, whom he places hugging each other; the mother who places herself next to the father, with Luca in her arms and her hands tightly holding those of Enrica and Sandro; Luca, who unwaveringly places everyone in a circle as if on a merry-go-round; Sandro reconstructs a family situation that shows everyone engaged in something that interests them, but within a space the he circumscribes with a circle of chairs, and in the end explains: "I would like everyone to have their own freedom, but knowing that the others are there and that they love him." Enrica situates the parents back to back, surrounded by the children, and then she explains: "I would like mom and dad to remain in contact, in order to continue to maintain their presence, which is essential for us."

After the "game", the verbalisations, and the comparisons between the various needs expressed by the members of the group, the family leaves with a sense of ease and reconciliation.

4.4 Step 4

The sense of fullness with which the previous session ended is still perceptible on the faces and in the bodies of the family members. Luca no longer seeks out the table to do his drawings. He, too, sits in the circle, situating himself between his mom and dad. Sitting still for him is a feat. Every now and then he gets up and takes a turn around the room but then returns to his seat. Enrica seems present and attentive but also relaxed and smiling. Sandro fools around and thinks up jokes, which elicit comments and laughs from all of the family and from the therapist, too.

It seems useful to be able to open this session asking the family to initiate a free discussion, without specific indications on the part of the therapist. Spontaneously, the family decides to speak about what happened over the course of the three meetings already experienced. The father provocatively asks the others: "It seems important to me to talk about what we are doing. How is it working here so far? At the beginning I was apprehensive about you, kids; even if we, your mom and I, were sure that it would be useful. But what do you say?'

It is as if Sandro has already thought and considered this: "I was sure that you were going to reproach me for hitting Luca, and I was worried. Instead, well, we hardly talked about it. . .. And I was glad about that."

Luca interrupts him: "Yeah, we didn't talk about it also because you stopped hitting me." And he laughs. And immediately the parents confirm this, having noticed a regained atmosphere of peace in the house.

Enrica says in astonishment: "I was sure that it would be a waste of time. Instead, we did and said a lot of important and good things, which helped to improve our relationship."

The parents every now and then look at each other, showing harmony and satisfaction. The mother highlights: "Like dad said, we were sure that coming here would help us. Now maybe we've understood that so many of the tensions we felt – as well as the ones between Luca and Sandro – were born out of silence. Your father and I now know that we should have spoken more and in a better way about our separation. Instead, we felt guilty."

"Or maybe we were too embarrassed, confused . . ." adds the father.

The mother resumes: "Our distress wasn't only expressed through the fights between Sandro and Luca, but also through Enrica's silence" – the girl nods – "and through the sense of mine and dad's impotence." She sighs. "Now we know that it's always necessary to say what we're feeling, and what we want. It won't solve all the problems, but it's a good way to confront them."

Sandro resumes speaking, and smiling, turns to Luca. "Yeah, but don't think that now everything's been resolved and that you can raise hell in my room! If you get me angry, I'll let you have it!" He gets up from his chair, and walks over to his little brother threateningly, but instead of hitting him, he hugs him. The two laugh and tickle each other.

The therapist feels that the experience is coming to an end. He highlights the salient points of the journey that he has shared with the family and expresses a sense of well-being and pleasure that he is now feeling, observing the family nucleus, and intuiting – beyond the masks – the tranquil and satisfied faces of each of them. As a final "game", he suggests that each one should express in one word their current state of mind, and that this will represent their farewell at the end of the therapeutic activity.

Father: "Calm"
Mother: "Confidence"
Enrica: "Nostalgia"
Sandro: "Curiosity"
Luca: "Desire to play".

5. Conclusions

The crisis stemming from the Coronavirus pandemic has contributed in a huge way to the broadening of intrafamilial tensions, because of the measures of social distancing, which have accentuated the difficulties of contact between the family and the network of outside contacts. The constraint of the quarantine, by which individuals had to stay confined within their own house for days, weeks, and sometimes months, has furthermore put a strain on the family equilibrium, and the family's spontaneity of contact has become a measure of its mental health: where the contact is forced and continuous, it is natural that distress and conflict develop. And if the family is already suffering from a precarious fluidity in the relationships internally and externally, it is understandable how Covid may have produced a huge number of anomalous situations, with outbursts of aggressiveness and/or a development of relational pathologies, which to this day still require help and treatment.

The tools that our model offers to the therapists that exercise it are all seeking the same objective: to experience relationships with awareness and confidence in themselves and in life – an objective that can only be achieved if the therapist pursues it – by living in the first person the ethical dimension of the contact – and if he/she is able to "fall in love" with the family with whom he/she is working.

Notes

1 "There are two pivotal concepts that concern the family as an organism: the synchronic one of the *co-creation of the contact boundary* as the achievement (more or less spontaneous) of the intentionality of contact between the individuals and with the therapist, and the diachronic one of the relational ground of the experience represented by the *evolutionary context,* from the experience of the family linked to its history (which includes the family life cycle)" (Spagnuolo Lobb, 2013, p. 198).
2 This paragraph follows the work model with the family developed by Margherita Spagnuolo Lobb (2013) and illustrated in Chapter 8.
3 American artist (1882–1967), leading exponent of the American realist artistic movement.

References

Bogliolo, C. (2012). *Fare ed essere terapeuta. Dubbi e domande nella conduzione della psicoterapia relazionale* [Doing and being a therapist. Doubts and questions in conducting relational psychotherapy]. Milano: FrancoAngeli.

The Family Studies and Research University Centre of Università Cattolica in Milan, Human Highway. (2020). *La Famiglia al tempo del COVID-19* [The Family in the time of COVID-19], https://centridiateneo.unicatt.it/famiglia-ricerca-famigliacovid-19 #content.

ISTAT – Istituto Nazionale di Statistica. (2020). *Il numero di pubblica utilità 1522 durante la pandemia (periodo Marzo-Ottobre 2020)* [The 1522 public utility number during the pandemic (period March-October 2020)], www.istat.it/it/archivio/250804.

Loi, D., & Pesce, F. (2021), *La violenza di genere e domestica durante l'emergenza da Covid 19* [Gender and domestic violence during the emergency by Covid 19], https://welforum.it/il-punto/laumento-delle-diseguaglianze-in-tempo-di-pandemia/ la-violenza-di-genere-e-domestica-durante-lemergenza-sanitaria-da-covid-19/2021.

Perls, F., Hefferline, R. F., & Goodman, P. (1994). *Gestalt therapy: Excitement and growth in the human personality*. New York: The Gestalt Journal Press, or.ed., 1951.

Sampognaro, G. (2016). Working with the developmental age in Gestalt therapy. In M. Spagnuolo Lobb, N. Levi, & A. Williams (Eds.). *Gestalt therapy with children. From epistemology to clinical practice* (pp. 169–190). Siracusa: Istituto di Gestalt HCC Italy Publ. Co., www.gestaltitaly.com.

Sampognaro, G. (2021). *I piccioni di Skinner* [Skinner's pigeons]. Lecce: Youcanprint.

Spagnuolo Lobb, M. (2013). *The now-for-next in psychotherapy: Gestalt therapy recounted in post-modern society*. Siracusa: Istituto di Gestalt HCC Italy Publ. Co., www.gestalt italy.com.

Spagnuolo Lobb, M. (2016). Gestalt therapy with children. Supporting the polyphonic development of domains in a field of contacts. In M. Spagnuolo Lobb, N. Levi, & A. Williams (Eds.). *Gestalt therapy with children. From epistemology to clinical practice* (pp. 25–62). Siracusa: Istituto di Gestalt HCC Italy, www.gestaltitaly.com.

Spagnuolo Lobb, M. (2018). Aesthetic relational knowledge of the field: A revised concept of awareness in Gestalt therapy and contemporary psychiatry. *Gestalt Review, 22*(1), 50–68. DOI: 10.5325/gestalt review.22.1.0050.

Tolstoj, L. (1877). *Anna Karénina*. New York: Thomas Y. Crowell & Co.

Chapter 14

Gestalt Psychotherapy and Ageing[1]

Alessandra Merizzi

1. Introduction

The chapter presents some reflections on the application of Gestalt therapy (GT) to the work with older people (OP), including a view on the challenges brought by the Covid-19 pandemic.

To begin with, the changes that can occur in the process of the self in relation to the environment will be analysed: what happens to the id, ego, and personality self-functions as we age. Part of the background considered will include aspects of vulnerability, how OP face states of frailty, and how they may ask for help and engage with the helper.

Then the needs that might lead to the first contact with the professional, the therapeutic resonance and risks for impasse, and what the co-creation of a "relational dance between patient and therapist" might look like (Spagnuolo Lobb, 2017) will be explored. To this end, common aspects related to self-growth and possible "healing" through the therapeutic relationship will be analysed.

2. Ageing in the Field of the Covid-19 Pandemic: An Important Opening Statement

The spread of the new coronavirus brought a lot of attention to the older population, highlighting the level of ageism in our societies. All of us read newspapers headlines, comments on social media, and witnessed the lack of interest towards nursing homes in the UK, Russia, and other 'civilised' countries by their governments. Vulnerability in later life was markedly highlighted as a weakness and as an inevitability. I question: what messages are younger generations going to internalise, and how will these affect their own ageing in the future? How are these statements affecting OP by reinforcing their own negative stereotypes and feelings of being a burden on society?

After two years of the pandemic, the consequences of restrictions, isolation, and overburdened health services have become visible to us all. In general, we have seen a deterioration in the physical and mental health of many OP.

DOI: 10.4324/9781003313335-17

3. Ageing and Its Rich Background

3a. The Body, Cognition, and Experience of Self – Id-Function

In general terms, growing older implies a process of slowing down. Biologically and biochemically, the speed and quality of production of new cells and other mechanisms becomes reduced. This means that the body needs more time to move, to balance, to think, and so on.

But not every aspect of our physical abilities declines. Regarding the experience of self, it is important to consider how our nervous system may be affected by the passing of time.

Age-related changes in the brain's structure and function can vary significantly across individuals. The senses and sensorial perception are affected by ageing, thus if we cannot hear or see well enough, the stimulus from the environment cannot be fully captured or processed by our perceptive abilities (Craik and Salthouse, 2008).

Other obstacles are found at the level of attention: the capacity to multitask, performed through divided attention and working memory, is affected by the slowing down of the processing speed (Harada et al., 2013). This means that we are somehow forced to pay attention to what we are doing in the here and now, as it can become increasingly difficult to hold various thoughts and actions simultaneously.

Since many people are unaware of these changes as they occur, an attempt to carry on multitasking will affect the retention of information in the short-term memory storage. The information is not processed well enough to be stored, or it may be processed in the short-term memory, but the 'need' or attempt to multitask won't allow enough time for the information to be properly stored (Salthouse, 1996).

The slowing down of information processing also means that all the abilities classified as 'fluid intelligence', for instance, the ability to learn new things and solve problems in an abstract way, can decline. On the other hand, the abilities classified as 'crystallised intelligence', which are related to accumulation of knowledge and experience, will improve.

The peculiarity of our memory is that whilst we can still increase our knowledge, it may become challenging to retrieve words from our inner vocabulary, and we may need more time to accomplish the retrieval task. However, it is often the case that not enough time is allowed to pass, and our anxiety may increase and block the process altogether.

Many of these aspects play a part in making a change to the experience of the process of self at the basic level of the id-function. The variety of this change can be great, especially when common age-related chronic diseases such as arthritis appear. Therefore, the range of body experiences and the way the self will be present at the contact boundary with its id-function could be seen as a spectrum, where, on the one extreme, there are individuals who are ageing well and who are only affected by minor changes; on the other, there are individuals who develop co-morbid illnesses and so become disabled and extremely vulnerable.

Lieberman and Tobin (1983) emphasised the difficulties of OP in acknowledging their own change in, for example, physical appearance. This is experienced at all levels of self-function, so this complexity deserves separate analysis.

During the pandemic, many felt older, as if the ageing process had gone faster than normal. The prevailing experience at the id-boundary was related to breathing, the narrowing of the space in which to move being often indoors, smelling the same odours, feeling the heartbeat faster, and other signs of anxiety, fear, sadness, and distress. The restriction of movement, the stillness, sitting down for longer, the prevalence of visual stimuli on electronic devices, as well as experiencing a lack of physical presence and stimuli have all contributed to the acceleration of the ageing process.

Often, clients deny their body experience, constantly pushing it into the background, and we do a large amount of body work to raise awareness at the level of the id-function. I think it is important to keep an open and curious attitude to explore how our older client experiences the changes mentioned previously, including the more recent experience of the pandemic.

Once accepted, a positive aspect of slowing down may be that it elicits a greater focus on the present moment. In our practice, we often work to slow down the experience that is co-created. We invite the person to decrease the speed of body movements, to take time to explore the therapeutic process, and to linger with the emotions that arise (or with the silence).

The "being slower" of an older client may then become a blessing rather than a curse. Through this exploration, negative age attributions may emerge. Then it is important to challenge the false belief by using "metacognitive" exploration, such as focussing on the "how come". The word "ageing" can easily become a label with counter-effects like those of psychodiagnostics labels.

3b. Ageing Stereotypes and the Process of Self: The Ego-Function

This topic opens another discussion regarding how ageing stereotypes may affect the process of self and ultimately the therapeutic encounter. The scientific literature offers plenty of studies showing the powerful, both positive and negative, influence ageing stereotypes play in how we physically age in holistic terms; Levy and colleagues have observed attributable changes in various aspects, such as memory, hearing, cardiovascular problems, and even the development of Alzheimer Disease biomarkers (e.g., Levy *et al.*, 2006, 2009, 2016).

Levy's (2009) theory on Stereotype Embodiment states that stereotypes "(a) become internalized across the life span, (b) can operate unconsciously, (c) gain salience from self-relevance, and (d) utilize multiple pathways". The process for which stereotypes are embodied has two directions: from childhood to old age (over-time) and from the society to the individual (top-down).

I would like to add an aspect to this theory based on mirror neurons and inter-personal neurobiology findings (Gallese *et al.*, 2007), and in line with the GT theory of self (Perls *et al.*, 1951). Firstly, I would suggest a broadened concept of "top-down" direction which also includes family and close relationships. Whereas, as Levy reports, in the outside world, children are exposed to subliminal messages, within the family environment and neighbourhood, children witness the way adults relate to their elders as well as the way OP relate to each other and their self-attitudes.

Children are an active part of the environment and very quickly respond to these interactions, often by imitating and identifying with the loved and inde-structible parent. Given that our Western culture has a predominantly negative view of ageing, it is likely that the stereotypes internalised by children are of such a quality; however, this will also depend on the quality of intergenerational relationships in that family environment. The language of these messages is both verbal and non-verbal, part of the relational co-creation in the family field. While societal subliminal messages are passively internalised, the ones coming from the family environment are bodily experienced, part of a relational interaction and therefore actively internalised. This might explain how, despite the prevalence of ageist stereotypes at the societal level, some people introject positive ones. This might also explain how stereotypes become embodied and not only stored as semantic categorisations.

To illustrate how ageing stereotypes become part of co-created relational situ-ations, I use the self-fulfilling prophesy cycle (Figure 14.1). The following exam-ple attempts to represent a common scenario in which an old lady attributes her memory difficulties to ageing as she believes this to be the only cause (stereo-type); she will then assume a passive attitude towards her difficulty, in coherence with her belief that ageing is inevitable and so are memory problems; her daughter internalises similar stereotypes since these beliefs have been shared in the family intergenerationally; she will then respond to her mother with a comment, congru-ent with her internalised stereotypes, which will reinforce her mum's negative belief. This cycle will multiply and become trigenerational when children are part of the relational field.

Certainly, similar cycles, already part of the background of our clients, can silently become part of the therapeutic encounter.

The ego-function of self plays an active role in the way stereotypes become part of the co-created relational situation, by attempting to make and reinforce meaning from the input given by the id-function (confusion, forgetfulness) and the personality-function ("I am old").

The messages that *virally* spread during the Covid-19 pandemic can reinforce such negative cycles. According to Levy (ibid.) and as illustrated in the figure hereafter (Figure 14.2), these messages go from society to the individual, thus they are enacted and embodied in the close context of the family or adjacent com-munity. From the "top" level we find first the decisions of governments such as of the United Kingdom, which initially counted no deaths from the virus in nursing

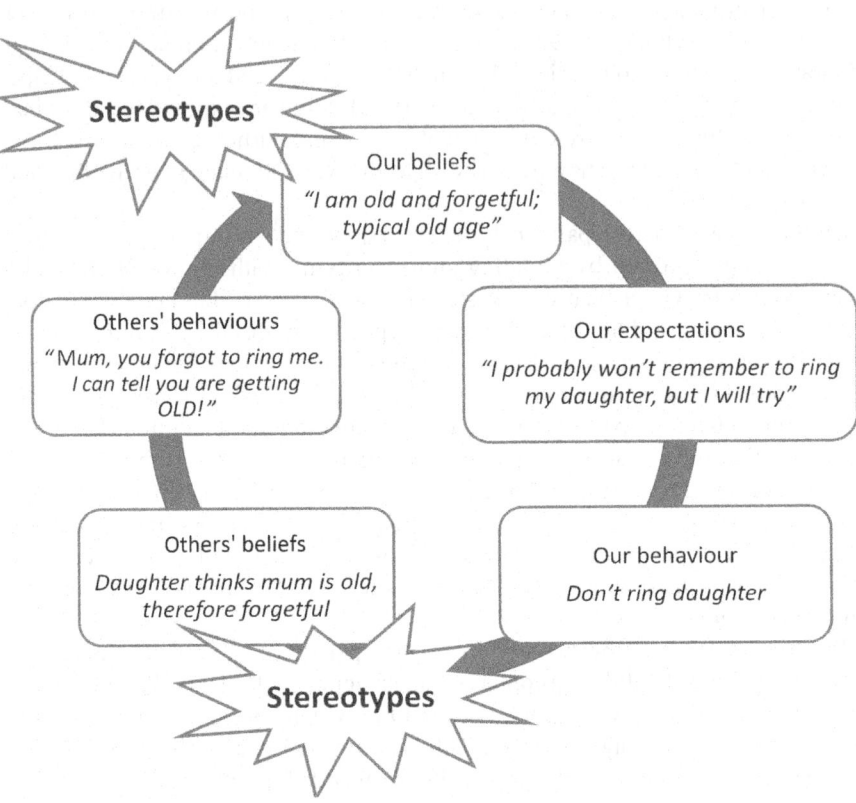

Figure 14.1 The self-fulfilling prophecy cycle and ageing stereotypes

homes, or Russia, which forced people over 65 to stay at home, without considering the practical consequences, then the many attacks in social media that highlight the equation that ageing equals frailty and uselessness, hence a "burden on society". These messages can influence family dynamics by triggering introjected ageism stereotypes which are played out in various ways by adults towards older family members, for example by becoming overprotective, or at the other extreme, by becoming neglectful. As a result, OP respond either passively (similarly to the previous example) or in a rebellious and oppositional way. In any case, the activation of introjected ageism would shake their background, since there is a forced identification with a negative and demeaning image of ageing.

3c. Identity Changes and the Crisis of the Personality-Function of the Self

It is impossible to identify a specific age that states when a person becomes "old". Health services have generally a "cut-off" age of 60 or 65. However, with

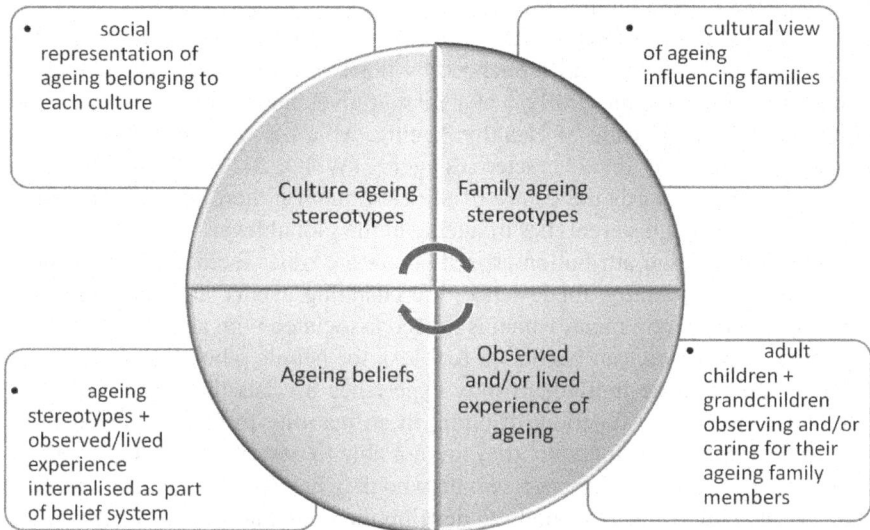

Figure 14.2 The cycle of self-fulfilling prophecy and stereotypes of aging

higher life expectancy and increased wealthy living, many people feel young at 60. Some individuals would attribute the start of this stage of life to retirement. Others would attempt to deny it entirely, driven as they are by the expectations of society and by their own negative ageing stereotypes. I have observed that people around me tend to say that they are "old" when they start experiencing some type of limitation: aches, reduced motor or cognitive speed, and so on.

Our attitude towards ageing can significantly shape who we will become. A passive identification with the limits of ageing will transform our experience of self at the contact boundary with the other. This process for some people may start during their 30s or 40s, and it is mainly experienced at the id and ego-functions (through focussing on bodily experienced limitations and making comments on this with someone else using age attributions). These experiences will complete an integration at the personality-function when an age-attributable life-changing event occurs, for instance the retirement. The person's identity will then change to "I am old" or to "I am still young, and I have nothing to do with OP". These two polarities are extremes of a continuum of a wide range of experiences in terms of ageing identity changes.

In my working experience, I have found that clients who identify themselves at the personality-function with the "I am old" extreme tend to be very passive, difficult to engage, and tend to co-create a depressive situation in which nothing can be done. At the other end of the spectrum, clients whose personality-function takes on the "I am still young" extreme of identity, tend to be active and ener-getic, but at the same time, difficult to engage; they are fearful of being urged to compromise aspects of their risky lifestyle, for instance when they miss sessions due to injuries caused by hazardous sport activities. The latter extreme has been reinforced in the last decade by the promotion of Active Ageing, a policy framework published by WHO and influenced by positive psychology. The Covid-19 pandemic brought, paradoxically, a change that gives hope: in January 2021, the WHO declared the decade of Healthy Ageing, which is a view on ageing that embraces the diversity that characterises ageing (WHO, 2021). It is thus the first attempt to move towards the centre of the continuum hitherto described, which may help to challenge stereotypes of ageing at the global level.

Along with the age attribution aspects, there are other factors that contribute to the renewal of identity, for instance, life changing events such as retirement. The experience of retirement, which is indeed associated with ageing and shaped by ageing stereotypes, can become a real loss for people whose major focus in life was career. These individuals may experience a crisis that expresses itself at the level of the ego-function, resulting in an inability to renew their identity through the personality-function: they are not able to describe who they are now, and instead they focus their narrative onto who they have previously been. Retirement can also offer the opportunity to develop the grandparent role, which might pleasantly renew the personality-function experience with a sense of playful connection, responsibility, and of being the expert and the wise one.

Another important life-changing event is related to the necessity for a member of a couple to become caregiver of the other, which role implies the loss of the loved partner as they were before, the loss of their retired couple life with future plans together, plus the loss of the sense of self, sometimes up to the point of nullifying oneself to completely dedicate to the other. This change can become so dramatic that it goes beyond transforming the identity from being a partner to a caregiver. This may reach a level where the process of self is lost into a complete confluence with the other: even at the ego-function level, the person is not able to speak about themselves; instead, their narrative will only give space to their "cared for".

In short, later in life, there are events that require a significant adaptation of our self-process. Depending on introjected ageing stereotypes and the type of life-changing events that will occur, a person's experience of self may be compromised to the point where they experience confusion, bewilderment, and an identity crisis.

3d. Gains and Strengths of Ageing

Despite the challenges previously underlined, literature shows that getting older offers some advantages. For instance, most OP experience emotional stability and affective well-being at least until they reach the age of 80 (e.g., Carstensen *et al.*, 2000, 2010).

The Socioemotional Selectivity Theory states that OP respond to the perception of limited time and predicted endings by prioritising emotionally gratifying experiences in the present rather than focussing on future rewards (Carstensen, 2006).

Differently, the Life-span Theory of Control suggests that OP have decreased capacity to control their environment, and therefore they would prefer the use of secondary control strategies, such as emotion regulation, to adapt to given circumstances instead of changing the situation with primary control strategies (Heckhausen *et al.*, 2010).

Other authors argue that OP seem to become more skilled in emotional regulation processes through life experiences; for instance, they may have better expertise in predicting emotional effects of future events (Scheibe *et al.*, 2009), acquire better adaptation of emotion-regulatory strategies to situational demands (Blanchard-Fields, 2007), and experience an effortless emotion-regulatory process (Scheibe and Blanchard-Fields, 2009).

Emotional regulation in older age can thus be considered a strength, one that is present at the id-function.

Charles and Piazza (2009) underline that this strength can become less available when the individual is exposed to prolonged negative experiences. Their Strength and Vulnerability Integration Model suggests that age related physiological vulnerabilities decrease the ability to regulate high levels of emotional arousal, and when this becomes sustained, in time, there are increased risks for the individual's health. When OP seek therapeutic help related to their low mood or anxiety, it is likely that they are in a prolonged stressful situation and that they have lost contact with their emotional-regulatory strength. For instance, after one year of pandemic, residents of care homes that were severely affected by the virus were afraid to leave their rooms and enter the communal area (Trabucchi, 2021).

However, this strength may still be in the background. In my clinical experience, I have been pleasantly surprised to discover this quality when it becomes more figural, as it enhances the level of engagement and quality of contact.

An outcome of the improvement of the emotional-regulatory process is the increase of ability in conflict resolution and management of negative emotions. Recent studies showed that OP tend to adopt passive emotion-regulation strategies such as walking away from a situation (e.g., Blanchard-Fields *et al.*, 2007). The awareness that they cannot change the other has increased. They tend to prioritise harmony, use these disengagement strategies effectively to reduce emotional distress and report greater satisfaction from social interactions with a higher level of positive affect (Luong *et al.*, 2011). Therefore, the changes in emotion-regulation support a better-quality engagement at the ego-function, allowing the person to be fully present when experiencing positive interactions and to withdraw in a functional way when conflicts arise.

Additionally, Hess (2005) observed that OP are better in making judgements when choosing a social partner. The knowledge that comes from experience and the becoming wise are strengths of ageing which may become available at the personality-function. This becomes part of the person's life story, for which a selected recall often gives pleasure to people, particularly when sharing it with others. An advantage of a younger therapist may be that the intergenerational encounter facilitates the exploration of this aspect, allowing the older client to experience the wise aspect of her/his personality. When negative experiences prevail in the current life, it is rewarding to counterbalance these through the expression and acknowledgement of the person's rich background. This may also elicit a counterbalance of power in the therapeutic relationship as the client can feel like the "life expert". At times, though, such co-creation can become part of transference and countertransference dynamics that may need attention (Merizzi, 2019).

3e. Becoming Frail and the (In)ability to Ask for Help

Ageing predisposes one to higher levels of vulnerability for which several people will develop various types of health conditions. Unlike younger generations, OP from the current cohort seem to have difficulties with asking for help and accepting it. A strong internalised message of people in their 70s/80s is "if I ask for help, I am weak"; moreover, when experiencing psychological distress, the message becomes "if I ask for help, I am mad". When the symptoms become overwhelming, it will then become more acceptable for them to seek out their general practitioner and take medical prescriptions such as antidepressants.

This internalised message may be reinforced by the current socio-cultural aspects of our Western society. Families and communities are increasingly disintegrated, with families divided by broken relationships, and with many public spaces either removed and/or privatised. The geolocation of family members has become global. As a result, people are pulled apart from one another and are left to communicate only through the media. OP, who are already exposed to the loss of partners and friends, have diminishing relational contact with their family members, and a lack of support from services and from their community. This is also reinforced by the stigma attached to ageing, which provides a worthless image of older age. The outcome of getting older in such an environment is an increased risk of becoming isolated and experiencing loneliness. Therefore, the experience of reaching out may be accompanied by the feeling of being a burden, then the need for help is denied to avoid this feeling. When OP approach therapy, these characteristics in the background may still play a part in the therapeutic encounter, for instance, by lowering the level of engagement. The therapist may hear comments such as "I am wasting your time here".

Overall, the experiential ground of an older client may feel shaky and unsafe and may drag energy away due to an experience of feeling powerless, at a standstill, or stuck in the void. However, there is also potential. There are strengths. And the void is fertile. It is important in therapy to take small steps together with kindness and gentleness and "dance" exploring the ground.

4. Dancing With the Frail and Wise

4a. Why Do OP Seek Therapy?

Drawing upon the multiple aspects previously discussed, it becomes evident that there is an incidence of specific psychological issues, which are distinct to this stage of life. Considering the current cohort of OP, clients accessing low intensity mental health services or private professionals may present with historical and never-treated psychological distress, such as anxiety, depression, or unprocessed traumas. Others may develop psychological symptoms for the first time in relation to their current situation, for instance in response to isolation or multiple bereavements

For some people, retirement brings challenging times, not only in terms of their personal adjustment to it, but also in terms of the couple relationship since the couple may have to make important adaptations and seek therapy to learn how to cope with their new marital situation.

When OP develop disabilities, they may access specialised support, whilst their family caregiver may look elsewhere for help when not supported by the same health service. The work with older caregivers may be challenging as they tend to: a) seek support when they are already overwhelmed by stress and demands; b) do not identify themselves as a "client", in that the "client" is their loved one; c) strongly focus attention on their loved one rather than on themselves.

In older age, anyone can experience adverse events to which one may creatively adjust by dangerously withdrawing from reality, retroflecting and self-harming through drugs and alcohol abuse, or conversely, adapting by projecting and becoming aggressive towards others. Generally, OP experiencing such high levels of distress, presenting a diagnosable personality disorder or psychosis, tend to access crisis centres and be seen in inpatient settings.

Considering that the *zeitgeist* of forthcoming ageing generations is different from the one of the current cohorts, the listed reasons for therapy may change in the future.

4b. When the Therapy Begins: Resonance Versus Impasse

I meet Norma. It is our second session. Norma feels anxious and low in mood. She lives on her own as she lost her husband five years ago. Her children live in various parts of the country. The nearest is 40 miles away. She has a few friends that meet regularly for coffee; however, she recently decreased her attendance. Her sister lives in Yorkshire and, until recently, she loved to take the train to visit her.

Norma says "I cannot get the train anymore. I am afraid to get lost. Going to town and meeting my friends is also becoming difficult". Norma is in her 70s. Her mother died of dementia, and she is very concerned that she is developing the same. Norma received a diagnosis of Mild Cognitive Impairment (MCI). Whilst she shares this information with me, I also feel worried for Norma; the question:

"is she developing dementia?" pops into my head. The anxiety circulates between us.

At this point, I may decide to share my feeling. My concern may be reinforced by the belief that dementia is common in OP and if her mother had it, there is a risk that she will inherit it.

How is the sharing of my worry going to support our therapeutic encounter? We may explore the anxiety in the field, part of our co-creation, and with creative indifference notice what emerges.

However, my resonance with Norma's concerns is underpinned by my own ageing stereotypes, which I rationally try to undermine through learned scientific updates (e.g., Di Nuovo *et al.*, 2020). Norma's feeling is also influenced by her own stereotypes, which are strongly reinforced by the memory of her ill mother. Narrative therapy authors Milton and Hansen (2010) report that practitioners become bewitched by their clients' negative stories of ageing. I see Norma's and mine as a co-creation that is influenced by ageing stereotypes which are part of the therapist's and client's field, and therefore become part of the co-created ground. The effect of this 'spell' may set in motion the self-prophesy cycle presented earlier and may transform the resonance of the therapist into feelings of pity and powerlessness, limiting the quality of contact and the now-for-next. This co-created experience can then lead to an impasse in the domain of "intentional resonance" (Spagnuolo Lobb, 2017). The contact boundary between the therapist and the client becomes desensitised due to the prevalence of emotional responses attached to stereotypes of ageing, the latter acting as introjects. The risk is then, as Spagnuolo Lobb describes in her model (2013, 2017), the co-creation of a depressive field.

I tell Norma: "I am feeling anxiety in my chest and my breathing is shallow. Yours seems so too." And then I add: "I am aware of the risk of you developing dementia just as your mum did. I am also aware that not everyone with an MCI will develop dementia and that memory difficulties can be related to many things including feeling anxious, low, and to dealing with stressful events. *(short silence)* How do my words land on you?" Norma takes a moment to respond "Mmh. *(silence)* That is how I feel . . . anxious, low, and stressed by my worries." Then she adds: "Do you mean that my memory problems are perhaps linked to the way I feel and that they are not necessarily the beginning of dementia?" I nod. I notice her eyes opening wider as she looks at me more intensely, a feeling of hope started to emerge and overcome our co-created anxiety. She smiles at me. "I see you smiling at me. How is your breathing now?" Norma replies "Oh, I can breathe better." "Me too," I respond.

In the act of sharing some facts from my knowledge of MCI, I challenged our introjected stereotypical beliefs. It was then possible to re-attune to each other and reopen our co-created dance.

4c. The Dance Can Begin

Exploring the "how come" of a belief is a useful way to enter the introjected stereotypes, see the individual for who they are, and work on the feelings emerging from those memories in the here and now. The resonance of the therapist and the co-created experience of reciprocity may allow a sense of safety to be re-embodied by the client. In working with OP, the therapeutic dance may create an opportunity to enhance the awareness of the emotional and relational feelings, to experience enough support for the acceptance of one's limits and to explore the often-unseen possibilities.

Norma and I are now aware that there is still anxiety over the likelihood of developing dementia, at times becoming figural and at times staying in the background. But we know that this is not the only possible future for her.

Norma's recollections unlocked the memory of loss, stress, and sadness at having taken care of her mother, only to see her leave for a nursing home. In reporting the following dialogue, I refer to Norma with N and to me with A.

N: "I don't want this happening to me or my children."
A: "I feel the weight of your memories, Norma, and the concern for your future."

Norma cries, looking away and covering her eyes. I let her be with her tears and lean over slightly with my body. She seems to sense my increased proximity and slowly calms down. She makes eye contact with me again.

N: "I am sorry, I shouldn't cry."
A: "Tears are welcome here."
N: "I don't like crying in front of other people."
A: "You don't like crying in front of me?"
N: "No, I feel stupid, miserable . . . sorry . . . how can you do this job and hear this all day?"
A: "Well, I like my job, it feels good to help others. . .. You seem worried for me now, what about your worries?"
N: "I would like them to disappear. And the memory problems . . ."
A: "Let's focus on the worries now. Would you like to try something with me? (she nods). Repeat with me: I am Norma; I have memory difficulties; I worry because my mum had dementia; I do not have dementia; I am Norma, and I am not my mum; my life is different than hers."
N: "It feels good to say it."
A: "You know Norma, we cannot predict the future. Looking at the present, I can say that many things have changed in the last 10 years. It is possible to diagnose people with MCI . . . who knew what that was 10 years ago? And most importantly, now there is much more understanding of dementia and people with dementia can now live a better quality of life." (silence)
N: "I didn't know services have changed . . . but you are right, many things have changed since then . . . and anyway, I don't have dementia now. I have this mild thing. (silence) I am glad I am seeing you."

The work that followed was an exploration of Norma's difficulties in her daily life, the impact of memory problems on her relationships, and on her sense of self. We met for six sessions. The memory difficulties that shook Norma's sense of safety were still there. However, through our encounters, she was able to re-embody her confidence. By the end of the sessions, Norma restarted to travel by train and to go out more often to meet the people she loves.

4d. Reflections on Applying GT to the Work With OP

The example illustrated previously is of a clear and straightforward clinical case. Depending on the context in which a clinician works, the client's presentation may vary in complexity, and this will also have an impact on the therapeutic goals and expectations of the therapeutic work.

GT as a phenomenological and experiential approach works on procedural memory loops (Burley and Freier, 2004) which is resistant to ageing, even in the presence of Alzheimer's disease (e.g., Kawai *et al.*, 2002) and supports the formation of new memories over time (Brown *et al.*, 2009).

Pure Gestalt requires the therapist to begin the work by looking at anamnestic information as it emerges from the ground. Considering the complexity of an older person's ground, my approach is to actively bring ground aspects into the figure and carry out a proper anamnesis which can provide an initial understanding of factors that may influence the work; for instance, if a client is taking medications that can affect their cognition (e.g., Nevado-Holgado *et al.*, 2016). Additionally, it could inform the clinician of possible risks that need to be considered, and at times, immediately communicated to the appropriate services.

Considering what has been discussed to this point, the therapeutic goals that may characterise the work with OP are that of:

1. Accepting the process of ageing as it is for the individual, free from stereotypes.
2. Enabling the process of self to adjust and regulate to the situation, despite the possible coexistence of uncertainty and limitations.
3. Aiding the person in engaging with what is available in his/her own field with a renewed and open attitude.

To work towards these goals through the therapeutic dance, therapists should explore their own ageing stereotypes together with the client's ones, bringing these to figure as part of the co-creation. It is also important for the clinician to be present and become a receptacle for the suffering related to the losses, and then move towards an acceptance of what is no longer available to the person. When the person's life story becomes part of the co-created narrative, it may be useful to explore and value the person's strengths, which are resistant to time. "The therapeutic dance" (Spagnuolo Lobb, 2017) can become the means to bring strengths and values into awareness in the here and now. Exploring the resources available in their current field enable the person to emotionally regulate and make a conscious adaptive choice. Further attention goes to ending the therapeutic work, which will possibly be paced gently, depending on the level of loss and bereavement the person has been facing.

5. To End

This chapter is not exhaustive in terms of the multiple aspects that characterise the therapeutic work with OP nor of the theory upon which it is based.

The literature offers plenty of resources to gain a general understanding of gerontological psychology and of the psychopathology of ageing. Much more has yet to be written about applying GT to the work with OP. At the time of the writing of this chapter, Gestalt literature offers only a few contributions to the topic, with a shared view of the validity of the GT approach for OP (e.g., Meulmeester, 2013; Woldt and Stein, 1997).

The GT theory of self (Perls, Hefferline & Goodman, ibid) can offer a new perspective of the changes in ageing, of the person's transformative experience in relation to their environment, and informs on how ageing stereotypes are formed and maintained as a co-creation at the contact boundary. In terms of therapeutic work, the underpinning neurocognitive aspects of the Gestalt approach seem valid across the lifespan. In general, I support the view that GT can be applied following its basic principles. But at the same time, I wanted to be thorough by pointing out aspects that may require specific attention.

Woldt and Stein (1997, p. 182) state that: "A significant benefit related to therapeutic success with older adults is the opportunity for the therapist to begin unravelling unresolved personal concerns related to aging, disability, and death." It is surprising to discover the potential of therapeutic work with OP, emerging as a co-created dance that enriches both the client and the therapist.

Note

1   The chapter is 30% shorter than the original because of given page limits. Please, contact the author for a full copy.

References

Blanchard-Fields, F. (2007). Everyday problem solving and emotion – An adult developmental perspective. *Current Directions in Psychological Science, 16*, 26–31.

Blanchard-Fields, F., Mienaltowski, A., & Seay, R. B. (2007). Age differences in everyday problem-solving effectiveness: Older adults select more effective strategies for interpersonal problems. *The Journals of Gerontology Series B: Psychological Sciences and Social Sciences, 62*(1), P61–P64.

Brown, R. M., Robertson, E. M., & Press, D. Z. (2009). Sequence skill acquisition and off-line learning in normal aging. *PloS One, 4*(8).

Burley, T., & Freier, M. C. (2004). Character structure: A gestalt-cognitive theory. *Psychotherapy: Theory, Research, Practice, Training, 41*(3), 321.

Carstensen, L. L. (Ed.). (2006). *Social structures, aging, and self-regulation in the elderly*. New York: Springer Publishing Company.

Carstensen, L. L., Pasupathi, M., Mayr, U., & Nesselroade, J. R. (2000). Emotional experience in everyday life across the adult life span. *Journal of Personality and Social Psychology*, *79*, 644–655. DOI: 10.1037/0022-3514.79.4.644.

Carstensen, L. L., Turan, B., Scheibe, S., Ram, N., Ersner-Hershfield, H., Samanez-Larkin, G. R., Brooks, K. P., & Nesselroade, J. R. (2010). Emotional experience improves with age: Evidence based on over 10 years of experience sampling. *Psychology and Aging*. Advance online publication. DOI: 10.1037/a0021285.

Charles, S. T., & Piazza, J. R. (2009). Age differences in affective well-being: Context matters. *Social and Personality Psychology Compass*, *3*, 1–14.

Craik, F. I. M., & Salthouse, T. A. (2008). *The handbook of aging and cognition* (3rd ed.). New York: Psychology Press.

Di Nuovo, S., De Beni, R., Borella, E., Marková, H., Laczó, J., & Vyhnálek, M. (2020). Cognitive impairment in old age. Is the shift from healthy to pathological aging responsive to prevention? *European Psychologist*, *25*(3), 174–185. DOI: 10.1027/1016-9040/a000391.

Gallese, V., Eagle, M. N., & Migone, P. (2007). Intentional attunement: Mirror neurons and the neural underpinnings of interpersonal relations. *Journal of the American Psychoanalytic Association*, *55*(1), 131–175.

Harada, C. N., Love, M. C. N., & Triebel, K. L. (2013). Normal cognitive aging. *Clinics in Geriatric Medicine*, *29*(4), 737–752.

Heckhausen, J., Wrosch, C., & Schulz, R. (2010). A motivational theory of life-span development. *Psychological Review*, *117*(1), 32.

Hess, T. M. (2005). Memory and aging in context. *Psychological Bulletin*, *131*, 383–406.

Kawai, H., Kawamura, M., Mochizuki, S., Yamanaka, K., Arakaki, H., Tanaka, K., & Kawachi, J. (2002). Longitudinal study of procedural memory in patients with Alzheimer-type dementia. *No to Shinkei= Brain and Nerve*, *54*(4), 307–311.

Levy, B. R. (2009). Stereotype embodiment: A psychosocial approach to aging. *Current Directions in Psychological Science*, *18*(6), 332–336.

Levy, B. R., Ferrucci, L., Zonderman, A. B., Slade, M. D., Troncoso, J., & Resnick, S. M. (2016). A culture – brain link: Negative age stereotypes predict Alzheimer's disease biomarkers. *Psychology and Aging*, *31*(1), 82.

Levy, B. R., Slade, M. D., & Gill, T. M. (2006). Hearing decline predicted by elders' stereotypes. *The Journals of Gerontology Series B: Psychological Sciences and Social Sciences*, *61*(2), P82–P87.

Levy, B. R., Zonderman, A. B., Slade, M. D., & Ferrucci, L. (2009). Age stereotypes held earlier in life predict cardiovascular events in later life. *Psychological Science*, *20*(3), 296–298.

Lieberman, M., & Tobin, S. S. (1983). *Experience of old age*. New York: Basic Books.

Luong, G., Charles, S. T., & Fingerman, K. L. (2011). Better with age: Social relationships across adulthood. *Journal of Social and Personal Relationships*, *28*(1), 9–23.

Merizzi, A. (2019), Clinical supervision in older adult mental health services. *Working with Older People*, *23*(4), 241–250. DOI: 10.1108/WWOP-09-2019-0024.

Meulmeester, F. (2013). Risk of psychopathology in old age. In G. Francesetti, M. Gecele, & J. Roubal (Eds.). *Gestalt therapy in clinical practice: From psychopathology to the aesthetic of contact* (pp. 281–294). Siracusa: Istituto di Gestalt HCC Italy Publ. Co., www.gestaltitaly.com.

Milton, A., & Hansen, E. (2010). Moving from problems to possibilities with older people. In G. Fredman, E. Anderson, & J. Stott (Eds.). *Being with older people: A systemic approach* (pp. 161–80). London: Karnac Books Ltd.

Nevado-Holgado, A. J., Kim, C. H., Winchester, L., Gallacher, J., & Lovestone, S. (2016). Commonly prescribed drugs associate with cognitive function: A cross-sectional study in UK Biobank. *BMJ Open, 6*(11), e012177. DOI: 10.1136/bmjopen-2016-012177.

Perls, F., Hefferline, G., & Goodman, P. (1951). *Gestalt therapy: Excitement and Growth in the Human Personality*. Highland, NY: The Gestalt Journal Press.

Salthouse, T. (1996). The processing-speed theory of adult age differences in cognition. *Psychological Review, 103*, 403–428. DOI: 10.1037/0033-295X.103.3.403.

Scheibe, S., & Blanchard-Fields, F. (2009). Effects of regulating emotions on cognitive performance: What is costly for young adults is not so costly for older adults. *Psychology and Aging, 24*, 217–223.

Scheibe, S., Mata, R., & Carstensen, L. L. (2009). Yes, they can! Older adults accurately forecast emotional responses to wins (though not losses) in the 2008 US presidential election. *The Journals of Gerontology Series B Psychological Sciences and Social Sciences, 65B*(2), 135–44. DOI: 10.1093/geronb/gbp132.

Spagnuolo Lobb, M. (2013). *The now-for-next in psychotherapy: Gestalt therapy recounted in post-modern society*. Siracusa, Italy: Istituto di Gestalt HCC Italy Publ.Co., www.gestaltitaly.com.

Spagnuolo Lobb, M. (2017). From losses of ego functions to the dance steps between psychotherapist and client. Phenomenology and aesthetics of contact in the psychotherapeutic field. *British Gestalt Journal, 26*(1), 28–37.

Trabucchi, M. (2021). *Rsa, dopo il vaccino: "Riaprire sì, ma con prudenza e senza forzature* "[Rsa, after the vaccine: "Reopen yes, but with caution and without forcing"], www.redattoresociale.it/article/notiziario/rsa_dopo_il_vaccino_riaprire_si_ma_con_prudenza_e_senza_forzature_.

Woldt, A. L., & Stein, S. T. (1997). Gestalt therapy with the elderly: On the "coming of age" and "completing gestalt." *Gestalt Review, 1*(2), 163–182.

World Health Organisation. (2021). *UN decade of healthy ageing. 2021–2030*. www.who.int/initiatives/decade-of-healthy-ageing.

Chapter 15

Gestalt Psychotherapy in the Relationship with the Chronic Patient

Accepting and Supporting the Experience of Loss Through an Aesthetic Gaze

Alessandra Vela and Donatella Buscemi

To our patients, who bring us back to the importance of making contact with the sense of one's own limitations, by listening to one's own body.

To our patients, who remind us of the beauty of the trust in "sustaining" the other even in silence, communicating the most important thing the painful experience of the disease brings with it.

To our patients, who teach us about the security that is born in the sharing of pain, through the full presence and the attentive and engaged gaze of the other.

For M., for her curiosity, for her infinite love of life, for her melodious voice, for her unforgettable gaze.

1. A Missed Dinner: The Beginning of Therapy[1]

I want to go home. It's late. I'm starving and I haven't prepared dinner. But why wasn't I able to say no to Claudio, the most thoughtful (but also annoying) psychiatrist I know, when he suggested I take on this new case? I don't remember exactly now, but why did he give this referral to me? I only remember that it was about a woman of a certain age. And is that why he perhaps did not take into consideration the possibility of meeting with me online?

Finally the bell rings. Here she is! It couldn't be anyone else but her – extremely punctual. I open the door, and yes, it's her: tall, well-groomed, dressed with attention to the smallest detail. However with those thin legs . . . how are they able to hold her up! Looking at her, I already feel the pain coming my way . . . but I feel ready to begin this new adventure. For today, dinner can wait. M. enters my office for the first time on a late afternoon at the beginning of summer, when the pandemic seems to be letting up a little, after months of confinement through the first lockdown. The psychiatrist has referred her because he senses that he is not the right person for the case of M., and my specific competencies make me that person. I invite her to take a seat, and her story immediately takes shape in her melodious voice, accompanied by shallow and not very fluid

DOI: 10.4324/9781003313335-18

breathing, which I am able to detect, despite the presence of the mask. Her gaze is direct, her posture slightly stiff and revealing tension, specifically in the shoulders and chest, with little bodily ground in the lower part of her body. M. is 70 years old. She tells me that 2 years earlier, she discovered that she had a rare uterine tumour, for which she immediately underwent demolitive surgery and then chemotherapy and radiation therapy. After examinations, subsequent to the therapies, it seemed as if they could talk of the illness's remission, but instead, about a year later, pulmonary and bone metastases were detected. M. is currently in treatment at a centre in Milan, with an oncologist, to whom she sends quarterly medical reports of the tests, carried out in the Sicilian city where she lives. She is continuing oral chemotherapy on a daily basis, with the goal of controlling the known secondary lesions.

Completely immersed in my personal sensorial experience, and inspired by curiosity towards M., I allow some questions to take shape: why is M. seeking help two years after her diagnosis? Why a year after the discovery of the metastasis? What is her present emotional need? How much and how has the pandemic influenced her experience of the disease? While I try to make sense of these questions and almost at the end of our first session, a tear glides down my face upon hearing the story of her illness. Although realising that it comes down to "a spontaneous response to an actuality" (Perls *et al.*, 1994, p. 224), I do not have the time to ask myself if it's a good thing to get emotional with her on our first meeting. M. freezes, surprised. Her features soften. She assumes a more comfortable position in her chair, finally leaning her back into it. She sighs. I, too, sigh, and continue to tear up: her narrative is characterised by a sense of loss and the absence of expectation, unless it is one of: "we shall also fail together". Her malaise is powerful when she imagines a worsening of her illness, which will conclude with her no longer being autonomous, and once again hospitalised, an experience, which, this time, she will be forced to face alone. It is a very difficult image to accept and is not fully assimilated, just as her fear of death is extremely intense in that it will not let her be anymore with the people she loves.

But besides the content that M. is bringing to the session, what am I breathing in the field? Perls, Hefferline, and Goodman use the concept of the field to assert that the individual "constitutes a totality with the environment to which it relates" (Macaluso, 2020, p. 32). Our journey begins in a field characterised in essence by fear: my fear of not being up to working together, confirmed by the disappointment felt in discovering me to be younger than expected (it is now easier for me to understand the sense of inadequacy felt by Claudio, the psychiatrist, in the session with her), M.'s fear of loving life, and aware of her own distress in imagining herself in a struggle, given her need to be restful and unanxious in order to live. Therefore, from a field perspective, fear belongs to both of us. As Spagnuolo Lobb writes (2013, p. 82): "The field perspective in Gestalt psychotherapy invites us to non-dichotomous thinking . . . it is necessary to say that we are referring to a concept of a phenomenological, hence experiential field, which however is not a merely subjective reality."

What is our action within the field that has allowed us, despite the fear, to move towards the emergence of a sense of security, which might permit us to work together, towards the co-construction of a solid ground, at a point in life when the ground seems to have collapsed? I felt that my emotional sensitivity enabled a different organisation of the field to come about (Wollants, 2012), and in fact,

> the therapist sees the change in psychotherapy as a *unitary change* of both the client and him/her self. Their field changes, and not just the client's. The perception of the client and that of the therapist both change, and both these changes have to be taken into account.
>
> (Spagnuolo Lobb, 2016a, p. 264)

2. The Therapy Continues: The Encounter With Cancer

The person afflicted with a chronic illness must learn to live with the idea that undergoing treatment will not lead to recovery, and that the disease goes through an uncertain and unpredictable progression, often characterised by periods of greater well-being and by others of a sharpening of symptoms. And all of this will last for his/her whole life. The patient has to continuously find a new way of adapting to the altered conditions, reassess his/her own habits, come to terms with the changes of his/her own body, ones which often lead to progressive disability.

And often, even the therapist has to "reassess his/her own habits". Just think about how often, with these patients, it may be necessary to abandon the classic psychotherapy setting in order to offer them the only possible intervention – the home setting.

When we meet with a patient in Psychiatry, but also in Oncology (the discipline closest to Psychiatry, in the wait for a diagnosis that can bring one to the extreme boundaries of unspeakable and inexpressible pain), the way in which we look at each other, and greet each other, is important in creating, or impeding, a relationship; equally important is the harmony between the time of those giving care, and the time of those receiving care. (E. Borgna)

Chronic pathologies embrace all branches of medicine, but the incidence of cancer reaches numbers that are sadly very high, also thanks to the fact that the increase of oncological pathology is accompanied by a lowering of the mortality rate. And therefore, with the exception of those that survive this pathology, the majority are forced to live with it for a very long time, up until death.

The knowledge that a chronic disease has an evolution that involves mind and body has recently led to an in-depth exploration of the psychological aspects associated with it, and to the birth of a real scientific discipline: psycho-oncology. This discipline is attempting to improve attention towards the psychological and social impact of the disease both in the patient and his/her family, to integrate psychological treatment into the pharmacological and surgical treatments, to study the predisposition to the development of tumours, and therefore to act with prevention in early diagnosis, as well as during the progression of the illness.

This discipline is aimed at patients whose psychological malaise does not primarily depend on a psychopathological malaise but rather on the traumatising situation of the illness, and therefore the reflective consideration on this condition must necessarily be developed starting from the concept of *trauma*, generally defined as that condition where the individual feels distressed, disorganised, and relives in a continuous way "the sense of being impotent and vulnerable in the face of the threat to his/her overall health and physical being" (Sampognaro, 2017, p. 118), and is not able to face the situation using common strategies for solving problems.

After a few meetings, it is clear to me that M. made this request for psychotherapy because her creative adaptations, those she has put into practice up until now, are no longer effective and have led her to feel the fear of not being adequate, of not being interesting to others. The collective trauma of the pandemic has increased this fear to the limits of her endurance. She feels fallible – a new experience for her.

The oncological disease (and in general, chronic and terminal pathology) bursts into the life of a person, assaulting all aspects of his/her existence, from his/her corporeal condition to family and social relationships, to the organisation of daily life, to the possibility of thinking of oneself in the future, with the inevitable consequence of impacting one's sense of self, understood as a person's on-going process of experiencing the world (Spagnuolo Lobb, 2001).

The diagnosis of incurable disease disrupts the existential development of a person, whose perception is one of having had the connecting thread to the future broken. In Gestalt psychotherapy, the self is the process, the function, and the event of contact that integrates past experience with the solicitation of the present, in order to take a step into the future.

> The present is a passage out of the past toward the future, and these are the stages of an act of self as it contacts the actuality. . . . What is important to notice is that the actuality contacted is not an unchanging "objective" state of affairs that is appropriated, but a potential that in contact becomes actual.
>
> (Perls *et al.*, 1994, p. 153)

And this is what is happening with M., whose main experience in terms of her illness is one of disappointment but also of intense anger towards those doctors who had given her the possibility of thinking herself cured, of returning to a very much desired *status quo* prior to her illness. In order to fully understand the oncological patient's drama, it is necessary, in the first place, to know the significance that the illness assumes in that particular life context and how the patient assesses his/her own ability to face it, in relation to the goals, which he/she has set.

Who is M.? What expectations of life does she have at the moment of her diagnosis? M. is the mother of three adult daughters who are already working. One is married with two children whom M. adores. She was a teacher in a secondary school. She gave up her career as a school principal, a profession to which she aspired, to take care of her daughters when they were little. Her husband was very busy professionally. M. has always been the mainstay of her family, the reference point as well of her family of origin. However, on the social level, she is presently closed off. She rejects invitations from her friends and goes out less with the family. She has stopped going to the gym (where she did postural gymnastics). The amount of time she spends reading has diminished. Above all, she has stopped travelling, an activity she loved, because she has developed a fear of feeling sick far from home, both physically and in terms of her anxiety symptoms. These limitations already began to take shape prior to the lockdown. At the time of my meeting with her, her closing herself off from others is also a consequence of worries associated with the pandemic situation, important background to her anxious experiences.

The loss of vitality and of the stimuli to see people and to take care of her own future often characterises these patients, not only due to the complex circumstances of their health but especially because they are traumatised by their sickness. Obviously, all of this has consequences in every sphere of their life, in particular on the relationships with the people closest to them. M. is living what happens to all those who are affected by a chronic pathology: she is experiencing continuous losses.

This type of illness represents a traumatic event, which risks undermining a sense of personal integrity, causing extremely high levels of psycho-physical stress and frustration.

In my work with M., it is more and more evident that her anxiety is linked to the unexpectedness of what has happened following the diagnosis and its consequences – an anxiety "related . . . to a sudden and uncontrolled loss of ground security, that the self could not sufficiently foresee" (Spagnuolo Lobb, 2016a, p. 283).

When a person is facing the trauma of an incurable disease, which represents a threat to life itself, "there is a response of horror, panic, a strong sense of impotence, and a loss of control over things" (Cascio, 2013, p. 154).

M. is experiencing the need to work through the trauma that the diagnosis has generated. She has to be able to deal with the very strong link, which, at least until a few years ago, existed between the diagnosis of the tumour and death, because, in the face of a chronic illness (as opposed to a degenerative and nevertheless terminal one), it is necessary to reach a progressive adaptation in order to be able to cope with the stages that a long-term pathology brings with it. The therapeutic intervention must ensure a warm atmosphere of containment, "capable of giving a sense of welcome necessary for developing the security and confidence in the ability of the treatment" (Partinico et al., 2003–2005, p. 11).

From a neurobiological viewpoint, traumatic experiences, such as, for example, the diagnosis of a chronic organic illness, are associated with a dysregulation of the Autonomous Nervous System. This implies, according to the model of the polyvagal theory suggested by Porges (2017), that when the nervous system does not sense a safe environment, and therefore the functionality of the ventral vagus is reduced or absent, there is an increase in the activity of the Sympathetic Nervous System and of the dorsal vagal Parasympathetic Nervous System, or of both, or the reduction of sympathetic activity. In the first case, strategies of mobilisation, such as attack and escape behaviours, are promoted, and in the second, a bio-behavioural shutdown which would result in fainting spells, inhibition, and dissociation. In both cases, one runs the risk of considerable disorders on the physical, emotional, behavioural, and psychic levels, and the neural circuits which support social behaviour and regulation are involved in the health, growth, and recovery of energies, and thus the states of security are a prerequisite for social behaviour and also for having access to the higher cerebral structures, which allow human beings to be creative and productive (Porges, 2017). Finally, "for our physiology to calm down, to heal and grow we need a visceral feeling of safety" (Van der Kolk, 2014, p. 79).

Porges (2017) recognises the importance of taking care of the clinical environment since different characteristics of the medical environment trigger a sense of vulnerability and activate a defensive neuroception.[2] For example, medical settings often do not facilitate characteristics of social support, which we normally have in our daily life. Our clothes are taken away. We are placed in a public space, and there is no longer any predictability. Many of the characteristics which our nervous system uses to regulate itself and to feel safe are not available.

With the OMS declaration of March 11, 2020 on the state of the COVID-19 pandemic, such studies as these are beginning to stir great interest. This health and social emergency represents a further source of psychological distress for these patients and their families: in fact, whoever is suffering from a serious or critical illness, including cancer, has a greater risk of COVID-19 infection. In particular, subjects with oncological or onco-haematological pathologies, in relation to the immunosuppression state, are more subject to infections, whether bacterial, fungal, or viral, often taking on complicated forms (Bellani *et al.*, 2020).

The numerous restrictions of a health nature, among the measures put into place to combat the pandemic, have influenced treatment facilities, and as a result, regular oncological therapies (Bellani *et al.*, 2020). The patients in treatment reveal both the worry of not receiving the therapies scheduled for their illness and ambivalence towards these same therapies out of a fear of exposing themselves to the risk of contagion. We are witnessing an increase of generalised fear and anxiety, a sense of loneliness (with a possible reduction of compliance to therapies), and a fear of not receiving adequate care (Gregucci *et al.*, 2020).

The family members, on the other hand, express the fear of not being able to provide adequate concrete support to their loved ones and also of not being present in the helping process, in case of deterioration or death.

3. The Integrating and Regulative Function of the Self: The Somatic Experience in Oncology

"When the actuality is pressing, certain values oust other values furnishing a hierarchy of what does in fact marshal brightness and vigor in its execution. Sickness and somatic deficiencies and excesses rate high in the dominance hierarchy" (Perls *et al.*, 1994, p. 55).

The eruption of the disease and the unpredictability with respect to its evolution generate a change in the pre-existing figure/ground balance: the individual experiences a sudden loss of ground security. The self is no longer able to assimilate the change. "The ego-function is no longer in control of the ability to adjust creatively" (Spagnuolo Lobb, 2016a, p. 281).

When a chronic perception of danger becomes fixed, as in the case of M., the risk is very high that the disease will take the form of a rigid predominant figure, one that is impossible to force to retreat into the background to make way for new figures, necessary for personal growth. And if this process is functional for overcoming the first phases of a traumatic experience, it becomes pathological with the passing of time, because it prevents the rediscovery of vital energy required to stop focussing on what then becomes the only need present in the perceptual field of the individual (Cascio, 2013; Spagnuolo Lobb, 2016a).

And with me? How does M. wear her being a cancer patient in her relationship with me, her psychotherapist? How does she define herself in the face of a sense of the fragmentation and the destructuration of the family and social roles, subsequent to the surgery, the treatments, and today the experience of a pandemic?

In M.'s story, there are only sporadic, not particularly relevant episodes of anxiety. Today, she refers to intense sorrow and elevated anxiety. She knows that she is a woman possessed of fine resources. She sees herself as a determined, thorough, neat, sociable, and affectionate person. But in therapy, what gradually emerges is her need to have an alternative to that image of perfection, to know that she can surrender herself, and allow herself to become "little". I detect her gradual self-surrender and her willingness to show me her fallibility. She begins to recount that she feels at the mercy of the unpredictability of her clinical condition and of the progression of her pathology. She would like a response to this sense of loneliness that she is feeling.

How can one count on the bodily ground of a sick body? When an emotion emerges during therapeutic contact, does she feel it or does she desensitise it? Are her feet firmly resting on the ground? What are the bodily experiences generated by the illness? What are the repercussions of this "unreliable" body's experience – which, instead of supporting, becomes a continuous threat – on the id-function of herself? What weight does the sense of loneliness have, one that she feels in a time that negates the possibility of social contact? The first security to collapse for M. is that of her corporeal ground. It was by her body, after all, that M. was "betrayed", but it is her body that she has to care for, subjecting it to therapies and frequent "intrusions". During our sessions, M. occupies her space with me without showing a full sense of bodily rootedness, while breathing shallowly.

The occurrence of disease introduces a discontinuity in the existential journey, a discontinuity which "obliges" the body to emerge from the ground, and aggressively makes it a figure. It is a body which exposes its own vulnerability; from this sudden collapse of the bodily ground, the contact with the "next", towards which life aspires, fades away (Spagnuolo Lobb, 2013).

The body is the preferred organ of contact, and it tells the history of its contacts and the new features of the current ones: the body is what pre-eminently gives us the idea of being individuals, "the knowledge of the person I am cannot set aside the body that supports me and allows me to accumulate experiences, connections, abilities, peace, love, memories that enrich my life" (Schnake, 2003–2005, p. 95). It is clear, therefore, how the diagnosis destabilises the ground of the self's assumed securities: "The tumour activates the fantasy of an internal, invisible, alive, unkind, persecutory enemy while one is in a state of total impotence" (Partinico et al., 2003–2005, p. 10). The diagnosis of the disease showcases a no longer efficient body, one no longer capable of carrying out the intentionality of contact.

One is faced with an altered image, whose adaptation is a task involving grief over the loss of one's own identity, on both a cognitive and affective level (Morasso and Lagostena, 2004). This confusion alters the delicate relationship between self-support and hetero-support: the internal senses of security and fullness are directly proportional to the sense of being able to entrust oneself to the environment. Suffering does not belong exclusively to the patient but to the entire field out of which it emerges: it calls into question the health professional involved.

The Gestalt therapist who encounters cancer finds him/herself thus fluctuating between the experience of his/her own body and the experience of the other's body; there is no other possible way to do this, as Frank argues (Clemmens et al., 2013, p. 15): "it is necessary 'to lend our body' to the patient, offer our embodied self as a support in the relational field".

It is through the instrument of the body that M. asks for help: it is thanks to it that she can acquire new awareness and a new integration of the self, able to support the organism in its various processes of interaction with the environment, and in the act of entrusting herself to it.

An organic illness can bring about bodily desensitisation for the purpose of defence, and so it is necessary to be careful in the facilitation of body awareness. Allowing these patients to enter into contact with the other and with the environment, and enhance the awareness of their own bodily self, ostensibly denied up until this moment, is the way in which the psychotherapist supports the now-for-next, the involvement of the self in the development of the intentionality of contact, and giving sense to their own life.

4. The Disease's Progression: Responding to the Pain of the Field

Parallel with our ongoing psychotherapeutic process, the fact should not be overlooked that oncological disease is not a static event but rather gradually evolves and therefore new needs of a physical, psychological, and spiritual kind may continually come to the surface, ones that change with the state of the disease and the state of the consciousness of the diagnosis. A few months after our first meeting, M. comes to the session very dazed: a new metastasis has been identified as well as the slow progression of the others. What follows from this news is a change in chemotherapy. M. ends up again without hair, without the possibility of taking up once more her customary daily activities, already limited by the pandemic, with the same energy and the same desire – a situation which was slowly and gradually developing. M., devoid of energy, is not able to experience anything other than the pain of the loss of her identity and role, and other than the changes in her personal habits and lifestyle. All images and sensations remain frozen at the moment of the diagnosis of this new metastasis.

> Give sorrow words. The grief that does not speak whispers the o'er-fraught heart and bids it break.
>
> (W. Shakespeare)

With the chronic patient, it is often necessary to support some concrete actions of the diagnostic-therapeutic process imposed by the disease. It is necessary then, in any setting, for us to intervene, "to dialogue" with the world dealing with the patient's pathology. At a certain point, with the approach of her health check-ups, M. shares her anxiety over the thought of having an MRI. We work together to identify, through imagination techniques, a safe place in which to take refuge whenever anxiety gets the upper hand during the procedure. We also work on her breathing and the ability to stay focussed on it, with a view to reach a state of relative relaxation during these anxiety-inducing and painful experiences.

M.'s requests begin to change: from the need to control her symptoms and to preserve her personal dignity threatened by the continuous interruptions of her being in the world, to the search for sustenance on the part of the environment, which she asks to take full responsibility for her pathology with her overall state of suffering – an environment which, however, is today experienced in an ambivalent way.

The work with M. has been going on for months, when, in a moment of great angst, she confides to me that initially she felt wary about our process, but also eager to be accepted by me, and not feel abandoned when facing up to her fragility. My tears during our first session made the difference. That moment, so full of great humanity, was precious to her: she felt completely understood in her confrontation with pain, and did not perceive any type of pity.

That experience of openness was an example of the Gestalt modality that Macaluso (2020) defines as "spontaneous therapeutic action", in which "the relationship is co-created through moments of mutual recognition and intimate contact, in which the therapist becomes involved in a personal and authentic way" (p. 34). Perls, Hefferline, and Goodman state that

> within the spontaneous experience there is no separation between the plan and the goal. We do not act on the basis of a plan or on a preliminary evaluation

of the situation, nor in terms of a final objective. We proceed gradually, as the action develops, in an immediate and intuitive fashion. And satisfaction comes not from achieving specific results, but from performing the action itself. We feel a sense of pleasure, of satisfaction, which is intrinsic to the action itself.

(Spagnuolo Lobb, 2016b, p. 79)

It is through this type of contact experience that it is possible to achieve that reciprocity that entails "being truly heard and seen by the people around us" (Van der Kolk, 2014, p. 79).

Despite the fact that traumatic experiences, endured with incurable diseases, have a profound impact on people's lives, often generating a great deal of angst,

it is possible to mobilize the human capacities for resilience, and for the preservation, which belongs to human beings as a living species, of their strong vocation towards the future, towards the next step . . . something which humanity cannot do without, in order to avoid the feeling of "dying".

(Cascio, 2013, p. 153)

For this to be possible, it is important that we, in our role as psychotherapists, create a secure ground by means of our gaze, our voice, and our facial expression: "traumatized human beings recover in the context of relationship: with families, loved ones, AA meetings, veterans' organisations, religious communities, or professional therapists. The role of those relationships is to provide physical and emotional safety" (Van der Kolk, 2014, p. 210). In fact, the human brain appears as a social brain, organised from birth to reflect others, to create significant connections with them, by means of experiences of interdependence (Molinari and Cavaleri, 2015).

These experiences, during the COVID-19 pandemic, have been possible as well in the psycho-oncological context, through psychological interventions carried out by means of virtual technology, with the implementation of psychological telephone help lines aimed at identifying the psychosocial needs of the patient and the family, for the purpose of beginning or continuing individual or group psychotherapeutic interventions. The positive side to this crisis is that, even though the pandemic is devastating to the nervous system, it has turned out that, during a unique moment in history, we have had the tools that allow us to connect with each other even when we are obliged to be isolated. The polyvagal perspective can help us to understand how the nervous system has received incompatible demands: the necessity of avoiding contact with the virus through social distancing prevents the fulfillment of the biological imperative of connecting with others in order to feel calm, safe, and secure. Avoiding being infected triggers a strategy of chronic mobilisation but social involvement that usually provides security, regulation, and well-being signals a threat. The possibility of undertaking online therapy allows us to respond to this dilemma, since being there has been made possible by providing, by means of reciprocal facial expressions and vocal intonations, opportunities for social connection and security (Porges, 2020).

But what kind of security is possible for someone who every day asks herself "how long will this disease let me continue to live"? And "live with dignity"?

M., during our work together, gradually recaptures the ability to "love" life again. She allows her family members to help her whenever she feels very tired, with a new confidence in their presence, and in their way of taking care of her. She begins to trust. It is very complex work, directed towards the acceptance of the greatest "rip-off" of her existence, and aimed at finding some sense to life despite this rip-off: living with her sickness, which she always mentions as the cause of the huge limitation to the love to be expressed towards the people dearest to her. We work with M. to give a sense to what has happened, to provide space for the expression of her emotional experience connected to loss, grief, death, and to be able to build together a "different" life plan.

5. The Final Encounters: The Boundaries of the Therapeutic Process

The journey into oncological disease "is certainly a journey of acceptance of our basic condition of being human: the encounter with limitation, with vulnerability, with uncertainty, with the wearing down of the body, and therefore the encounter with time, and with the pain of detachment" (Fabbrini, 2003–2005, p. 82). And it is during this journey that the psychotherapist, above all, must ask himself specific questions:

> *Which field?* It is a field in which one is faced with death, in which one often remains as if paralysed in present *time*, where pain does not allow one to consider future possibilities, and where the past ends with exercising an inhibiting influence on the present;
> *Which phenomenological observation?* Which body does one observe? Which intentionality is the body expressing when entering into contact? Often, one notices a sensation of encountering bodies experienced as being "always on the alert", suspended bodies;
> *Which self?* In the work in oncology, one often finds oneself listening to experiences and interrupted stories, a consequence of energy blocked by the news of the disease, of an incomplete figure, and of a disoriented moving within the environment.

Thus, the therapeutic intervention with the oncological patient:

> Foresees a *conscious use of the senses*: the support through body language allows one to welcome the damaged body and give back the perception of its own identity, the reconfirmation of its value, dignity, and human dimension;

Is directed towards a *reduction of bodily tension*, facilitating sensitivity to stimuli coming from the environment, from the outside, so that the ego-function may be able to find again the ability to creatively adjust (Spagnuolo Lobb, 2016a). This allows the illness, at least in part, to recede into the ground, in order to leave space for emotions and actions focussed on all of his/her current needs rather than only those connected to the pathology: he/she begins "to move";

It is a process that requires *sudden changes of rhythm* for the new physical complications, for the tests coming closer and closer, for the new organic difficulties that in some way deeply influence even the psychotherapeutic relationship. This is necessary for adding new meanings to the experience, for discovering new perspectives, or for glimpsing possible changes.

Finally, the clinical goals of the work are:

To support a process of integration of the disease into one's own life and one's own bodily experience;

To respond to the sense of loneliness that is felt: to reassure the patient and his/her family members during the many moments of discomfort and confusion, which inevitably they will encounter during the course of the illness, problems that become intensified at that moment in which they will feel left alone, and do not know how to cope with the destabilising symptoms and the fear of death;

To "sustain" the patient with great humanity; the therapeutic relationship is, above all, a gesture of humanity.

When we work with patients afflicted with chronic illnesses, we are called on to be a safe and secure ground in the face of their terror, in order to go through together whatever unknown, interrupted, and extremely variable forces appear during the therapeutic process.

Dwelling on our cancer is an attitude, that concerns the present and the future. The disease disrupts everyone's plans, but we have to be better and not lose the desire to plan, but simply modify the objective.

(U.M., oncological patient)

This evening I didn't hear the bell ring. M. is not here . . . It will be sad to go and make dinner.

Notes

1 The patient was in therapy with Dr. Vela; the theoretical-clinical reflections of this present work are the result of the shared cooperation of the two authors.
2 For a more in-depth study of the concept of neuroception, see Porges, 2017.

References

Bellani, M. L., Gritti, P., Scarponi, D., Serpentini, S., & Torta, R. (2020). *Relazioni psicologiche e psicopatologiche rispetto all'emergenza Covid-19 nei pazienti oncologici e onco-ematologici e nelle loro famiglie* [Psychological and psychopathological relationships in relation to Covid-19 emergence in oncologic and oncohematologic patients and their families]. Corso FAD "Emergenza sanitaria Covid-19 e Psico-Oncologia. Competenze da integrare nella pratica clinica", organizzato da Istituto Superiore di Sanità – Servizio Formazione – e Federazione delle Società Medico Scientifiche Italiane (FISM).

Cascio, A. R. (2013). Fenomenologia dell'evento traumatico nella psicoterapia della Gestalt [Phenomenology of the traumatic event in Gestalt therapy]. In P. A. Cavaleri (Ed.). *Psicoterapia della Gestalt e neuroscienze. Dall'isomorfismo alla simulazione incarnata* (pp. 153–163). Milano: FrancoAngeli.

Clemmens, M. C., Frank, R., & Smith, E. (2013). Esperienze somatiche e disfunzioni emergenti: un dialogo [Somatic experiences and emerging dysfunction: A dialogue]. *Quaderni di Gestalt, XXVI*(1), 9–28. DOI: 10.3280/GEST2013-001002.

Fabbrini, A. (2003–2005). La morte, per esempio . . . [Death, for instance . . .]. *Quaderni di Gestalt, 36/41*, 81–85.

Gregucci, F., Caliandro, M., Surgo, A., Carbonara, R., Bonaparte, I., & Fiorentino, A. (2020). Cancer patients in covid-19 era: Swimming against the tide. *Radiotherapy and Oncology, 149*, 109–110.

Macaluso, M. A. (2020). Deliberateness and spontaneity in Gestalt therapy practice. *British Gestalt Journal, 29*(1), 30–36.

Molinari, E., & Cavaleri, P. A. (2015). *Il dono nel tempo della crisi. Per una psicologia del riconoscimento* [The gift in the time of crisis. For a psychology of recognition]. Milano: Raffaello Cortina Editore.

Morasso, G., & Lagostena, A. (2004). L'assistenza psicologica al malato terminale [Psychological care of the terminally ill]. In M. Bonetti, M. Rossi, & C. Viafora (Eds.). *Silenzi e parole negli ultimi giorni di vita* (pp. 163–181). Milano: FrancoAngeli.

Partinico, M., Conte, E., & Mione, M. (2003–2005). L'esperienza del morire come ultimo importante atto del vivere umano [The experience of dying as the last important act of human living]. *Quaderni di Gestalt, 36/41*, 9–23.

Perls, F., Hefferline, R. F., & Goodman, P. (1994). *Gestalt therapy: Excitement and growth in the human personality.* New York: The Gestalt Journal Press.

Porges, S. W. (2017). *The pocket guide to the polyvagal theory. The transformative power of feeling safe.* New York: W.W. Norton & Company, Inc.

Porges, S. W. (2020). The COVID-19 Pandemic is a paradoxical challenge to our nervous system: A polyvagal perspective. *Clinical Neuropsychiatry, 17*(2), 135–138.

Sampognaro, G. (2017). La scrittura autobiografica come strumento di empowerment [Autobiographical writing as a tool for empowerment]. In M. Bongiovanni and P. Travagliante (Eds.). *La medicina narrativa strumento trasversale di azione, compliance e empowerment* (pp. 118–128). Milano: FrancoAngeli.

Schnake, A. (2003–2005). Presenza e attualità dell'approccio gestaltico olistico alla malattia [Presence and relevance of the holistic Gestalt approach to disease]. *Quaderni di Gestalt, 36/41*, 91–100.

Spagnuolo Lobb, M. (2001). The theory of self in Gestalt therapy. A restatement of some aspects. *Gestalt Review, 5*, 276–288. DOI: 10.5325/gestaltreview.5.4.0276.

Spagnuolo Lobb, M. (2013). *The now-for-next in psychotherapy: Gestalt therapy recounted in post-modern society.* Siracusa, Italy: Istituto di Gestalt HCC Italy Publ.Co., www.gestaltitaly.com.

Spagnuolo Lobb, M. (2016a). Self as contact, contact as self. A contribution to ground experience in Gestalt therapy theory of self. In J.-M. Robine (Ed.). *Self. A polyphony of contemporary Gestalt therapists* (pp. 261–289). St. Romain la Virvée, France: L'Exprimerie.

Spagnuolo Lobb, M. (2016b). La conoscenza relazionale estetica: una proposta gestaltica di linguaggio terapeutico nella società contemporanea [Aesthetic relational knowledge: A Gestalt proposal for therapeutic language in contemporary society.]. *PNEI Review*, *2*(6 Suppl.), 71–85.

Van Der Kolk, B. (2014). *The body keeps the score*. New York: Viking.

Wollants, G. (2012). *Gestalt therapy. Therapy of the situation*. London: Sage.

Chapter 16

For Whom the Bells Do *Not* Toll

The Processing of Bereavement in Our Time

Carmen Vázquez Bandín

1. Introductory Considerations

> Noa Pothoven, the seventeen-year-old girl who requested euthanasia in the Netherlands because of having suffered post-traumatic stress and depression, dies (BBC, June 5, 2019).

> A twenty-year-old Belgian woman requests and is granted euthanasia because of being depressed for years
>
> (CNN, July 3, 2015)

When we hear this type of news on television, we cannot help but react with surprise, incredulity, and with a range of feelings that revolve around "the soul" and the conscience. What circumstances of isolation and loneliness are reflected in these reports, which are only a few of so many examples that we can find in daily newscasts? And this is the case, to say nothing of the suicides, the homicides committed within families, the massacres or terrorist attacks. Where is our society heading? Is a cult of death beginning to take shape, or is it life, the most precious possession that we have along with health, which has ceased to be important?

The world, especially in the West, has changed substantially in less than 30 years. No one is sure about where these changes are taking us, nor what the final result will be, because, for now, we are immersed in uncertainty and bewilderment. This obviously also influences the way in which we currently experience three basic processes of human existence: trauma, loss, and grief. As I have already said on other occasions (cf. Vázquez Bandín, 2013), these three human experiences are characterised by a common denominator, which is suffering. Even if we could continue to define and differentiate these three experiences,[1] it is clear that in our present liquid and postmodern society, something has changed in our coping processes.

In 2000, Zygmunt Bauman (2000), in *Liquid Modernity*, even though he was not the first nor the only one to emphasise the ongoing change in the cultural and social paradigm, in some way began to speak about themes such as "emancipation", "individuality", "space-time", "the work culture", and "community". Years

DOI: 10.4324/9781003313335-19

earlier, Lyotard (1979), in *The Postmodern Condition*, had also examined the destiny of thought at the threshold of the computerisation of society, of the state – and the reason for being – of culture and its changes. Modernity and postmodernity are concepts that are being used especially in the human and social sciences, and they help us to understand some characteristics of our societies and the transformations that we are undergoing (compare Spagnuolo Lobb, 2016, 2017).

Taking this into account, I will concentrate on certain changes in this chapter that have characterised today's society and culture, and therefore psychology and psychotherapy, in particular with respect to the experience of loss and bereavement in western culture. Secondly, I will speak about some specific forms of grief, like those due to a child not yet born, those due to suicide, and to pathological grief. As my final input on the subject, I will refer to how the Gestalt model, based on the field and on the dialogic relationship, can be a truly fitting form of support and psychotherapy in situations of bereavement today.

In this chapter, suffering, loss, and bereavement will not be discussed as strictly individual processes, as if each one of us were an island punished by the tidal waves of misfortune, without any connection to anyone or anything beyond ourselves. Although loss may undoubtedly have a profound personal significance, it is worth remembering that the human being is not an isolated entity, and that "there is no single function of any animal that completes itself without objects and environment" (Perls *et al.*, 1994, p. 4), including feelings or thoughts. And this relationship of the individual with his surroundings is not only physical but also social,

Consequently, it is important to highlight the central position occupied by the relationship with others, in the context of suffering, caused by bereavement. Suffering does not exclusively belong to the individual, nor does it belong only to the environment (compare Perls *et al.*, 1994; Spagnuolo Lobb, 2001, 2003, 2005; Vázquez Bandín, 2008, 2010, 2014) but to both. It is a suffering of the contact boundary, of the "between". It is a suffering of the relationship.

2. The Present World in Which Bereavement Takes Place

2.1 The Virtual Reality and the Trap of Social Networks

Society has become liquid. The fluid dance between figures and grounds, in which the individual interacts with him/herself and with others in a constant process of updating his/her experience, has been lost. It has rigidified. Placed before a constantly liquid background, the individual no longer has a ground to support him/her. One permanently takes root in this uncertain ground, thus generating coalescing modes of contact, or conversely, one tenses up in order to avoid sinking into nothingness, and in this way, becomes isolated from others, excessively setting oneself apart, losing oneself and the other, by creating a separate reality and separate values in an egotistical way, which makes one incapable of making enriching contacts.

In this scenario, grief, loss, and death are almost regarded as a social, personal, and familial failure, which has to be expelled from the essence of the human being.

We can think of the current interest of the individual towards social networks as a creative adaptation, which unfortunately adds more isolation and unreality to our way of life. In this isolation in which individuals are immersed, social networks are an instrument for the creation of "one's own community", but what is really being generated is a "substitute" community, in which social skills are not necessary. They are areas of comfort, where a true dialogue does not exist since the created community is adapted to the individual, and so there is no controversy or conflict. Consequently, the "collective" gets selected on the basis of one's own requirements and can easily be chosen or eliminated with a simple click of the mouse, while the "emotional capital" is measured by the number of contacts accumulated in the different Facebook, Twitter, and Instagram accounts.

The "dialogue", therefore, that occurs within the social networks is none other than a place in which to comfortably close oneself off and "listen to the echo of one's own voice." At present, belonging to a social network can, on the one hand, help to alleviate a sense of loneliness, which the individual is suffering, because of the scenario of the great individualisation in which one is living; on the other hand, it constitutes a *real trap*, since it does not truly represent a person's enhanced socialisation.

Within social networks, one can find stories of people experiencing a terminal phase, or who talk about death or of someone's funeral, transforming death and bereavement into a spectacle unrelated to any personal feeling. In this way, a person's life takes place in a global society but without a fixed identity, forcing one into a continual dependence on the presence of "another" who validates one's identity and allows one to "be seen."

Isolation, excessive individualisation, lack of references, negation of any principle of authority, the "protocolisation" of illnesses, the pursuit of one's own happiness, the "psychopathologising" of states of mind, work productivity, and many others, constitute the life context into which we will now introduce some bereavement processes in the present world. To begin with, I will refer to a situation in which grieving "is not possible" because of "social efficiency", which denies the suffering of the loss of a loved one. Death, as such, is again relegated to hospitals or to funeral homes and is becoming a mass spectacle.

2.1.1 The First Case: Striking Down the Experience of Death[2]

Alberto, at fifty years of age, receives the news that his mother is in a delicate state of health, in a critical situation. When he arrives at his mother's house, he ascertains that not only is her situation delicate but that she is living through the final phase of an illness, described as "terminal". His first difficulty arises from this medical term. The difficulty resides in the fact that the medical diagnosis –

whose relevance and precision is not in discussion – puts him face to face with the requirement of merely waiting for the death of his mother. In these circumstances, the life that remains to be lived by "his" mother is greatly altered by an objective and appropriate diagnosis. Alberto is faced with a situation in which his mother is still alive, but he is "forced" to "think" of her approaching and inevitable death. What hell! That "hell" is an obstacle to be leaped over if he wishes to live without submitting prematurely to his mother's future death. If someone is tormented by an anticipated death and is "forced" to feel it, then he can no longer live. In Alberto's case, he ventures to live that delicate moment with his mother in a pleasant and even sometimes entertaining way. This allows them to manage their sadness not in loneliness but in a fully shared way.[3] Alberto arrives at the moment in which he has to face the cruel event of his mother's death, a person he loved. Having to cope with the fact does not equal thinking that it will happen. At this point, he is living his specific experience of death in its reality. He has little time to realise that the organisation of the funeral has already begun at a breakneck pace. The funeral parlour[4] has already established the timing and has made it binding. Once an agency is responsible for the memorial service, it imposes the timing, the places, and even the disposition of the body of the deceased. Alberto, who has already experienced a "traditional" funeral in the past, shared by the community, in which the neighbours had a place as important as the relatives, is seeing how the days of the wake have now been reduced to a few hours. In a context of absolute negligence, he has even had to argue with the funeral parlour's employees that were about to close the coffin without even notifying the relatives and friends of the deceased. As in a television show, it is necessary "to move onto something else", and accept the logic of a time without memory, without sympathy, without sorrow, without paying homage to the people one loves.

And the surprises for Alberto have not yet ended. He accompanies the body of his mother to the cemetery, but here, too, there is an additional moment of tension. His mother, of Jewish origin, is cremated and her ashes gathered and placed in an urn. There is no time for graves or for inscriptions,[5] or for evaluating whether to subject the body of a deceased woman, of Jewish origin, to the fires of a crematorium.

This example, narrated with a certain amount of irony, shows how society tries to avoid mourning as a social act of farewell and honour for those who die, as well as an act of group support for those experiencing loss.

2.2 Some Gestalten of Bereavement

In previous articles (compare Vázquez Bandín, 2008, 2013), I have spoken more specifically about the processes of bereavement, of the various phases and therapeutic supports necessary for the comfort and assistance of adults. I refer the reader to these articles in order to have a generalised view of the subject matter and the specific therapeutic interventions from a Gestalt perspective.

In this context, I wish to concentrate on grief relative to more specific losses, such as the mourning for *a son's suicide*, the mourning for *an unlived life*, and *pathological bereavement*. Even though these forms of grieving have always existed, they play a role of paramount importance in these postmodern times, and generally speaking, are not the subject of reflection.

2.2.1 The Second Case, Grieving the Suicide of a Son: "I Only Want to Know Why"

I find Rosa in the waiting room of my office. We know each other because she took some training seminars with me years ago. She is an educator and works in a school as a guidance counsellor. She is a woman of fifty, short and plump, with white hair. I remember that she was a serious woman, very professional and responsible. She is married and a mother of two sons – Felipe, the eldest, and Pedro, the younger son, 25 years old, who has recently died by suicide. This is why she has called me, to request a meeting with me.

Rosa and I look at each other before saying hello. I see that she is despondent and I feel deeply compassionate for her. We both "pull ourselves together" as if "nothing has happened." But we both know that I know what has happened. I am aware of and surprised by my cold manner, and I think "this is the field and my aesthetic resonance."

Once in my therapy space, I realise that she is sitting very straight, leaning very energetically against the back of the chair. It takes her a few minutes before beginning to speak. I respect her silence and I feel myself . . . I am waiting, contained, respecting her timing. I lightly draw breath. And then I take in air with deep breaths.

Rosa sighs and begins to speak while staying in her own world.

R.:   Truthfully, I don't know why I've come here. What we cannot rectify, we cannot rectify, and the less you speak about it, the better it is.

T.:   *(Silence on my part) (I do not wish to break the containment; she is like a volcano about to explode).*

Rosa looks at me out of the corner of her eye and continues:

R.:   *But I have no one with whom to talk about Pedro and about what has happened. Julio, my husband, has urged me to make this pact of silence . . .*

I evaluate her comment and sense great difficulty in feeling her desire, her need, and I respond:

T.:   *And you, what is it you need now?*

Our eyes meet and I see that she is beginning to tremble all over. Her stiffness is beginning to shatter, but she breathes deeply and again becomes composed.

R.: *I don't know what I need (she says softly). If I only knew why he did it . . .*

Her voice is imploring me, and I am extremely moved. I would like to have the words to comfort her and to answer her question, but obviously, I do not have them, and I feel an enormous sense of impotence.

Again silence, but this time, it is a silence that I feel separates us, distances us from each other.

T.: I do not have an answer to your question – I tell her – but I would like to know how you are feeling in this moment.

R.: *I don't want to talk about myself. I don't want to know how I am. If I analyse myself, I'll fall apart, I'll disappear. I am overwhelmed by my heartache and I am crying non-stop.*

She is not able to continue and before she is able to finish what she is saying, she shivers and bursts into tears with a muffled cry, and then sobs. She reminds me of a child, alone and defenceless.

She cries for a while and speaks through gritted teeth about her loss, about her surprise at what her son did, about her immense sorrow, from which, she says, "she will never recover." And between each sob and whisper, she monotonously repeats: "Why? Why?"

It seems that Rosa needs to pay attention to her husband's suggestion, to remain "isolated" from the facts and from their pain. But this is contained within her by means of muscular hypertonia, which blocks the letting go of her emotions and feelings.

In this first session, Rosa and I unblocked her "rigidity". I do not try to blend in with her, by comforting her or encouraging her to express her emotions. I just simply accept her. I accept how she is with me and her situation. I look for a way to be present with her, with my five senses. I hope and confide that my presence will allow contact to be made in a spontaneous and intentional way. This respect-ful presence breaks her blocked state and allows her to be with me. As the book of our founders states: "when neither flight nor removal is possible, the organism has recourse to blotting out its own awareness, shrinking from contact, averting the eyes, clamping teeth" (Perls *et al.*, 1994, p. 121), and this is what Rosa does continuously.

Accepting the death of a loved one is difficult and even more so if it is a son, because according to the law of life, we take for granted that he will survive us. This "why, why?" typical of bereavement, is an attempt to substitute with rationality the emotional pain, the suffering that includes a loss. The horizons of a person in mourning are destroyed. The sense of a timeline is altered. One experiences with bewilderment "the presence of an absence". All the functions of the self are altered.

For a certain period of time, Rosa decides to come weekly to psychotherapy, because "the grief, confusion, and suffering are prolonged, for there is much to be destroyed and annihilated, and much to be assimilated" (Perls *et al.*, 1994, p. 139).

2.2.2 The Third Case, Mourning a Life Not Lived: "My Unaccepted Son"

It could seem that the death of an unborn child should not give rise to grief, but it is not so. The death of a foetus during pregnancy, or of a baby during the delivery, or a few days after the birth, is often a subject that is overlooked by the professionals and even by the parents, who do not understand why they are feeling so deeply affected. It is necessary to explore the significance of perinatal loss from the viewpoint of the parents, in particular of the mother. When a loss during pregnancy occurs, life and death journey together.

Laura is a young woman of 24. She has been in therapy for around six months. The reason for consulting me is her apathy and absence of interest in life in general. Laura seems to be a resolute and decisive person. She defines herself as "modern and active". When I ask her to explain what she means by "modern", she answers: "I am trying to cut out all social and family messaging and the introjections that have always stifled me." She says it too quickly, and creates in me this sense of "flight", as if she is running away from something of which she is not conscious. I share this sensation of mine with her.

T.: *When you say "take away all social and family messaging" I have the sensation that you may be running away from something, as if there were something you do not want to be aware of. ... Is there something that echoes within you about this, something that resonates within you?"*

L.: *I don't know (while she is saying this, her face changes colour. She becomes pale, and her breathing accelerates). There is something that I have never told anyone, but which doesn't bother me . . . I think. I had an abortion over a year ago. I was pregnant, but not with a permanent partner, and I wasn't able to take care of a baby. . . . But it was a clear-cut decision. . .. I didn't think that it would affect me, but now that you're asking me, I realise that my heart aches, and I feel bad.*

She says these things without stopping, almost without breathing, without taking a break. But as her monologue progresses, her voice gets lower and lower, and her eyes stop looking directly at me.

T.: *It strikes me that you have stopped breathing and that your words have lost strength. I would like to ask if you could exhale hard towards me.[6] Blow air towards me.*

Laura and I have established a good relationship in these months of therapy. She says yes and prepares herself for this experiment. She sits straighter in the chair (a form of self-support), takes a breath and blows it at me; at first timidly, and then she repeats the action more forcefully, looking at me without batting an eye.

She does not have time to ask or tell me anything. Her face again changes colour and expression. She seems filled with emotion and the tears begin to fall down her cheeks. I, too, am filled with emotion.

T.: *What is it that is bothering you, Laura? What are your tears saying to us?*

L.: *I don't know why, but I can't seem to free myself of my dead child, the abortion that took place a year ago, when I decided that I didn't want to have a child.*

I am struck by her expression "my dead child" and I tell her.

T.: *I get goose bumps when I hear you say "my dead child" and I feel a deep sorrow and sense of despondency.*

L.: *It hurts. It hurts a lot that I didn't have it! But you know what? I wasn't ready to take care of a baby!*

I hear her voice. It seems like the voice of a little girl. She fluctuates between sadness and anger.

T.: *What do you feel now?*

L.: *Anger, a lot of anger, and I feel that it is against me, and also against my parents. I don't know why they brought me up the way that they did!*

I think that this may be an introjection, which "is avoiding" her feelings and her relationship with me.

T.: *I'm losing you now. . .. Can I do something to make you come back here, so that we can be together in this?*

My words trigger tears again. She is immensely emotional. When she calms down a bit, she says to me:

L.: *Your words have touched my heart. No one has ever said anything like that to me. And I understand that this is what I do when something overwhelms me. I feel alone and I run away. . .. I feel that this is what I did with the abortion. The news stunned me, and the only way I was able to escape was by aborting. . . . At home there were only rules, but no type of support, of comfort.*

In this session, we went "beyond" the contact model that Laura has introjected, and we were able to rediscover each other in the here and now of our encounter. Our encounter allowed her to understand her contact style in difficult times. She will often go back to this style of hers because Gestalt therapists do not perform "miracles", but she was capable of having a new experience, and gradually she will become more flexible. The function of mourning came to light and with it her suffering and sorrow.

Laura had "reified" her pregnancy without feeling that it involved a new human life. She had repeated her usual strategy of running away from difficulties and not seeking support or comfort in such a vital situation. Based on her family history, she was used to growing up without parental support, without understanding, assailed and criticised as she was by the introjections that had governed her upbringing.

This bereavement, besides being included in the section of "lives not lived", could also fit into the category of "complicated" bereavement, as a "delayed" bereavement, or at least a "denied" one. Sometimes, one thinks that when one makes the decision not to have a baby, this does not entail a bereavement, but obviously, it is not so, as this example demonstrates.

2.2.3 The Fourth Case, Complicated or Pathological Bereavement: "I Refuse to Live Without Him"

As I have said before, if a death is sudden, traumatic, as with homicide, suicide, a road or work accident, a perinatal death, etc., the psychological distress is greater than that related to an anticipated death. When a person disappears and his body is not found, there are many difficulties for the family members in beginning the process of bereavement.

Horowitz *et al.* (1980) define complicated bereavement as one in which the intensity reaches such a level that the "person is overwhelmed, resorts to maladaptive behaviours, or stays endlessly in this state without advancing in the process of bereavement towards a resolution."

We can categorise complicated or pathological bereavement into four groupings:

* *Chronic bereavement*: has an excessive length of time[7]; it never reaches a satisfying conclusion, and the person suffering from this is aware that he/she cannot find closure.
* *Delayed bereavement*: also known as inhibited, suppressed, or postponed. The person has an insufficient emotional reaction at the moment of loss. This can be attributed to the absence of social support, to the need to be strong for someone else or something similar, or to the feeling of being overwhelmed by the extent of the losses. In a future moment, the person can experience the symptoms of grief, sometimes for a subsequent loss; the symptoms can be disproportionate to the loss in progress.
* *Exaggerated bereavement*: the person experiences an intensification of normal grief. He/she feels overwhelmed and resorts to maladaptive behaviour. The person is aware that his/her symptoms are related to a loss. The main psychiatric disorders materialise, ones that arise after a loss. Examples of this include bereavement-related depression, anxiety in the form of panic attacks or phobic behaviours, alcohol or other kinds of substance abuse, and post-traumatic stress disorder.
* *Disguised bereavement*: the person experiences symptoms and behaviours that cause difficulties, but he/she has no awareness, nor does he/she recognise that they are associated with loss. They can appear as physical symptoms (psychosomatic illnesses, etc.) or maladaptive behaviours (inexplicable depression, hyperactivity, etc.).

In the DSM-IV[8] a major depressive disorder is not diagnosed in the presence of symptoms that last less than two months after the death of a loved one. This evaluation criterion was removed from the DSM-5,[9] for various reasons, especially in order to eliminate the idea that bereavement lasts only two months, when most professionals recognise that the time period for grieving is in general 1–2 years. In the second place, it was removed because it is recognised that grieving is a serious factor in psychosocial stress and can provoke a major depressive episode in a vulnerable individual.[10]

My opinion is that, independent of the given diagnosis, depression due to a "delayed" grief shows, on the phenomenological plane, characteristics very different from any other form of depressive suffering. The figure that emerges in this form of suffering is the loss of a beloved person with whom the patient was united in a deep emotional bond.

Before presenting an extract from a session, Table 16.1 shows some reactions due to this "continuing" bereavement that becomes stagnant in the refusal to experience it, as if processing it involved "abandonment" and an "absolute forgetfulness" of the loved one, because this is the principal fear that infuses this form of suffering.

Riccardo, a 42-year-old man, asks me for an appointment. He lives in another city, but he insists on doing psychotherapy with me. When I go out to meet him in the waiting-room, I find a poorly-shaven and distracted man with big circles under his eyes.

As soon as we sit down in the therapy office, he says to me in a tired voice: "I can't take it anymore. I have been tormented for three years by the death of my son and living is unbearable." His voice is monotonous, "tired", almost as if he has repeated these words like a mantra throughout these years. I am amazed and feel pressured by the urgency of his comment, which contrasts a little with the sluggishness in his shape, his movements, and his attitude.

Riccardo tells me that three years ago his seventeen-year-old son died in a motorcycle accident, and since then, he is no longer able to find any peace. "I can't, nor do I want to recover peace-of-mind," he insists. I am struck by the end of his sentence, this "I don't want" full of strength and conviction, despite his anguish.

Table 16.1 Possible grief complications

Physical reactions	Changes to the immune response, adrenal cortical activation (ulcers, HTN), increase in serum prolactin levels (with menstrual disorders), increase in growth hormones (with diabetes, HBP), death due to cardiac problems.
Psychological/Psychiatric reactions	Depression/mania, schizophreniform reaction, images of anxiety and phobia, post-traumatic stress syndrome, behavioural disorders, toxic substance abuse.

He also tells me that he has been pursuing a pharmacological form of therapy for the last three years because he was diagnosed with depression. He is an entrepreneur of a prosperous business, but during these last years, there has been more time spent neglecting his work than working at it; and the business has suffered: "But it doesn't interest me!", he says to me. He eats little and poorly. He sleeps badly, and relations with his wife, mother of his son, are deteriorating. "She, the mother of Santiago, seems to have reacted well; she remembers him with melancholy but she is feeling alive again. I, on the other hand . . ." I sense a certain amount of reproach in his words, or . . . envy. . . . He admits that he does not allow himself to be consoled or supported. And the more he is told to make an effort to emerge from the situation, the more he becomes adamant about not doing anything and sinking into his pain, sadness, and isolation.

Riccardo clearly has the profile of a practical and resolute man, even though at this moment he does not reflect that. He has been an entrepreneur and a fighter besides launching a company and getting good results. "I'm a self-made man," he says to me. I think that his self-centred contact style is feeding a retroflexive way of being in the world and is consuming him. It is as if he has applied his stubbornness and wilfulness to putting an end to his life. I base my reasoning, as always, on the fundamental theory developed by Perls et al. (1994, p. 241 ff.).

Progress in therapy has been slow and prolonged. Riccardo has never missed his weekly appointment, despite the distance from the city in which he lives. Perhaps this has softened his stubbornness and allowed him to "feel taken care of and understood by me."

> Emotional suffering is a means of preventing the isolation of the problem, in order that working through the conflict, the self may grow in the field of the existent.
>
> (Perls *et al.*, 1994, p. 140)

I felt deep tenderness and compassion for him and for his manner of suffering. I continued to remind myself in each session that Gestalt therapists do not "eliminate the symptoms"; rather they assist the process with their presence. They follow along with their five senses open, in each and every here-and-now that they co-construct in every second of their relationship, even when they are dealing with a journey through a desert full of fears and reproaches, in which it seems that the earth's fertility will never appear with new green shoots. I had to use all of my "Gestalt faith" (cf. Perls et al., 1994, p. 123), trusting in the fact that at every step we made, there would always be a ground beneath our feet.

Presently Riccardo has made peace with life. He has created an NGO, aimed at helping parents who have lost a child in a tragic way.

3. Bereavement in the Pandemic

We have seen three "special" forms of bereavement, depending on the object, but independently of the specific nuances of each type, we have to clarify that each person undergoing the grieving process is unique and it is this unique person that we assist.

It seems appropriate to highlight a special form of bereavement, which has to do with the current pandemic, in which a relevant figure has been – and continues to be – the millions of deaths that COVID-19 has brought with it, leaving families and friends to experience what I have called a "suspended bereavement" (cf. Vázquez Bandín, 2020).

I call it "suspended" because it is not postponed, denied, or blocked, but caused by special health measures (no hugs, no attendees, or only a small group at the burial and funeral, etc.). The persons in mourning were forced to "put aside" their sadness, and they didn't have anyone around with whom to share their pain. They did not have a social ground on which to lean.

This is not the place to speak at length about the special characteristics of the therapeutic work with these patients, but I would like to point out some key elements to take into consideration in the therapeutic work with persons undergoing this type of suspended bereavement.

The first task is therefore to create, to co-create between the patient and the therapist an emotional and narrative bond which allows for the processing of grief. This bond is an interplay between patient and therapist, which enables the co-creation of a "between" that exists in the present, in the here-and-now of the relationship. The patient needs "another" here-and-now, which allows him the experience of "hearing himself speak with someone" who is there for him/her.

Other therapeutic tasks are:

- Allowing the patient to speak, and providing empathic listening, which allows him/her to grasp the specific vicissitudes of the loss; while, on the phenomenological plane, the therapist focusses on facial expressions, tone of voice, and on the aesthetic relational knowing.
- Focussing the therapeutic work on the present moment of the situation into which the patient has fallen.
- Knowing in detail how the patient's day is organised (shopping, personal hygiene, meals, sleep) in order to give support and to coordinate possible compromises.
- Knowing what family and social supports he/she currently has.
- Recommending to the patient the possibility of writing some kind of "journal" about his pain and grief, but only if he/she wants and likes to write. This allows one to be with the patient in an "implicit" way in the solitude of his/her home.

The aim of these specific tasks, in "suspended" bereavement, is to make it easier for the patient to become rooted in the "here-and-now" of his/her situation. This rootedness allows him to follow the successive phases of working through grief as a process in itself, since "there are regulating reactions of the organism itself, such as crying and mourning, that help restore equilibrium if only we allow them to" (Perls *et al.*, 1994, p. 53).

A fragment of the beginning of a therapeutic process may serve as an example:

Irene comes into my office after having made an appointment over the phone. She is 42 years old and has lost her husband because of COVID-19, four months ago, right in the middle of the lockdown.

We greet each other through our masks. Her body is stooped and her head is lowered. I immediately feel sadness and weariness. We sit down. She collapses onto the couch and says to me:

"Thank-you for seeing me. We all seem plague-ridden now."

She doesn't give me time to say anything, and begins to recount the absurd way in which she lost her husband. Her narration is monotonous. She always looks towards the floor, as if she has told this story to herself over and over again. How she left him at the door of a hospital in Madrid because they did not let her enter. And how, afterwards, she was not able to speak to him on the phone or to acquire some information from someone about his health. She did not have any more news or information about him until, four months later, they called her to tell her that "the ashes of her husband were in Jaén – 400 kilometers from Madrid – and that they were bringing them to her home."

While I listen to her slow and monotonous story, my heart aches and at the same time I feel a deep anger. It is as if I do not have before me a human being but a rag doll, who is not even capable of crying or registering her existence.

"Terrible," I say to her, "but how did you live through this period of distress and anxiety?"

She looks at me without understanding my question. I need, I want to have a human being beside me. Even if it is a human being who is suffering.

I repeat more precisely:

"And when you left your husband at the hospital, what did you do? How have you lived through these months?

She seems to make a superhuman effort, and, with great difficulty, little by little, she tells me about some minute moments in those four terrible months. Tiny daily details. . . . Her face changes, and suddenly, she begins to sob uncontrollably. Despite her sorrowful weeping, I breathe a sigh of relief. Irene is once again a human being!

Nevertheless, in the same way as I have pointed out the forms of suffering, which correspond to a grief that is verbalised or not, I would also like to highlight that the Gestalt therapist does not try to "dig" into the patient's past in order to find something that we could consider as some kind of bereavement. I would like to mention here that, as Gestalt therapists, we work with the here-and-now of the ongoing situation, oriented towards the ensuing moment (the "next"). It is not our responsibility to create works of "archaeo-psychology". Nor is it our job to explore the past in search of traumas and grief as a way of satisfying our need to find work "material". Perls *et al.* remind us of this: "The past and every other fixity persist by their present functioning" (1994, p. 69).

Within the Gestalt approach, we can find useful information on the theme of bereavement,[11] even if we cannot say that there is a vast literature on the subject.

4. Conclusion

Those who know me are aware of my interest in the theme of death, of bereavement, and of the suffering that goes with it. I have been harbouring this interest from well before the appearance of my own losses and bereavement. I would like to thank Margherita Spagnuolo Lobb for allowing me the opportunity to share my knowledge and especially my feelings and experiences on this subject.

We live in turbulent times, in which traditional paradigms are undergoing radical transformations. We do not know where these changes will lead us, but wherever they lead us, the experience of mourning and suffering for our deceased loved ones will always be at the center of our hearts, this being a characteristic of our humanity. Our primitive ancestors did it, just as the Egyptians, the Greeks, and the Romans did! In the entire evolution of our history, suffering connected to grief has been based on our love of others, the people we love.

I would like to conclude with a thought from Derrida (2003, p. 20), who speaks of the field without naming it, and without defining bereavement, clarifies how it is impossible if devoid of love. We can speak of compassion, of awe, and of other reactions, but *for there to be grief, it is necessary that there be love.*

> The law that governs the relationships of every subject with a deceased friend (or beloved person) – that is, with death and love – is a structural and universal law, an "inflexible and fatal law: of two people who have loved each other, there is one who will see the other one die." . . . When death comes, it is not only the end of this or that particular life, but the "end of something absolute." Thus, there is no bereavement possible. But since the absence of grief makes the person left go mad, only a state of melancholy permits the integration into one of the other's death and the continuation of life.[12]

So be it! *Ab imo pectore!*[13]

Notes

1 *Trauma*: Psychic trauma is usually defined not only as an event that profoundly threatens the well-being (or life as well) of an individual, but also as the consequence of that event in the system or mental structure or in the emotional life of the individual. *Loss*:

an absence, being deprived of something which was once possessed; loss does not always signify death and, therefore, in this present statement, we are only and exclusively referring to a significant loss that leads to a traumatising situation. Psychological bereavement is the state and the process which follows a loss due to the death of a loved one (Vázquez Bandín, 2013, p. 298).

2   This text is drawn (and adapted) from an article by Sladonia A. (2006).

3   Sadness, like every other feeling, is the expression of a field, so another is necessary, or the absence of that other, in order to feel and express it. "An emotion is the integrative awareness of a relation between the organism and the environment" (Perls *et al.*, 1994, p. 186).

4   Since the middle of the last century, funeral "enterprises" have transformed the death of someone into an occasion for manufacturing a new object of postmodern society: the industrial and commercialised corpse, another object, like every other.

5   Jacques Lacan (1984) in his pioneering study, *Family Complexes,* studied the place on a tombstone which deals with, in certain circumstances, the inscription of the name and surname of the deceased person.

6   When I see that the breath is withheld, sometimes, if I consider it appropriate, I suggest to the patient to blow hard as a way of "releasing" the air in a relational way (compare Frank, 2001).

7   The average length of bereavement is in general from 6–24 months, but in 10% of cases it persists beyond 24 months, and, sometimes, becomes chronic (compare Bonanno and Kaltman, 2001).

8   Compare American Psychiatric Association (2000).

9   Compare American Psychiatric Association (2013).

10   The ICD-10 uses the Z63.4 code to refer to normal bereavement (disappearance or death of a family member) within the factors that influence the state of health and contact with the health services, the problems relative to the support group, including family relations, and it includes, in adaptation disorders, (F43.2) the grieving reactions of any length of time considered abnormal for their manifestations or content (Díaz Curiel, 2011).

11   Compare Bate (1995); Sabar (2000); Clark (1982); Francesetti (2011, 2015); Lasaja (2014); Rudman and Leibig (2016).

12   Author's translation.

13   From the Latin: "With all of my heart!"

References

American Psychiatric Association (APA). (2000). *Diagnostic and statistical manual of mental disorders* (4th ed.). Text revision. Washington, DC: Psychiatric Association.

American Psychiatric Association (APA). (2013). *Diagnostic and statistical manual of mental disorders* (5th ed.). Washington, DC: Psychiatric Association.

Bate, D. (1995). Closing the last Gestalt. *The British Gestalt Journal, 4*(2), 134–136.

Bauman, Z. (2000). *Liquid modernity.* Cambridge: Polity.

Bonanno, G. A., & Kaltman, S. (2001). The varieties of grief experience. *Clinical Psychology Review, 21,* 705–734.

Clark, A. (1982). Grief and Gestalt therapy. *The Gestalt Journal, 5*(1).

Derrida, J. (2003). *Béliers. Le dialogue ininterrompu entre deux infinis, le poème* [Aries. The uninterrupted dialogue between two infinities, the poem]. Paris: Galilée.

Díaz Curiel, J. (2011). Estudio de variables asociadas a la psicoterapia grupal en los procesos de duelo patológico [Study of variables associated with group psychotherapy in pathological grief processes]. *Revista de la Asociación Española de Neuropsiquiatría*, *31*(1), 93–107.

Francesetti, G. (2011). Lutto ed esperienze depressive reattive [Bereavement and reactive depressive experiences]. In G. Francesetti & M. Gecele (Eds.). *L'altro irraggiungibile* (pp. 127–134). Milano: FrancoAngeli.

Francesetti, G. (2015). The presence of absence: Mourning and reactive depressive fields, In G. Francesetti (Ed.). *Absence is the bridge between us* (pp. 138–145). Siracusa: Istituto di Gestalt HCC Italy Publ. Co., www.gestaltitaly.com.

Frank, R. (2001). *Body of awareness. A somatic and developmental approach to psychotherapy*. Highland, NY: Gestalt Press.

Horowitz, M. J., Wilner, N., Narmar, C., & Krupnik, J. (1980). Pathological grief and the activation of latent self-images. *American Journal of Psychiatry*, *137*(10), 1157–1162.

Lacan, J. (1984). *Les Complexes familiaux dans la formation de l'individu* [Family complexes in the formation of the individual]. Paris: Navarin.

Lasaja, E. (2014). A journey to motherhood: Postpartum depressive experiences. In G. Francesetti (Ed.). *Absence is the bridge between us* (pp. 225–245). Siracusa: Istituto di Gestalt HCC Italy Publ. Co., www.gestaltitaly.com.

Lyotard, J.-F. (1984). *The postmodern condition: A report on knowledge*. Minneapolis: University of Minnesota Press (or. ed., *La Condition postmoderne: Rapport sur le savoir*. Paris: Éditions de Minuit, 1979).

Perls, F., Hefferline, R. F., & Goodman, P. (1994). *Gestalt therapy: Excitement and growth in the human personality*. New York: The Gestalt Journal Press, ed.or. 1951.

Rudman, M., & Leibig, C. (2016). Aging and beauty, living and dying. In M. Spagnuolo Lobb, D. Bloom, J. Roubal, J. Zeleskov Djoric, M. Cannavò, R. La Rosa, S. Tosi, & V. Pinna (Eds.). *The aesthetic of otherness: Meeting at the boundary in a desensitized world, proceedings* (pp. 297–302). Siracusa (Italy): Istituto di Gestalt HCC Italy Publ. Co., www.gestaltitaly.com.

Sabar, S. (2000). Bereavement, grief, and mourning: A Gestalt perspective. *Gestalt Review*, *4*(2), 152–168.

Sladonia, A. (2006). La muerte en los tiempos de la postmodernidad [Death in the times of postmodernity]. *Revista Digital Universitaria*, *7*(8), 2–10.

Spagnuolo Lobb, M. (2001). The theory of self in Gestalt therapy. A restatement of some aspects. *Gestalt Review*, *5*, 276–288. DOI: 10.5325/gestaltreview.5.4.0276.

Spagnuolo Lobb, M. (2003). Therapeutic meeting as improvisational co-creation. In M. Spagnuolo Lobb & N. Amendt-Lyon (Eds.). *Creative license. The art of Gestalt therapy* (pp. 37–50). Wien and New York: Springer.

Spagnuolo Lobb, M. (2005). Classical Gestalt therapy theory. In A. L. Woldt & S. M. Toman (Eds.). *Gestalt therapy. History, theory, and practice* (pp. 21–39). Thousand Oaks, CA: Sage Publications.

Spagnuolo Lobb, M. (2016). Psychotherapy in post modern society. *Gestalt Today Malta*, *1*(1), 97–113.

Spagnuolo Lobb, M. (2017). Psychotherapy in post modern society. *Gestalt Today Malta*, *1*(2), 45–55.

Vázquez Bandín, C. (2008). *Buscando las palabras para decir* [Looking for the words to say]. Madrid: Asociación cultural Los Libros del CTP.

Vázquez Bandín, C. (2010). *Borradores para la vida* [Drafts for Life]. Madrid: Ed. Asociación cultural Los Libros del CTP.

Vázquez Bandín, C. (2013). Loss and Grief. Sometimes, just one person missing makes the whole world seem depopulated. In G. Francesetti, M. Gecele, & J. Roubal (Eds.). *Gestalt therapy in clinical practice. From psychopathology to the aesthetics of contact* (pp. 295–315). Siracusa, Italy: Istituto di Gestalt HCC Italy Publ. Co., www.gestaltitaly.com.

Vázquez Bandín, C. (2014). *Sin ti no puedo ser yo* [Without you I can't be me]. Madrid: Ed. Asociación cultural Los Libros del CTP.

Vázquez Bandín, C. (2020). Only the living can witness the passing of death: Mourning in times of pandemic. *The Humanistic Psychologist*, *48*(4), 357–362. DOI: 10.1037/hum0000225.

Afterword

Santo Di Nuovo[1]

This volume, edited by Margherita Spagnuolo Lobb and Pietro Andrea Cavaleri, has gathered together theoretical and methodological chapters and applied studies on Gestalt psychotherapy in different clinical fields. It constitutes a concrete example of what has been asserted for a long time in the research on clinical intervention. In this field, the generalisation of the results cannot depend on the outcomes of single separate studies, but rather it develops out of how much a theoretical model can amplify its own radius of intervention, and thus it is strengthened and corroborated the more there are applied possibilities that have been verified as effective in different contexts.

Therefore, it follows as important that the Gestalt psychotherapy method has achieved this notable effort of pointing out their own epistemological and clinical coordinates and then declining them in various contexts, especially where psychic suffering and the need for support emerge today with greater urgency.

The theoretical model presented in the first part of the volume finds application in the second part, in multiple sectors of clinical intervention that characterises the work of the psychotherapist.

Aesthetic relational knowing, reciprocity, anthropological perspective, and phenomenology are theoretical and methodological criteria that have been used for the concrete reading of cases, and the data sheets and clinical procedures presented in this volume have illustrated and facilitated this application.

The fields of application are numerous and cover the entire range of life psychopathologies: childhood suffering, critical family issues, conflictual relations in couples and the consequences for children, complex traumas – among which there is abuse – in pre-adolescence, autism, social withdrawal, addiction, ageing and mental deterioration, chronicity and the experience of loss, and the processing of grief.

The concept of psychopathology has been revisited from a "situational" point of view. From this perspective, it is the "situation", not the single individual, that causes a state of suffering to emerge. Here we are dealing with a perspective vision very dear to Gestalt psychologists, who, already from the Thirties, had broadened the concept of experience to the forces present in the field. It is Kurt Lewin, in fact, who states that one cannot isolate a person from their environment.

DOI: 10.4324/9781003313335-20

The main novelty of this book is that it provides concrete clinical tools for intervening in the "situational" experiential field, which is created in the here-and-now and includes the therapist.

Attention to the neurobiological basis is paid but accompanied by an appropriate use of the phenomenological method, which blunts the risks of reductionism always lying in wait in the behavioural neurosciences.

The editors have intended to celebrate the 70th year of publication of the book *Gestalt Therapy* by rereading the foundations of this method in a relational key, and it seems to me that this goal has been fully realised, with the aid, as well, of the illuminating comments of two elders of Gestalt psychotherapy, such as Erving Polster and Gary Yontef.

The integrations derived from the challenges of the pandemic – which constitutes the natural "ground" of all the work – have increased the social value of this effort of reflection and therapeutic recommendation, aiming not only to reduce malaise but to enhance resiliency, and therefore the well-being of individuals and social groups in all fields in which it is threatened today.

This volume offers a Gestalt therapy view on different situations of suffering; a vision which includes the therapist themself, the tools useful for the modification of the person's experiential field and of the contextual ground from which it emerges. It also proposes integration of a work group, synergistic and interactive, and in its turn, integrated within an international context: two other qualities of the book which I would like to highlight.

And this is only the first volume of a pair, because the editors are promising another one, which will try to reorganise the broad range of psychopathologies in the light of the collective social trauma resulting from the pandemic. We eagerly await it, in the certainty that the Gestalt therapy approach to theory and practice in clinical psychology will have so much that is useful to tell us from this perspective as well.

Note

1   Professor Emeritus of Psychology, University of Catania; President of the Associazione Italiana Psicologia (Italian Association of Psychology)

Biographical Notes

Editors

Margherita Spagnuolo Lobb, PsyD, Gestalt Psychotherapist, director since 1979
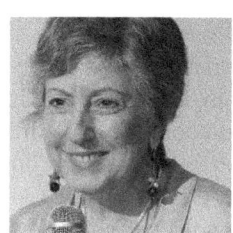
of the Istituto di Gestalt HCC Italy (Siracusa, Palermo, Milano), post-graduate school of psychotherapy accredited by the Minister for the Universities; she leads International Training Programs in Gestalt Development and Psychopathology and for Supervisors. Full Member: NYIGT, SPR, GTA. Past-President: EAGT, FISIG, SIPG, FIAP. She has authored more than 250 scientific publications, has edited 9 books, and has written *The now for next in psychotherapy. Gestalt therapy recounted in post-modern society* (2013), translated into 11 languages. She is editor of the Journal *Quaderni di Gestalt* (since 1985), and of the *Gestalt Therapy Book Series* (Routledge). She has received the Lifelong Achievement Award from the Association for the Advancement of Gestalt Therapy (AAGT) (Toronto, Canada, 2018) and from the Regional Council of Psychologists of Sicily. www.gestaltitaly.com; margherita.spagnuolo@gestalt.it

Pietro Andrea Cavaleri, PhD, PsyD, Gestalt Psychotherapist. Trainer at post
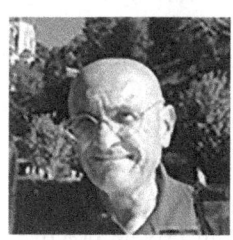
graduate School of Psychotherapy of the Istituto di Gestalt HCC Italy. He has taught at the University of Palermo, at LUMSA University and at the Pontifical Faculty of Educational Sciences "Auxilium". He has been psychologist-in-chief at the Public Health Service of Caltanissetta, and counsellor for social policies of the same city. He has authored *La profondità della superficie (The depth of the surface)* (FrancoAngeli, 2003), *Vivere con l'altro (Living with the other)* (Città Nuova, 2007) and with Molinari, *Il dono nel tempo della crisi (The gift in time of crisis)* (Raffaello Cortina, 2015). He has edited the book *Psicoterapia della Gestalt e Neuroscienze (Gestalt Therapy and Neurosciences)*.

Contributors

Donatella Buscemi, PsyD, Gestalt Psychotherapist. She works at the Casa Rosetta Association as Clinical Director of the Family Counselling Center. She also works with patients affected by degenerative neurological diseases and gambling. She is lecturer at the Pontifical Faculty of Educational Sciences "Auxilium". She has published articles and the book, *L'amore oltre l'eros. I legami affettivi nel quotidiano* (*Love beyond Eros. Affective bonds in everyday life*) (Città Nuova, 2013).

Paola Canna, PsyD, Gestalt Psychotherapist and trainer, Family Mediator at the "Il Metalogo" School of Mediation and Systemic Counselling of Genoa. For twenty years, she has been working in private practice in Padua, with individuals and couples. She currently works as a family mediator in collaboration with lawyers of the Padua court. She has published articles on Gestalt mediation. She has been a member of the Editorial Committee of the Italian Journal of "Ethics for the Professions" for psychological matters.

Elisabetta Conte, Psychologist, Psychotherapist, International trainer and supervisor. She teaches at the Graduate School of Psychotherapy of the Istituto di Gestalt HCC Italy in Milan, and was for many years co-coordinator of the Venice branch of the same Institute. She teaches Gestalt psychotherapy in other countries in Europe, Ukraine and Russia. She is in private practice in Venice with individuals, couples and groups. She has published numerous articles in the field of psychotherapy and is on the editorial board of the journal "Quaderni di Gestalt."

Marialuisa Grech, Psychiatrist, Gestalt Psychotherapist, Medical Director at the U.O. addiction and alcohology service APSS Trento – Simple structure of territorial coordination residency and prevention. Trainer at the Istituto di Gestalt HCC Italy, in Milan. Member of the national executive of the scientific society FederSerd, regional vice president.

Michele Lipani, PsyD, Gestalt Psychotherapist. He has been working as a psychotherapist with children, adolescents, and families for more than thirty years at the Childhood Neuropsychiatry Unit of the Public Health Service of Caltanissetta. He collaborates as a trainer with the Istituto di Gestalt HCC Italy. He has published several articles on psychological distress in developmental age.

Alessandra Merizzi, PsyD, Gestalt Psychotherapist, specialised in Psychogerontology since 2009, currently researcher at the National Institute of Health and Science on Aging (INRCA-IRCCS) and psychotherapist in private practice. Active member of the Manchester Gestalt Centre, Treasurer of GPTI, Board Member of Gestalt Publishing Ltd, member of EAGT Editorial Board (newsletter); member FPOP and SIPG. Leads workshops and lectures on ageing internationally.

Rosanna Militello, PsyD, Gestalt Psychotherapist. Trainer at Istituto di Gestalt HCC Italy. Professional Expert of the Judge and Consultant of the Public Prosecutor's Office – Court of Palermo. Lecturer at the Pontifical University of Education Sciences "Auxilium". International trainer in Russia, Ukraine, Georgia, and Mexico City. She has published articles on abuse, maltreatment, and the management of traumatic relationships, in books and professional journals published by FrancoAngeli.

Maria Mione, PsyD, Gestalt Psychotherapist, she works in private practise, individual and couples therapy, in Venice (Mestre) and Turin. International Gestalt therapy trainer and supervisor, mainly for the Istituto di Gestalt HCC Italy. She is author of various publications in the clinical field. She's a member of the Editorial Board of the Italian Journal *Quaderni di Gestalt*.

Antonio Narzisi is Head Psychologist and Researcher in Developmental Neuroscience at IRCCS Stella Maris in Calambrone (Pisa). His clinical focus is on Autism Spectrum Disorder and Neurodevelopmental Disorders. He is referent for Autistic Spectrum Disorder of the Department of Psychiatry and Childhood Psychopharmachology of IRCCS Stella Maris (Pisa, Italy). He is Adjunct Professor of Psychology at the University of Pisa. He is the author of numerous publications in peer-reviewed journals.

Santo Di Nuovo, graduated in Philosophy and in Psychology, is emeritus professor of Psychology at the University of Catania, and President of the Italian Association of Psychology (AIP) and of the Italian Network of Psychological Associations (INPA). He is co-editor of the international Journal "Life Span and Disability". Since 1974 he has produced over 350 publications, including 35 books. Among the articles, 80 were published in international scientific journals or volumes. His main scientific interest is in methodology of research and in procedures and techniques of assessment. He was engaged in several researches on the evaluation of outcome and process of psychotherapy. In 2017 he obtained the Award of the Italian-American Association of Psychology (IAPS) as Distinguished Italian Psychologist.

Manuela Partinico, PsyD, Gestalt Psychotherapist, Family Mediator. Supervisor at the Istituto di Gestalt HCC Italy, FISIG associate trainer and contract professor at the University of Padua, Faculty of Psychology. She works as a psychotherapist in private practice in Vicenza and Padua with individuals, couples, and as a family mediator. Expert in oncohematology and palliative care, she has collaborated for many years with the Public Health Service. She is the author of numerous publications relating to couple psychotherapy, family mediation, pain management, and palliative care in national and international volumes and journals. manuelapartinico@hotmail.com

Giancarlo Pintus, PsyD, Gestalt Psychotherapist, teaches "Gestalt Psychotherapy in Addictive Experiences" at the Istituto di Gestalt HCC Italy. International trainer in Russia, Ukraine, Serbia and Georgia. He works as a psychotherapist privately, in agreement with the Italian health system and private organisations. He has been a researcher at the Psychiatric Clinic of the University of Pisa, CEFPAS of Caltanissetta, University of Edinburgh, and Assistant professor at the University of Enna "Kore". Author of articles and books on addiction in Gestalt psychotherapy.

Erving Polster received his Ph.D. degree from Western Reserve University in 1950. In 1958, he became first faculty Chairman of the Gestalt Institute of Cleveland and remained in that position until 1973, when he and his wife, Miriam, moved to San Diego. There they formed the Gestalt Training Center-San Diego, where for 25 years they taught gestalt therapy to students from all over the world. He has traveled internationally since 1968, giving lectures and workshops and presenting at conferences. Polster is co-author, with Miriam Polster, of Gestalt Therapy Integrated, published in 1973. He also has written *Every Person's Life Is Worth a Novel* (Norton, 1987), *A Population of Selves: A Therapeutic Exploration of Personal Diversity* (Jossey-Bass, 1995), *From the Radical Center. The Heart of Gestalt Therapy*, authored together with Miriam (GIC Press, 1999), *Uncommon Ground. Harmonizing Psychotherapy and Community to Enhance Everyday Living* (Zeig, Tucker & Theisen, Inc., 2006), *Beyond Therapy. Igniting Life Focus Community Movements* (Transaction Publishers, 2015) and, in the GTBS, *Enchantment and Gestalt Therapy. Partners in a Communal Awakening* (Routledge, 2020). His major interests have long been the transformation of psychotherapy as a curative process into psychotherapy as a communal source of orientation and guidance.

Giuseppe Sampognaro, PsyD, Gestalt Psychotherapist. He works at the Public Health Service in Siracusa, in the Department of Psychiatry and Childhood, and is trainer at the Istituto di Gestalt HCC Italy. Freelance journalist, he is an editor of the international journal *Quaderni di Gestalt*. He has published essays, novels, and short story collections.

Silvia Tosi, Psychologist since 1989 and Gestalt Psychotherapist since 1998, she is an international trainer at the Istituto di Gestalt HCC Italy and an EAGT accredited supervisor. For more than twenty years she has been working as a psychotherapist with children, adolescents, and families, both privately and in collaboration with the public service and schools. She is author of articles on developmental psychotherapy and serves on the editorial boards of the journal *Quaderni di Gestalt* and of the *Gestalt Therapy Book Series* (Routledge).

Carmen Vázquez Bandín, Ph.D., Gestalt Psychotherapist, ECP holder. International Gestalt Therapy trainer and supervisor. Founder and director of the Centro de Terapia y Psicologia – CTP in Madrid, Spain. Full member and past President and honorary member of Spanish Association for Gestalt Therapy (AETG); member of European Association for Gestalt Therapy (EAGT); New York Institute for Gestalt Therapy (NYIGT); European Association for Psychotherapy (EAP); World Council for Psychotherapy (WCP); IGTA; IAAGT. Specialised in the processes of mourning and grief. Co-director of the Gestalt therapy publishing company: Los Libros del CTP. Author of books, chapters and papers on Gestalt therapy. Translator into Spanish of books and papers about Gestalt therapy, including the foundational book: "Gestalt Therapy: Excitement and growth in the human personality".

Alessandra Vela, PsyD, Gestalt Psychotherapist, she is part of the training staff of the Istituto di Gestalt HCC Italy, and is assistant in the "Advanced International Training: A Gestalt therapy field approach to development and psychopathology". She has received a scholarship for the project "Oncological Networks – Oncological Rehabilitation" at the Public Health Service of Agrigento. She works in private practice and in the Clinical and Research Center in Psychotherapy HCC Italy. She is a member of SIPG (Italian Association for Gestalt Therapy), of SIPO (Italian Association for Psycho-Oncology), where she is also chair of the regional department of Sicily, since 2018. She serves on the editorial board of the journal *Quaderni di Gestalt*.

Gary Yontef, Ph.D., A.B.P.P., Fellow of the Academy of Clinical Psychology and Diplomate in Clinical Psychology (A.B.P.P.) has been a gestalt therapist since training with Frederick Perls and James Simkin in 1965. Formerly on the UCLA Psychology Department Faculty and Chairman of the Professional Conduct Committee of the L.A. County Psychological Association, he is in private practice in Los Angeles. He is a past-president of the GTILA and was longtime chairman of the faculty. He has been on the editorial board of the International Gestalt Journal (formerly The Gestalt Journal), associate editor of the Gestalt Review, and editorial advisor of the British Gestalt Journal. He is a co-founder of PGI. He has written over 50 articles and chapters on gestalt therapy theory, practice, and supervision and is the author of Awareness, Dialogue and Process: Essays on Gestalt Therapy.

Appendix

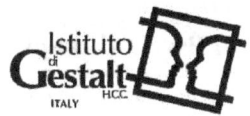

Recognized by the Italian Minister for Universities
(DD.MM. 9/5/1994 - 7/12/2001 - 24/10/2008 - 28/04/2011)

Post-Graduate School of Psychotherapy
Siracuse, Palermo, Milan
Director: Margherita Spagnuolo Lobb
www.gestaltitaly.com

CLINICAL DATA SHEET

Adapted from Spagnuolo Lobb M. (Ed.) (2001) Psicoterapia della Gestalt. Ermeneutica e clinica. [Gestalt Therapy: Hermeneutics and Clinical] Milan: FrancoAngeli, pp. 155–157 (translated by S. Benini and Lynne Rigaud)

Patient _____   **Date**_____

Place of birth _____

Address _____   **Phone nr** _____

Referred by _____

Therapist's first impressions of the patient:

- **Outer appearance**: (2–3 immediate adjectives)

- **Relevant physiological aspects**: current diseases; breathing; posture and character armor (muscular stiffening due to retroflections); grounding, muscle tensions, direct or avoiding eye contact, facial expressions; sleep-wake rhythm; eating habits; flexibility/adaptation abilities of the body processes.

- **Medications:** does the patient take medications? If so, what medication are they currently taking? Have they taken medications in the past?

- **Other specialists?** Have they been treated by other specialists? If so, when?

Recognized by the Italian Minister for Universities
(DD.MM. 9/5/1994 - 7/12/2001 - 24/10/2008 - 28/04/2011)
Post-Graduate School of Psychotherapy
Siracuse, Palermo, Milan
Director: Margherita Spagnuolo Lobb
www.gestaltitaly.com

1. Anamnesis

1.1 Family of Origin

- *Structure* (draw here the family tree)

- *Atmosphere of the family* (description of the relationships inside the family: relaxed/tense; warm/cold; aggressive/avoiding conflict; accepting/dismissive)

- *Relationship between siblings*

- *Relationship between parents* (avoiding conflicts? aggressive and accusatory?)

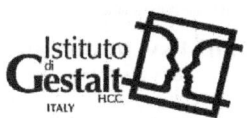

Recognized by the Italian Minister for Universities
(DD.MM. 9/5/1994 - 7/12/2001 - 24/10/2008 - 28/04/2011)

Post-Graduate School of Psychotherapy
Siracuse, Palermo, Milan
Director: Margherita Spagnuolo Lobb
www.gestaltitaly.com

- *Relationship between parent and children* (mention in particular: preferences/impartiality, respect of generational boundaries)

- *Relevant events in the life cycle of the family* (deaths, relocations, abortions, accidents, hospitalisations, separations, various traumas etc.)
  Always note the date in which the patient mentions the event for the first time.

- *Myths, secrets, taboos of the family of origin*

1.2 Current Experience

- *Current family* (if existing, describe its structure, atmosphere, and relevant events)

Recognized by the Italian Minister for Universities
(DD.MM. 9/5/1994 - 7/12/2001 - 24/10/2008 - 28/04/2011)

Post-Graduate School of Psychotherapy
Siracuse, Palermo, Milan
Director: Margherita Spagnuolo Lobb
www.gestaltitaly.com

- ***Social adaptation*** (describe life style, daily organisation, relationships, work or study)

1.3 Symptom (What Kind of Suffering Does the Patient Bring and What Kind of Narrative Do They Offer?)

- ***Diachronic perspective:*** history of the symptom (or suffering): when did it begin, what was going on in the patient's life? How did they attempt to cope with it? Did they feel the attempt was successful? What was their perception of the organism/environment relationship while trying to cope with the suffering? In what critical moment of the personal and transgenerational life cycle did the breakdown take place? What kind of environmental and personal support was lacking? It is important to highlight the close correlation between environmental and personal support.

- ***Synchronic perspective:*** description of the current symptom (or suffering). How does the patient speak about it? Describe the id-functioning and personality-functioning with respect to the description of the symptom: the "here and now of the narrative", the way the self is constituted here and now in the words of the patient.

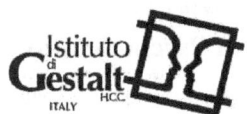

Recognized by the Italian Minister for Universities
(DD.MM. 9/5/1994 - 7/12/2001 - 24/10/2008 - 28/04/2011)

Post-Graduate School of Psychotherapy
Siracuse, Palermo, Milan
Director: Margherita Spagnuolo Lobb
www.gestaltitaly.com

2. Figure and Ground Formation

2.1 Ground (Description of What We Grasp of the Ground of the Patient, of How They Fit into Their World)

- *Id function*: describe how the patient makes contact through their body, how they move in the environment, how they breathe; the ground

- *Personality function*: verbal copy of the self, how does the patient describe themself

- *Polyphonic development of domains*: in the here and now of the session, look at the development of the patient. When do we sense them to be fluid, spontaneous and present at the senses, or when do we sense them to be not fully present and we feel the boundary is desensitised? How does the patient integrate introjecting, projecting, retroflecting, and confluence in the contact with the therapist? Describe what the patient has learned in their life in terms of domains, their "habitual" ways of fitting into the world, what "protecting resistances" they have learned in time; i.e. how have they learned to introject in the past?

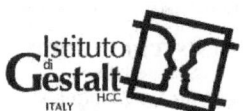

Recognized by the Italian Minister for Universities
(DD.MM. 9/5/1994 - 7/12/2001 - 24/10/2008 - 28/04/2011)

Post-Graduate School of Psychotherapy
Siracuse, Palermo, Milan
Director: Margherita Spagnuolo Lobb
www.gestaltitaly.com

2.2 Formation of the Figure

Ego function (ability of the patient to orient them in the contact and to make choices. Describe the modality of contact with the therapist)

Describe the "dance steps" between patient and therapist: they express the unique co-created relationship

3. Diagnosis

3.1 Descriptive Diagnosis

• *DSM-5 Criteria*

3.2 Gestalt Therapy Diagnosis – Aesthetic Relational Knowing: Empathy and Resonance

Aesthetic criterion: grace (as good form), rhythm (as emotional regulation), fluidity (as movement) + vibrating of the therapist (in which expression of the patient does the therapist feel the vibrant drama?)

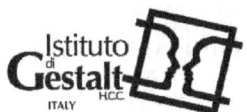
Recognized by the Italian Minister for Universities
(DD.MM. 9/5/1994 - 7/12/2001 - 24/10/2008 - 28/04/2011)
Post-Graduate School of Psychotherapy
Siracuse, Palermo, Milan
Director: Margherita Spagnuolo Lobb
www.gestaltitaly.com

- *Phenomenological and field criterion:* description of the experience of the field and of the movements. How do the therapists describe their own experience of making contact with the patient? How do the patients describe their own experience of making contact with the therapist? What feeling does the therapist get from the field that is created in the session?

- *The anxiety comes mainly from* . . . (what situation triggers the anxiety)?

3.3 Intentionality of Contact to Be Supported in the Therapy (Therapeutic *Now For Next*)

- *In order to calm the anxiety* and allow the spontaneity of the physiological and relational processes to emerge, it is advisable to . . . ?

- *At an individual level*: messages that should be encouraged or avoided

- *At group level*: encourage activities . . . and avoid . . . (social life and/or group therapy).

Recognized by the Italian Minister for Universities
(DD.MM. 9/5/1994 - 7/12/2001 - 24/10/2008 - 28/04/2011)
Post-Graduate School of Psychotherapy
Siracuse, Palermo, Milan
Director: Margherita Spagnuolo Lobb
www.gestaltitaly.com

4. Clinical Diary

Describe the relevant features of each session.

Index

Note: numbers in *italics* indicate a figure

abuse iii, 2, 75, 269; alcohol 193; 231; family 136; institutional 139; substance 173, 165, 178, 260; trauma of 143
abused child 137
abuse within abuse 139
addiction 49, 54; Carla's story of 174–176, 179–181, 183–187; clinical treatment of 183–184; gestalt psychotherapy and 173–174; gestalt psychotherapy, neurosciences, and 174–175; persistent trauma of ground experience and 173–187
addiction therapy 178–183; aim of 181–183; self-definition as challenge for 185
addictive behaviour 178
addictive experience: field of, 177; onset of 175
addictive object 181
addictive substances: chronic use of 183
adolescence: A's testimony 150, 153; autism and 149; complex trauma and 136; COVID-19 and 114; denial of (Laura's case) 123 (box); insecurity of 161; intake and abuse of substances associated with 178; shame and (Lidia's story) 142; social challenges associated with 149
adolesecent experience 161
adolescents: asking for help by 178, 180; boy self-isolating in room (example) 26, 28; Carla as 175; in eclipse 159–170; depressive dimensions of 163; family field and 165–167; family setting and 208; Francesca's story 193, 194;

Gestalt clinical work on, 140; growth phenomenon of 173; *hikokomori* (social withdrawal) among 160; "injured" 136; permanent anxiety among 163; reclusion and retreat of 160–161; reluctance to see a therapist 162; sense of emptiness among 161; social withdrawal among 160, 163–170, 171n3; *see also* social withdrawal
adolescent social closure 2
"adolescent wife" 197
aesthetic attitude: experience of oneself via 8
"aesthetic clues" 196
aesthetic competence 134
aesthetic criteria 85, 92, 169, 171n4
"aesthetic elements" 196, 198
aesthetic emotions 134, 140, 144n1
aesthetic expression 154
aesthetic feeling of therapist 81
aesthetic field coordinates 101, 103
aesthetic gaze 187, 238–249
aesthetic knowing 100
aesthetic model 133, 133
aesthetic relational knowing 2, 75, 183, 186, 196, 199; accessing 196; attunement established via 168; definition of 14, 195; defining 131n3, 134; as elective Gestalt tool 134, 138, 144n1; four cardinal points including 191; Gestalt therapy diagnosis, implemented by means of 82, 92, 109; how to draw on 194–196; reciprocity and 20–38; separated parenting of high conflictuality, mediation using 129; of therapist 216

aesthetics: as tool of therapeutic
    knowledge 11, 113
aesthetic tools 7
affective bonds 200, 208
affective certainties 176
affective co-regulation 200
affective exhanges 127
affective life 31
"affective neurosciences" 72
affective processes 27, 196
affective relationships 88, 191
affective self-regulation 200
affective traumas 73
affective well-being 228
ageing: background of 223–230; becoming
    frail and the inability to ask for help
    230; COVID-19 and 222, 228; dancing
    with the frail and the wise 231–235;
    gains and strengths of 228–230; Gestalt
    therapy and 222–235; Norma's story
    231–234
ageing stereotypes 224–226, 226, 227,
    228, 232, 234
ageism 232, 226
Ammaniti, M. 100, 203
analogic apperception 75
anamnesis 22, 81, 82–83, 87–88, 103,
    104, 234; worksheet 277 (Appendix)
anhedonia 9
anxiety 14, 27; addiction and 174–175,
    183, 185; adolescent 161, 163, 164,
    168; ageing and 224, 229, 231–233;
    angst and 178; A's testimony regarding
    feelings of 151–152; child 180;
    co-created ground and 194; COVID-19
    and 99, 100, 224; Francesca (example)
    194; generated by intense closeness
    24; managing 170; Matteo (example)
    159; me-with-you experience without
    109; M's story 244; Nino (example)
    107, 109–110; permanent 163;
    phenomenological and field criterion for
    93; polyphonic generation of domains
    and 27, 84, 107; pyschopathology and
    25; seeking help with 229, 231; social
    149; social withdrawal as response
    to 162, 167; Sofia (example) 169;
    therapeutic now-for-next and 93, 110;
    ways of expressing 166; within contact
    between therapist and client 33, 85
anxiety disorders 9, 23, 120; A's diagnosis
    with 150, 153; severe 36

apathy 100, 258
Arendt, Hanna 20
ASD see Autism Spectrum Disorder
Asperger, H. 147
Asperger's syndrome 147
assistances 26
attachment 1; addiction and 183;
    earned-secure 203n10; dysfunctional
    pathways of 186; psychophysiological
    studies of 27; secure 100, 176
attachment and "recognizing oneself"
    203n10
attachment theory 27, 31
attunement 33, 35, 170; aesthetic relational
    knowledge and 168; emotional 216;
    resonance and 85, 92, 101, 109,
    134, 137
aut-aut 51, 54, 74
Autism Spectrum Disorder (ASD)
    147–148; A's story 150–154;
    camouflage effect in 148–149;
    camouflage effect to élan vital 150–153;
    Gestalt therapy and 147–155

Bauman, Zygmunt 49
Beebe, B. 76, 199
being-with: of client 32; of client and
    therapist 32, 36, 37, 84; composite way
    of 213; the environment 21; suffering of
    101; through the body 28, 102
Benjamin, J. 76, 199
bereavement: change, processed and feared
    as 173; chronic 260; complicated or
    pathological 260–262; "continuing"
    261; delayed 260; disguised 260;
    exaggerated 260; family life cycle
    including 208; normal 266n10;
    pandemic (COVID-19)-related
    263–265; pathological 256, 260–262;
    professing of 252–265; psychological
    266n1; seeking therapy for 231, 235;
    "suspended" 263–264
bodily certainties (id-function) 186
bodily conditions of safety 27
bodily containment 120
bodily desensitization 89, 100, 119
bodily energy 124
bodily enthusiasm 26
bodily experience(d) 153, 168, 171n2,
    225, 227; clinical goals related to 249;
    id as way the body experiences its
    situation 13

bodily expressions xvi
bodily felt manner 14
bodily ground 89, 239; lack of (therapist notes on) 106; of sick body 244; sudden collapse of 245
bodily memories 28
bodily processes 10, 26–27; blocked 31; therapist notes on 86, 103
bodily reactions 186
bodily schemas 28, 171n6
bodily sensations 8
bodily sense of self 22
bodily structure 82
bodily tension, reduction of 248
body: aesthetic knowing of and by 100; of Aylan Kurdi 46; being-with through 28, 102; empathetic vibrations of 195; feeling the experience of the other in one's own body 68; "forgetting to be a body" 55; ground (psychotherapeutic) in relationship to 21, 51, 83; id and id-functioning as a way the body experiences its situation 13, 90; integration of body, emotions, words, experiential field enabling 143–144; kinesthetic resonance and 108–109; mind/body dualism and unity 72–73, 74; as object 52; as psychological object xvi; reality of 201; "reasons of the body" 30; Sartre on xvi; supporting intergration of emotion, words, and 133–144; theories of attachment/regulation in relationship to 27; trauma and 73
body awareness, developing 94
body language 152
borderline client 34
borderline functioning 2
borderline perception 107
borderline society 207
Brentano, F. 70
Bromberg, P. 74

camouflage effect: ASD and 148–149
camouflage effect to élan vital: ASD and 150–153
cancer, encounter with 240–243, 244, 245, 249; see also oncology
caregiver/child 32, 33
Cavaleri, Pietro Andrea: anthropological model of Gestalt therapy of 46–63; Yontef's response to anthropological model of 67–69; see also together-with

childhood: A's recollections of 150, 153; diagnoses received during 148; education 99; difficult iii, 2, 35; personality development and trauma in 137; stereotypes and 224; trauma linked to 75; world of 100
childhood malaise, case of 103, 114
childhood development 100
childhood myth: narcissism and 162–164
childhood pathology 101
childhood suffering 3, 90, 106, 269; psychotherapy and 99–115; treating by supporting ground of parental experience 122–130
children: aggressiveness betwee siblings 105; autistic 32; caregiver/child relationship 32, 33; condition of children in today's world 99–101; as "digital natives" 114; experiences of 2; fragmentation and uncertainty in 120; Gestalt approach to 100; Gestalt mediation between parents and 121; non-grounded sense of agency in 11; parent/children relationship 105; play in therapy with 113; psychotherapy for 112; relational disorders of 100; relationship between parents and 88; spontaneity of 56; struggle to focus in 9; suffering of being-with in 101; violence against women and 119; see also adolescents; creative adaptation
children of broken relationships 119–131; Gestalt mediation to treat 130–131; separation experience of 122–127; treating children's suffering by supporting ground of parental experience 122–130
Children's Apperception Test 111
circular dynamics 200, 203n19
clinical data sheet 3; anamnesis 82–83, 87–88; clinical diary 94; clinical example 85–94; clinical log 85; diagnosis 85, 92–94; diagnostic and clinical areas 82–84; figure/ground formation 83–84, 90–92; Gestalt psychotherapy and experience and 81–95; significant physiological aspects 82
closed-door therapy 136
co-agent 59
co-completion 154
co-constructed presence: with patient and therapist 38

co-construction of solid ground 240
co-constructors 59
co-created contact process, unfolding of
    167
co-created experiences: of a "between"
    in the present 263; between adolescent
    and therapist 168; between child and
    caregiver 102; between child and
    therapist 112; between client and
    therapist 23, 30–31, 73, 263; contact
    and help 11; at/of contact boundary
    134, 209, 235; of contact experience 85,
    100; of depressive field/situation 227,
    232; of experience of reciprocity 233;
    the field and 29–31, 110, 191, 220n1;
    field of therapeutic relationship 14; of
    figure and ground 25, 82; of geniune
    recognition 182; of "patient time" 138;
    process of 100; of "relational dance
    between patient and therapist" 222;
    of relational phenomena 85, 225; safe
    ground 10; of self and boundaries of self
    24; sense of security 7; of spontaneous
    therapeutic action 246; of stories 113;
    of therapeutic relationship 81; of third
    shared field 71
co-created field 195, 196; affective
    processes in 196; co-regulation of
    reciprocal recognition and 75–76;
    experience of contact in 201; family
    in therapy 216, 225; Perls and
    Goodman on 201; regulatory quality
    of 198; sharing experience of 202;
    sphere of recognition of 198;"third
    dimension" of 198; of transference and
    countertransference dynamics 230
co-created ground, experience of 194
co-created narrative 234
co-created relational field 177;
    phenomenological observation of 128
co-created space 210
co-created space-time 134
cognition: the body and experience of self
    and 223–224
collective trauma 58
co-management of daily life 119
co-mediators, with children 122
    (Case no. 1, box)
co-morbid illness 224
complex trauma: defintion of 136;
    neurobiology of 140; in preadolescence
    133–144; shame in 142–143

complicated bereavement 260; see also
    bereavement
co-parent 128, 129
co-regulation in the couple 200; co-created
    field and reciprocal recognition
    75–76; mutual recognition and 199; of
    therapeutic relationship 36
couple conflict 3, 122, 190; aesthetic
    relational knowledge in 194–196;
    impact of COVID-19 pandemic on 191;
    Francesca and Giuseppe as example
    of 190–202; four cardinal "Gestalt"
    points for orientation in couple's field
    191; Gestalt intervention and 191–202;
    mutual recognition and co-regulation
    in 200–202; "natural"-ness of 199;
    normalcy of 122; separated parenting
    and 128–130; space for recognition in
    190–202; struggle for recognition and
    196–200; see also crisis; jealousy
COVID-19: ageing during the era of 222;
    as amplifier of vulnerabilities 119;
    couple's tensions intensified by 217;
    global scientific and political failure in
    response to 58; as health, social, and
    psychological emergency 243; impact
    of 7; parents' relationship with children
    changed by 99; psycho-oncological
    context of 243, 247; as symptom
    of collective planetary diseases 59;
    viral messaging during 225; WHO's
    declaration of decade of Healthy Ageing
    288; see also crisis
creative accomodations with the other 7
creative adaptation 90, 101; addiction as
    form of 177; children and 100, 101, 134,
    208; experimenting with 112; flexibility
    of Gestalt approach in terms of 155; M.
    (example of) 241; Perls and Goodman
    on 57, 62, 63n13; relational strategy and
    134; social networks as 254; spontaneity
    of 100; symptom as 83, 101
creative adaptation of the self: post-
    traumatic reaction as 136–139
creative adjustment in a difficult situation,
    psychotherapy as 24, 26
creative adjustments 27, 31, 170, 200; with
    the other 38; self and 201, 244
creative differentness 34
creative disinterest 61
creative energy 56
creative Gestalt 28, 102

creative indifference 232
creative sense of the possible 67, 69
creative solutions 68
creative vitality 186
crisis: couple 181, 190, 191, 192; economic 197; emotional 209; family 217; generational 9; Coronavirus/health 15, 61, 219, 247; modern era of preacrity as 49; refugee 26; world crisis and Gestalt therapy 67–69
crisis centres 231
crisis of personality-function of the Self 226–228

Damasio, A. 72
dance: beginning the dance (in aged populations) 232–234; between figures and grounds 253; between therapist and patient 7, 84, 85, 134, 222; co-created 235; the field and the dance 23–24; flow with caregivers, 101; as hermeneutic figure of therapeutic change 3; with parents 180; spontaneous 23; with significant figures 137; therapeutic 233, 234
dance of reciprocity 14, 20, 25; co-creation of 81; model 32–36, 76
"dance of the swords" 186–187
"dance of the words" at contact boundary 185–187
"dance steps" model 2, 33, 82, 84, 166; co-creative of contact between child and caregiver 102; between therapist and patient 91–92, 108–109
dancing with the frail and the wise 230–234
death: accepting 257; ageing and 235; from COVID-19 263; cult of 252; fear of 10–11, 63, 100, 239, 249; loss and 266; mass spectacle of 254; suffering and 265; terminal illness and 242, 243; tragic 193; of unborn child 258–263; see also bereavement
depression 9, 149, 231; diagnosis of 262; due to delayed grief 261; inexplicable 260
depressive decline 159
depressive disorder 161; major 260–261
depressive field, co-creation of 232
depressive mood 34
depressive suffering 261
Derrida, Jacques 265

Descartes' error 72
Descartes, René 72
desensitised society: lack of ground in 8–10
desensitisation 9,11, 14; bodily 89, 119, 124, 245; corporeal and emotional 120; of couples 199, 200; of feelings and emotions 168; perceptive and emotional 99; repetitiveness as sign of 35; individualism and 49; of parents to their children 106, 114; as response to global complexity 47–49; of self 55, 62; sensory apathy and 100; substance abuse/addiction and 174, 175; to suffering 46; suffering of being-with and 101
developmental ability, latent 58
developmental approaches 148
developmental blocks 31
developmental breakdowns 149
developmental challenges, age-related 160
developmental complexity 28
developmental paths 165
developmental phase 110
developmental processes: fragile grounds and 164–165; greater attunement to 170; recovery of 167
developmental task of self-definition 178
developmental themes of autonomy and dependence 178
developmental theories 154
developmental trajectory 148
diachronic perspective 83, 88, 102, 106, 279
dia-gnosis, etymology of 15n1
dialogical competence 22
dissociation: adaptive strategy of 73, 75, 136; in couple conflict 200, 203n6; habitual narcissistic 7; as relational disorder in children 100; as result of failure of recognition 76; structural 74; trauma and polarity conflict and 73–74, 75
distress 119, 121, 124; addicts in 185; in children 111, 121, 208; clinical data sheet to document 81; couples in 119; Edoardo (example) 124 (box); families in 219; parental 99; psychological 148, 230, 231, 243, 260; trauma and 241; see also stress
distressing experience 137
drafting of the agreements 129–130

Duess Fables 111–112
dummy complex 174

ego-function/ing: adolescent 169; ageing
   stereotypes and process of self in
   224–227, 228, 229; A.'s account of 153;
   Carla 186; clinical data sheet 84, 91;
   disease and inability to adjust creatively
   244, 248; formation of figure and 91;
   losses of 84, 171n8; of self 194, 225
élan vital: ASD and 150–153
embodied empathy 30, 195
embodied experience 134
embodied mind 71
embodied pain 127
embodied self 245
embodied sense of security 9
embodied simulation 195
embodied stereotypes 224, 225
embodied suffering 100
embodied understanding 31
embodied words 134
emotional regulation 85, 92, 130, 281; in
   older age 229
emotional-regulatory process 229
emotional tolerance 139
emotivity, regulation of 168
environment: ability to count or rely on
   7, 38; ability to interact with 31; act
   of contacting 25; being-with 21; body
   in relationship to 72; centering of 15,
   59; "disinterestedness" in 61; family
   225; fear of contact with 9; organism
   and 13, 23, 29, 33, 51, 71; organism/
   environment contact 54; organism/
   environment field 3, 29, 30, 70;
   pandemic and 7, 9, 15; self and 23; self
   as function of organism/environment
   field 11, 28; work 48
epigenetics 32
Es-function 153
et-et 51, 54, 74; see also aut-aut
ethical crisis 15
ethical position: between individual and
   society 2
ethical position of the psychotherapist:
   post-pandemic period and 7–8
ethical values 8
euthanasia 252
experience of loss: accepting and
   supporting 238–249
experiential boundaries 8

experiential change 24
experiential condition of desensitization 9
experiential fields: between client and
   therapist 23; problematic 2
experiential fields of suffering 1
experiential ground, clinical concept of
   2, 16n3
evolution see human evolution
evolutionary perspective of relational
   psychoanalysis 12, 45, 82
evolutionary stalemate and vitality of
   human nature 55–58
evolution of civilization 47
evolution of sense of self 22
evolution of therapeutic journey
   (Lidia) 136
evolution of therapeutic process 85

familial failure 254
familial field 122, 128; see also family
   field
familial relationships 131
familial scenarios 121
familial security, ground of 130
familial subjection 209
family: clinical treatment of 207; current
   83; geolocation of 230; Gestalt family
   intervention, goal of 210–219; Gestalt
   therapy and 3, 207–220; as "prison"
   208; therapeutic session with 22;
   traditional 203n2; trying to understand
   68; unhappy 207
family dynamics 226
family field 82–83; phenomenological
   122; relational co-creation in 225;
   reorganization of 130; suffering of
   165–167
family gestalt 124 (box), 208
family history 83
family/individual plane 164
family law 119
family life cycle 88, 105, 130, 167, 208,
   209, 278
family messaging 258
family network, extended 136
family of origin 37, 82–83, 87–88,
   104–106; genogram 87; M.'s story 242
family/personal ground 164
family relationships: rupture of 120;
   violence in 190
family roles, destructuration of 244
family scenes 138

family security, sense of 112
family sessions 110, 113
family story 160
family ties 9
family therapy 2, 111, 166
female autism phenotype 149
female figure 129
female friend, sudden death of 192
female(s) 21; rise of social withdrawal
    among 171n1
field instrument *see* clinical data sheet
field: Aesthetic Relational Knowledge
    of 195; ageing in the field of COVID-
    19 pandemic 222; co-created
    experience and 29–31, 110, 191,
    220n1; concept of, in Gestalt therapy
    45n3; "dance" and the field 23–24;
    emergent clinical 7–15; experiential
    23, 59, 121, 143–144, 178, 216;
    experiential fields of suffering 1;
    Gestalt Institute HCC and studies in
    psychopathology and development in
    14; Gestalt field approach 121; logic
    of 127; of neurophenomenology xvii;
    Parlett's concept of 71; perceptual 51;
    phenomenological 71, 84, 133, 134, 140,
    177, 216; phenomenological approch
    to 195; relational 12; relational turning
    point in psychotherapy and 12–14;
    Robine's understanding of 71; shared
    phenomenological 24, 195; *situation* (as
    term) as opposed to *field* (as term) 13;
    situational 129; Spagnuolo Lobb on 71;
    therapeutic xvi, 36; therapist's feeling
    as part of 14; *see also* co-created field;
    depressive field; familial field; family
    field; organism/environment field;
    phenomenological field
field concept 2
field experience 24
field of action 53
field of encounters 2
field of experience 31
field of orientation 54
field perspective 25, 128
field theory 67, 68–69; Lewin 70
figure: addictive object as 181; body as
    245; co-creation of 25; in couple's
    conflict 192, 194, 195, 196; "dance"
    as hermeneutic figure of change 3;
    emergence of new 129, 130; formation
    of 84, 91, 108, 127; parental 180;

symptom as 182; therapist's perception
    of 30, 135
figure/background process 201
figure/ground dynamic 13, 82, 185, 210,
    212
figure/ground formation 13, 90, 83–84, 90,
    107–108
figure/ground relationship 1, 13, 30, 32,
    82, 102, 135; pandemic and 59
foreground 8
Frankfurt School 76
Frank, Ruella 27, 100, 115, 245
Fromm, E. xv

gains and strengths of ageing 228–230
Gallese, V. 72
Gestalt anthropology 51; global unrest and
    46–63; pandemic and 58–63
Gestalt field approach 121
Gestalt mediation 121, 122, 128–130
Gestalt mediatory process 121, 130
Gestalt model of parenting 131n4
Gestalt therapy *see* Perls, Fritz; Perls and
    Goodman model
Goodman *see* Perls-Goodman model
grief: delayed 261; as failure 254; normal
    260; as one of three basic processes
    of human existence 252; over loss of
    identity 245, 246; pathological 253,
    256; processing of 263, 269; suffering
    connected to 265; over suicide 256;
    symptoms of 260; over unborn child
    256, 258; working through 264
grief complications, possible **261**
ground: body and 51; building of 139;
    building together the sense of 33;
    defining 21; experiential 2, 16n3,
    83, 137, 140, 165; figure/ground
    dynamic 82; figure/ground formation
    90, 83–84, 107–108; figure/ground
    relationship 13, 30, 32, 59, 82, 102, 135;
    importance of 102; loss of 101–102;
    neuropsychological 154; pandemic's
    impact on 38; relational 83, 101, 113,
    138, 142; repairing the ground of
    parental experience 119–131; social
    10–11; solid 14; Wheeler on the
    importance of 13; why psychotherapy
    concerns itself with 21–23; working on
    the ground 10; working on the ground
    and on the dance 20–38
ground building 91, 92

ground experience 9; addiction and persistent trauma of 173–187; climate change and 11; clinical data sheet's documentation of 81; healing 15; id-functioning of 84; organization of domains in 28; social ground as 10–11; specific interpersonal support addressed to 31; therapeutic intervention on the 14; vitality of 25–26
ground of the parental experience, reparing 119–131

Hegelian thought 70
Heidegger, M. xv, xvi, 14
here-and-now: being-present in 131; being-there with child patient 134; of being-with the environment 21; of couple relationship 121; experienced by patient 28, 102; family in therapy 216; of mediation session 128; polyphonic development of domains and 84, 90; reality of 22; self and 83, 89, 154; of therapeutic contact 7, 10, 11, 14, 25, 85; "there-and then" and 142; vitality of contact and 139–142
Hiller, R. 149
Honneth, A. 75, 76
Horney, K. xv
human excitement 56, 57
human evolution 50–63; evolutionary stalemate 55–58; neurotic turn in 62; pitfalls of 51–53; regression in 53–55
humanistic ethic 37–38
humanistic tradition 7
humanization: of relationships 198; of work 58
human potentiality 61–63
human rights 47
Husserl, E. 7, 70, 75

identity: adolescent 178; devaluation of 126; of "drug addict" 176; loss of 245, 246; parental 129; personal 121; professional 197; renewal of 228; self-definition of 185; validation of 254
identity certainties 143
identity changes and crisis of personality 226–228
identity definition 150
identity development 149
id-function/ing: being-with through the body as 28, 102; as bodily certainty

186; bodily feeling and 168; body, cognition, and experience of self as 223–224; chronic depression as form of 169; clinical data sheet 84, 89, 90; ego-function of self in aging and 224; emotional regulation and 229
imagination 48; collective 59
imagination techniques 246
implict intentionality of contact 144n1
Implicit Relational Knowledge 30, 127
impotence: Lidia's story expressing sense of 143; self and 245; sense of 11, 33, 257; state of 245; of therapist 186
indifference 46; creative 232; cynical 47, 48; elite 49; perceptual 48; sensory apathy and 100
insecurity: adolescent 161; adult 176; fear and 126; pandemic and feelings of 38; states of 203n15; work 99
integration 22–23, 54–57, 62; between belonging and difference 202; complicated 50; of disease 249; effected by the self 201, 245; partial 51; process of 54; Strength and Vulnerability Integration Model 229
integration of body, emotions, words: experiential field enabling 143–144; preadolescence and 133–144
intentionality(ies) of contact 2, 22, 83; blocking 100; child suffering explained through 125; development of 26, 71; family 209–210, 213, 216; family members unable to acknowledge 106; formation of the figure and 84; frozen 134; fulfilling 28; grasping 213; implicit 144n1; loss of ground and 101–102; non-explicit 134, 138; now-for-next of the separated parenting and 129, 130; observation of 209; parental 3; recognizing and acknowledging 33, 38; restoring quality of 168; to be supported in therapy (therapeutic now-for-next) 85, 93, 110–111; unfinished 175
intentionality: of "adolescent wife" 197; being aware of 202; of "being-with" 32; blocked 166; communicative 153; couple's ability to differentiate 199; developing 202; disrupting 210; of "failed husband" 197; of the field 177; giving form to 201; implied 34; interrupted 186; lack of recognition of 25; now-for-next 183; phenomenology

of 74; of rasing a child 180; recognition of 26; separate 198; shared 24; supporting 31, 82, 112
intersubjective psychoanalysis 12, 76
intersubjective space 182
intersubjective viewpoint 127
intersubjectivity 32

Jacobs, Lynne 30
jealousy 190–192, 194, 196

Kanner, L. 147
Kant, I. 70; concept of synthetic unity 201
Kempler xv
Kurdi, Aylan 46

La Barre, F. 100
learning-narrative 201
Lewin, Kurt 70, 269
Lichtenberg, P. 47
Life Focus Groups 44
liquidity 207
liquid society 13, 61–62, 119, 252–253
losses: chronic pathology of continuous losses 242; grief relative to 256, 260, 269; suffering related to 234; see also bereavement; grief
losses of ego-functions 27, 94, 171n8
love: body and 245; death and 265; "falling in love" 220; Implicit Relational Knowledge and 30; pathological dependency on object of 182
loved ones 231; accepting death of 255, 257, 260, 261; loss of 228; support of 243
love of life 238, 248
love of others 265
lovers 56
"love story" with drugs 176, 178, 181, 187
"love strokes" 215

MacLean's triune brain theory 72
Maggio, Fabiola and Tosi, Silvia 100
malaise: child 101; childhood 103, 114, 120, 127, 140, 142, 153; family 207; M.'s experience with 239; psychic 12; psychological 241; psychopathological 241; reducing 270; social phobia as 3
males 21; autism spectrum disorder in 149; social withdrawal among 171n1
malevolent relationships 141, 142
MCI see mild cognitive impairment

Merleau-Ponty, M. 7, 70
mild cognitive impairment (MCI) 231
mourning: avoidance of 255; crying and 264; experience of 265; function of 259; sadness and 263; over suicide by a son 256; trauma of loss and 2; for an unlived life 256, 258–260; see also bereavement; grief
mutual synchronization 31

narcissism 170
narcissistic myth of childhood 162–164
narcissistic culture 38, 60
narcissistic disorder, diagnosis of 92
narcissistic experience 24
narcissistic society 9, 12, 164, 209
narcissistic solitude 7–8
narcissistic splits 32
neurobiology of addiction see neuroscience
neurobiology of complex trauma 140
neurobiology of relational sense of safety 26–27
neurobiology of relational trauma 71
neuroception 26, 45n4, 195, 203n15; defensive 243; before perception 74–75; phenomenology of 74; Porges on 26, 45n4, 74, 195, 243, 249n2
neurodevelopmental disorders 2
neurophenomenology xv, xvii; phenomenology and 70–72
neuroscience and Gestalt psychotherapy: addiction and 173–187
neurosciences 32; affective 72; behavioural 270; psychotherapy and 72; role of bodily exchanges between child and caregiver confirmed by 100
neurosis 2, 52, 74; anthropology of 50
neurotic adaptations 57
neurotic control over reality 61
neurotic perception 107–108
neurotics 52, 55
neurotic scission 54
neurotic split 62
neurotic turn 56, 62
neurotic turning point 54
normal 22: abnormal 178; "almost normal" adolescence 142
normal bereavement 266; see also bereavement
normalcy 8; of conflict 122
normal grief 260; see also grief

normality 55, 59, 178; experience of 60; illusion of 60
now-for-next: concept of 14; intentionality of contact to be supported in therapy (therapeutic now-for-next) 85, 93, 110–111; intuiting 183; limiting the quality of 232
now-for-next of separated parenting 129–130
now moments 138

oncological disease 241, 243, 245; journey into 248; psycho-oncological context 247
oncologist 239
Oncology 240; somatic experience in 244–245
Orange, Donna 11
organism and environment 13, 23, 29, 33, 51, 71
organism/environment contact 54
organism/environment field 3, 29, 30, 70; Gestalt intervention and the complexity of 191–202; self as function of 11, 2

pandemic: challenges of 15; collective trauma generated by 2, 9, 20; emergency and vulnerability intensified by 60; environment and 7, 9, 15; feelings of insecurity increased by 38; figure-ground dynamic in analysis of 59; human potentiality/reactions to 61–62, 63; onset of 1; see also COVID-19; crisis; post-pandemic
perception, feeling, intentionality, action, and narrative 202
perceptual deficit 48
perceptual field 51, 244
Perls, Frederick 70
Perls, Fritz: on activation of contact boundary 29; addiction and the "dummy complex" 174; anthropological theory of 51; contact modalities defined by 84; early principles and founding ideas of xv, xvii, 62; Freud contrasted to 51; Gestalt Therapy 1, 12, 21, 44, 50, 62, 201, 235, 265; "lose your mind and come to your senses" 23; on the patient making and finding themselves 185; Polster on 43–44; vitality concept and 24, 26; on vulnerability and suffering 61

Perls-Goodman model 23, 51, 74; pitfalls of 51–53; regressive responses and the neurotic turn 54, 55, 57
Perls, Laura 70
personality function/ing 9; ageing and 225, 227–229; chronic depression and 169; clinical data sheet 84, 89, 90; Es-function and (A.'s story) 153; Gestalt understanding of 121; renewal of (Luisa) 129; social/relational definition of the self as 186; see also Spontaneous Parental Personality Function (SPPF)
perturbing events 200, 203n15
phenomenological and field criterion 93, 109, 282
phenomenological analysis 201
phenomenological approach: GT as 234; treating children 100
phenomenological-experiential field 123
phenomenological field 24, 71, 73, 177; concept of 239; contextualizing the therapist's aesthetic emotions in 134, 140; definition of 131n2; family 122, 165, 216; insertion of patient into 84, 101; intiating therapeutic process from within 133; process of 165; shared 195
phenomenological field co-created in the therapeutic encounter 195
phenomenological field perspective 1
phenomenological/gestalt approach 155
phenomenological making of the body 168
phenomenological method 68, 270
phenomenological observation of the field 130
phenomenological observation of the co-created relational field 128
phenomenological perspective 70, 72, 73; moving away from subjectivitist reductionism and towards 154
phenomenological perspective of organism-environment field 155
phenomenological sensitivity 70
phenomenology 11, 67, 68, 269; diagnosis and (adolescent case studies) 160–161; Gestalt Theory (GT) and 70–77; neurophenomenology and 70–72; reality and 21; "under the radar" 72, 74
phenomenology of human relations 72
phenomenology of intentionality 74
phenomenology of neuroception 74, 75
phenomenology of perception 70, 74
phenomenology of relational field 12

"phenomenology of the contact boundary" 70
"phenomenology of the organism/environment field" 70
phobia 3, 261
play, staying in 30
Polster, Erving xv, 3, 270
polygenetic factors in autism 147
polyphonic development of domains 14, 27–28, *29*, 82, 84, 90–91, 101, 107; clinical data sheet (Appendix), 280; Spanguolo Lobb on 102
polyphony of competencies 213
polyvagal theory 26, 101, 243, 247
Porges, S. 10, 20; on neuroception and social engagement 195; polyvagal theory of 26, 101, 243; on 'under-the-radar" phenomenology 74
post-pandemic humanist ethics: paradigm of reciprocity in the training of psychotherapists for 37–38
post-pandemic world 26; conflict in couple relationships and opportunities still possible in 190–202; pyschopathological situations in 7–15; young people in 114
"post-traumatic elaboration" to Gestalt model 58
post-traumatic reaction 136–139
"post-traumatic processing" 15
post-traumatic stress disorder (PTSD) 252, 260
potentiality: concept of 56; faith in 57; human 61–62; new 63
preadolescence: gestalt therapy and complex trauma in 133–144
precocious interactive regulation 31
preconceptions 68
presuppositions xvi, 45n6, 216
private sphere 164, 173
process of self *see* self
prophecy, self-fulfilling 225, *226*, *227*, 232
psyche and symbol 63n11
psychobiological vulnerability 175
psycho-oncology 240, 247
psychopathological adaptation 57
psychopathological conditions xvi
psychopathological deficits 147
psychopathological malaise 241
psychopathological situations 1, 2, 24–25; in post-pandemic world, gestalt therapy in emergent clinical fields and 7–15

psychopathological risk 153
psychopathological symptoms 12
psychopathological ways of being 167
psychopathologizing 254
psychopathology 32; of ageing 235; child 140; concept of 268; as *creative adjustment in a difficult situation* 24; Gestalt Institute HCC Italy's research in 12, 14; historical background on emergence of 70; impact of pandemic on 270; as pathology of between-ness 115n5; *situations* in 1, 2; suffering of being-with 101–102; traditional 25
psychotic perception 107

Rank, Otto 61
reciprocity 2, 269; aesthetic relational knowing and 20–38; co-created experience of 233; "dance of the words" and 185–187; dominance of, in relation to the other 75; intra- and inter-dialogical 153; paradigm of 31–36; relational 177; *see also* dance of reciprocity
reciprocity between parents and children 121
reciprocity of presence 8
reciprocity of therapeutic contact 82
recognition: bond of 102; central importance of 198; conflict as space for 63n14; couples counseling as space for 190–202; in emotional bonds 63n15; exchange of 76; failure of 140, 174; genuine 178–180, 182; gift of 63n15, 75, 198; lack of 25; of movement-towards 34; mutual 47, 58, 129, 197, 198, 199, 200, 202; need for 175; of needs of others 15; policy of 63n15; promoting 177; reciprocal 75–76; search for 163; sphere of 198; therapy as experience of 184–185; three different modalities that trigger pathways to 75
recognition-breakdown-restoration 76
regression: as reaction to complexity 53–55
relational absence 123
relational co-creation: of family field 225; of sense of security 7
relational code of family life 210
relational compass 2
relational competencies 181
relational conflict 199

relational containment 120, 124
relational deficiencies, early 175
relational detuning of the adult 176
relational dysregulation 76
relational experience 209; basic 101
relational field 12, 126 (box); children
    as part of 225; co-constructed 177;
    co-created 128; difficult 101; embodied
    self as support in 245
relational fragility 61
relational ground 83, 92, 113; building
    138; importance of 101; solidifying of
    142; trust and 168
relational intervention 81
relationality xv, xvi; Heidegger on 14
relational keys of Gestalt therapy 1, 81
relational knowing see aesthetic relational
    knowing; implicit relational knowledge
relational mind 32, 37, 71
relational "music" 84
relational movements 33; Frank's work
    on 27
relational pathologies 220
relational phenomenon 85; disassociation
    as 74
relational product, perception as 71
relational reality 196
relational recognition see recognition
relational rootedness 3, 10, 93, 114;
    strong 182
relational schemas 28
relational school of psychoanalysis xv,
    12–14
relational security 9, 21, 174
relational sense of safety 26–27
relational suffering 31, 114; Gestalt vision
    of 165
relational surrogate 174
relational theory and practice 67, 69
relational trauma 71, 73; child therapists
    dealing with 149; early 137
relational turning-point in Gestalt
    psychotherapy 12–13, 23–24
relational way of knowing 82, 85
relational well-being 58
repair 58 76, 165, 199, 202
resonance: aesthetic 256; aesthetic
    relational knowing and 85, 92, 109;
    defined as contribution of therapist
    to situation 30; emotional 195, 216;
    empathy and 281 (appendix); having
    fun and experiencing 35; kinesthetic

108; mutual attunement and 92, 101,
    137; reciprocal 81; sensoriality and
    134; spontaneous 22; therapeutic 222;
    of therapist with situation shared with
    patient 24, 33, 168, 196, 233
resonance versus impasse (Norma's case)
    231–232
revitalising the contact boundary 24
revitalising the ground 182
revitalising the self 191, 200, 201, 202;
    addiction therapy and 178–180
Ricoeur, P. 75
Rizzolatti, G. and Sinigaglia, C. 72
rooted: mind rooted in the body 72; need
    to feel 10–11; possibility of feeling 20
rootedness: bodily 86, 244; in children
    130; in "here and now" 264; relational
    3, 10, 93, 114, 123, 182, 195;
    self-rootedness 14

safety: addiction therapy and perceiving
    the security and safety of the ground
    178–180; bodily conditions of 27;
    deficits in feeling of 101; neurobiology
    of relational sense of 26–27; Porges on
    20; sensation of 20; sense of 233, 234;
    visceral feeling of 243
Sartre, J.-P. xv, xvii
security: addiction therapy and perceiving
    the security and safety of the ground
    178–180; change and loss of 119;
    co-creation of sense of 7, 14; collapse of
    217; embodied sense of 9; emergence of
    sense of 240; ground of familial security
    130, 137; illusory sense of 58; internal
    senses of fullness and 245; lack of sense
    of 26–27; loss of ground security 124,
    242, 244; nascent 138; neuroception
    of 75; "normality," restoration of 59;
    physiological sense of 20; relational
    2, 9, 21, 142, 174; sense of 101, 176;
    sense of family security 112; sharing
    of pain 238; social and technical 56;
    ventro vagal sensation of 13; see also
    insecurity
security mechanisms 54
self: co-creation of 24; ego-functioning
    of 28; experience of 137; feeling of
    52; Gestalt theory of 63n10; Gestalt
    therapy's understanding of 13; human
    part of 62; integrative and regulating
    function of 244–245; lacking

functionality of 51; loss of parts of functioning of 25; as process of contact 31; of psychotherapist and of client 33; sense of 7, 11, 14, 22, 27, 32, 37; social 53; theory of 72
self-actualization 81
self as function of organism/environment field 11, 71
self-consciousness 91, 94
self-contempt 140
self-definition 26, 178, 185; boundaries of 187
self-disclosing 68
self-effectiveness 169
self-esteem 126 (box), 129
self-exclusion 163
self-functions 222, 224
self-fulfilling see prophecy
self-growth 222
self-harm 124 (box), 231
self-hatred 142
self-image 136
self-in-development 134
self-in-relation-to 20
self-in-the-making 143
self-in-the-world 14
self-perception 162
self-regulation: affective 200; between caregiver and child 27, 100; co-regulation and 202; of experiential field 23; of one's own child 8; organismic 23, 28; of situational field of contacts 23
self-regulative process 186
self-sacrifice 24
self-support 83; hetero-support and 245
self-surrender 244
sensoriality 134
separated parenthood 120, 130
separation experience 121; as boundary event 130; now-for-next in 129; suffering of children in 122–127
shame 10, 13; adolescent 163, 169; Giovanni and Maria, example of 197; giving adequate voice to 143; intimacy and 203n3; as relational message 163; risk of 37–38; surrendering 182; work on 142–143
situation, the: suffering and 269
situational being, human as 13
situational cries 52
situational demands 229

situational field 129, 186; experiential 270; of contacts 23
situational Gestalt therapy model 81
situational point of view 269
situational window iii, 2
slogans and stereotypes, going beyond 43–44
social efficiency 254
social ground 10–11
social networks 191; virtual reality and trap of 253–254
social withdrawal: adolescence and 159–171; adolescent transformation and 163; as cultural syndrome 164; as expression of suffering born of new narcissism 170; as Special Educational Need (Italy) 171n3; as symptom and problem to be resolved 168
soon to be xvii, 11; now-for-soon to be 34
Spagnuolo Lobb, Margherita xvii; on Gestalt theory of Self 63n10; Stern's influence on 195; see also aesthetic relational knowing; clinical data sheet; dance of reciprocity; now-for-next; soon to be; post-pandemic world
spontaneity 4; of children 56, 101, 110; concept of psychopathology and loss/lack of 14, 25; of contact 219; at contact-boundary 195; in contact-making 27, 33, 35; continuum from anxiety to 84; of creative adaptation 100; definition of 100; dormant 186; emergence of 85, 128; interrupted 25; losing 194; promoting 210; reciprocity at contact boundary and 185–187; spontaneous recuperating 110; restoring 111–114, 182; of self 181; split between deliberation and 74; supporting 36, 37, 93; towards the other 26
spontaneous creativity 203n12
spontaneous and vital presence of the Other 175
spontaneous "break-down" 76
spontaneous development of patient's intentionality of contact 71
spontaneous encounters with child's companions 165
spontaneous movement 7, 31, 33
Spontaneous Parental Personality Function (SPPF) 121, 126, 128, 130
spontaneous reaching 168
spontaneous resonance 22

spontaneous response to an actuality 239
spontaneous sense of self 2, 32
spontaneous therapeutic action 246
SPPF *see* Spontaneous Parental
    Personality Function (SPPF)
Stern, Daniel 30, 76, 100, 127,
    182; *see also* implicit relational
    knowledge; intersubjective space; now
    moments
stress: parental 165; psychological 230,
    260; psycho-physical 242; psychosocial
    261; responses to 27
subjectivity: body 143; full 71; own 76;
    sphere of 162; structuring of 102
support for separated parenting 128
suspended bereavement *see* bereavement
synchronicity 134
synchronic perspective 83, 89, 106, 279
    (appendix)
synthetic unity 201

therapeutic action 30, 186
therapeutic alliance 32
therapeutic art 187
therapeutic change 20–21
therapeutic contact 24; clinical data sheet
    and 85; reciprocity of 82
therapeutic insight 14
therapeutic intervention 14, 73, 194; child
    consultation as 111
therapeutic journey, evolution of (Lidia)
    136–139
therapeutic now-for-next *see* now-for-next
therapeutic process: client's letting go
    in 34; clinical log 85; initiating 133;
    moving-toward-the-other in 31; Nino
    113–114; parents as part of 112; three
    questions for 36; work model with
    child and 110–111; *see also* dance of
    reciprocity
therapeutic questions 112, 113
therapeutic relationship 3; adolescents
    and 170; development of 68; fear and
    courage as allies in 168–169; regulation
    of 36
therapeutic skills 27
therapeutic work, process of 134, 155;
    directed at youngsters 208
Thunberg, Greta 11
Tierney, S. 149

together-with 51, 54, 55, 67; *see also*
    aut-aut; *et-et*
transcendental philosophy xvi
trauma: addiction as 173–187; collective
    8, 9, 20, 58; complex 133–144; concept
    of 241; dissocation as adaptive strategy
    to 75; dissociation, polarity conflict,
    and 73–74; double 217; forgotten 192;
    illness as 241, 242, 247; of loss and
    mourning 2; of marital breakup 128;
    relational 71; social 119; treating 15; of
    war 12
trauma work 142
triadic model 127
triadic perspective on the field 71, 198,
    200, 202, 203
triune brain theory 72

vagus nerve 74, 243
virality: social 225
virtual reality 26, 47, 247; trap of social
    networks and 253–254
virus *see* COVID-19; pandemic
vital capacities 202
vitality: active expressions of 26; addiction
    and loss of 183; in children 162; client
    85; creative 186; dance of reciprocity
    and 32; different dimensions of 51;
    feeding 77; Gestalt therapy concept of
    24; of ground experience of client 25;
    of human nature 55–58; lack of 183;
    loss of 242; psychic malaise and 12;
    supporting 28, 62; unexpressed 164
vitality of contact, Here-and-Now and
    139–142
vulnerability 7, 142, 143; admitting and
    containing 164; adolescent 170; ageing
    and 222, 224, 230; of the body 245;
    COVID-19 as amplifier of 119, 190;
    emergency and 60–61; existential 102;
    experience of 61; psychobiological
    and social 175; sense of 243; serious
    forms of 120; strength and 61; *see also*
    Strength and Vulnerability Integration
    Model

Wheeler, George 71
Wollants, Georges 1, 12, 13, 14, 71

Yontef, Gary xiv, 3, 270